GRAPHIC GUIDE to INFECTIOUS DISEASE

GRAPHIC GUIDE to INFECTIOUS DISEASE

Brian Kloss, DO, JD, PA-C

Associate Professor
Department of Emergency Medicine
SUNY Upstate Medical University
Syracuse, New York

Travis Bruce, BFA

ELSEVIER

ELSEVIER

1600 John F. Kennedy Blvd.
Ste 1800
Philadelphia, PA 19103-2899

GRAPHIC GUIDE TO INFECTIOUS DISEASE   ISBN: 978-0-323-44214-5

Notices

Knowledge and best practice in this field are constantly changing. As new research and experience broaden our understanding, changes in research methods, professional practices, or medical treatment may become necessary.

Practitioners and researchers must always rely on their own experience and knowledge in evaluating and using any information, methods, compounds, or experiments described herein. In using such information or methods they should be mindful of their own safety and the safety of others, including parties for whom they have a professional responsibility.

With respect to any drug or pharmaceutical products identified, readers are advised to check the most current information provided (i) on procedures featured or (ii) by the manufacturer of each product to be administered, to verify the recommended dose or formula, the method and duration of administration, and contraindications. It is the responsibility of practitioners, relying on their own experience and knowledge of their patients, to make diagnoses, to determine dosages and the best treatment for each individual patient, and to take all appropriate safety precautions.

To the fullest extent of the law, neither the Publisher nor the authors, contributors, or editors, assume any liability for any injury and/or damage to persons or property as a matter of products liability, negligence or otherwise, or from any use or operation of any methods, products, instructions, or ideas contained in the material herein.

Library of Congress Cataloging-in-Publication Data

Names: Kloss, Brian T., author, editor. | Bruce, Travis, illustrator.
Title: Graphic guide to infectious disease / Brian Kloss, Travis Bruce.
Description: Philadelphia, PA : Elsevier, [2019] | Includes bibliographical
   references and index.
Identifiers: LCCN 2018006370 | ISBN 9780323442145 (hardcover : alk. paper)
Subjects: | MESH: Communicable Diseases | Infection | Pictorial Works
Classification: LCC RC111 | NLM WC 17 | DDC 616.9--dc23 LC record available at https://lccn.loc.gov/2018006370

Executive Content Strategist: James Merritt
Senior Content Development Manager: Kathryn DeFrancesco
Content Development Specialist: Angie Breckon
Book Production Manager: Jeff Patterson
Project Manager: Lisa A. P. Bushey
Book Designer: Patrick Ferguson

Printed in India

Last digit is the print number: 9   8   7   6   5

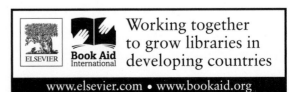

LIST OF REVIEWERS/ CONTRIBUTOR

CONTRIBUTING AUTHOR:

Hernan Rincon-Choles, MD, MSCI
Assistant Professor
Department of Nephrology and Hypertension
Cleveland Clinic Lerner College of Medicine of the
    Case Western Reserve University
Medical Director, Ohio Renal Care Group Huron
    Dialysis Center
Attending Physician, Glickman Urological and Kidney
    Institute

Topics written by Hernan Rincon:

Echinococcosis
Melioidosis
Granuloma Inguinale
Tularemia
Plague
Legionellosis
Scabies
Rabies
Ebola
Rift Valley Fever
Hanta Virus Pulmonary Syndrome
Hemorrhagic Fever with Renal Syndrome
Crimea Congo Hemorrhagic Fever
Colorado Tick Fever
Rocky Mountain Spotted Fever
Lyme Disease
Babesiosis
Ehrlichiosis
Anaplasmosis

GUEST REVIEWERS FOR DIAGNOSTIC TESTING:

Kanish Mirchia, MD
Department of Pathology
SUNY Upstate Medical University

Rochelle Nagales-Nagamos, MD, MBA
Department of Pathology
SUNY Upstate Medical University

Alexandria Smith-Hannah, MD, MS, MPH
Department of Pathology
SUNY Upstate Medical University

ACKNOWLEDGEMENTS

The authors would like to thank our friends, family, and all the staff at Elsevier for their support.

Thanks to Alex Seldes and Sabre Mrkva for being great friends and permitting us to draw Cleo with all those pediatric illnesses. Thanks to Karen Cyndari, MD/PhD candidate, for website development and support. Thanks to Kara Welch and David Rothman for assistance with the references and suggested reading section.

Very special thanks to Zubin Damania, MD, a.k.a. ZDoggMD, for making a cameo in our Zika Fever illustration; Mike Cadogan, MD, from the Life in the Fastlane Emergency Medicine website and blog for making a cameo in our Melioidosis illustration; and Jawad Kassem, MD, for making a cameo in our Middle Eastern Respiratory Syndrome illustration. Lastly, many thanks to Rob Guillory, Eisner Award-winning comic book artist for *Chew*, for his support and serving as a guest illustrator for our Avian Flu illustration. The guest appearances, celebrity cameos, and pop culture references contained in this textbook are intended to be works of satire and parody.

INTRODUCTION

Kloss and Bruce combine real medical education with comic book–style illustrations to create beautiful artistic images that enhance learning. Realizing that many medical professionals are visual learners, Kloss and Bruce enhance learning by breaking down complex medical conditions and diseases into illustrated scenes. As children of the eighties and with a passion for comic books, pop culture, nostalgia, and humor, their illustrations exceed boundaries set by other medical illustrations. *Irreverent*, *provocative*, and *unconventional* are terms that have been used to describe their campy, tongue-in-cheek approach to medical education. Their visual aids are colorful, comical, and boundary pushing, all of which make learning more fun and memorable.

Dr. Brian Kloss, a professor and emergency medicine physician, and Travis Bruce, a talented illustrator and designer, aim to educate physicians, physician assistants, nurses, medical students, and other healthcare providers using humor and comic book–style illustrations.

Their process is simple. First, Dr. Kloss pencils a rough draft of a medical syndrome, disease, or illness and hands it over to Travis. Travis then draws out the illustration and adds clarity and color. The end result is a helpful educational tool that is both comical and informative.

The dynamic duo has been collaborating since connecting at a house party in Brooklyn during the turn of the century. Their first educational product, *Toxicology in a Box*, was published by McGraw-Hill in 2013 and is available in Kindle version on Amazon.com. *Toxicology in a Box* is a set of 150 full-color flashcards geared toward teaching medical providers how to recognize and treat various toxic exposures ranging from the bizarre to the mundane.

Kloss and Bruce, in collaboration with Elsevier, are pleased to present their latest work: *Graphic Guide to Infectious Disease*. This body of text and illustrations represents 4 years of late nights, highly caffeinated beverages, deadline extensions, revisions, and more deadline extensions. While they're admittedly no Rick and Morty, they needed a few deadline extensions.

Their only request is that you loosen your collar, sit back, relax, and enjoy learning high-yield medicine via a truly unique medium. Welcome to Kloss and Bruce: Medical Education Through Comic Illustration.

Brian Kloss, DO, JD, PA-C
Associate Professor
Department of Emergency Medicine
SUNY Upstate Medical University

Travis Bruce, BFA
To learn more about us, please visit www.KlossandBruce.com

ABOUT THE AUTHORS

Brian Kloss, DO, JD, PA-C, is an Emergency Medicine Physician and Associate Professor at the SUNY Upstate Medical University and VA Medical Center in Syracuse, New York. He holds a Certificate in Radiologic Technology from Morristown Memorial Hospital in New Jersey, an Associate of Science in Chemistry from the County College of Morris, a Bachelor of Science in Physician Assistant Studies from Gannon University, a Juris Doctor for the University at Buffalo School of Law, and a Doctor of Osteopathic Medicine from UMDNJ-SOM (Rowan). He completed a postgraduate Physician Assistant Fellowship in Gastroenterology, is Board Certified in Emergency Medicine, and completed a Wilderness Medicine Fellowship at SUNY Upstate. Brian likes vintage video games, comic books, action figures, and old-school hip hop.

Travis Bruce is an artist, illustrator, and designer living in Queens, New York. He graduated with a BFA in illustration from the School of Visual Arts, with a focus on graphic narratives and children's books. Along with illustration, he has designed tabletop products and giftware for the past 15 years.

TABLE OF CONTENTS

PART 11 | OROPHARYNGEAL INFECTIONS

PART 12 | VIRAL

PART 13 | PARASITES AND PRIONS

PART 14 | BACTERIAL

BIBLIOGRAPHY AND SUGGESTED READING

PART 1

VIRAL HEPATITIS

Disease Name: **Hepatitis A**

Synonyms:	Infectious Hepatitis
Causative Agent:	Hepatitis A Virus (HAV)
Reservoir:	Humans
Incubation Period:	15-50 days; Average: 28 days
Geographic Regions Affected:	Worldwide

Description: HAV is a vaccine-preventable fecal-orally transmitted RNA virus that causes acute hepatitis. Hepatitis A is never chronic, is often asymptomatic in younger patients, and causes fulminant hepatic failure in <1% of cases. Risk factors include travel to endemic regions, ingestion of contaminated food or water (raw shellfish), work in day care centers (exposure to feces/diaper changing), close contact with infected patients, and men who have sex with men.

Signs and Symptoms: Typically, the younger the patient, the fewer symptoms he or she exhibits. Most infants will show little to no signs of infection, whereas most adults become symptomatic. Symptomatic patients experience nausea, vomiting, malaise, abdominal pain, and fever followed by scleral icterus and jaundice several days later. Symptoms often last for less than 2 months; however, the disease may be prolonged or can relapse over a 6-month period. Infection confers lifelong immunity.

Diagnostic Testing: Labs will reveal a hepatocellular pattern with ALT/AST elevations <1000, rising before an increase in bilirubin and alkaline phosphatase is seen. ALT, being more specific to the liver, is often higher than AST. IgM rises in acute infection, and IgG begins to rise in convalescence. Fulminant hepatic failure, a serious consequence of infection characterized by altered mental status (hepatic encephalopathy) and elevations of PT/INR, is more common in older patients and those with preexisting liver disease (chronic hepatitis B and/or C).

Treatments: Supportive. The disease is preventable by two doses of a vaccine given at least 6 months apart. Depending on the manufacturer, the second dose of the vaccine can be given up to 12 or 18 months after the first dose. Postexposure vaccine can be given in healthy persons aged 1–40 years within 14 days to prevent infection. Postexposure immune globulin is recommended within 14 days for unvaccinated patients with immunodeficiency, chronic liver disease, adults >41 years, and children <12 months old.

Pearls: There have been several food-related outbreaks of hepatitis A in the United States. Five hundred people became ill in 2003 after consuming salsa made with green onions at a now-bankrupt Mexican food chain restaurant.

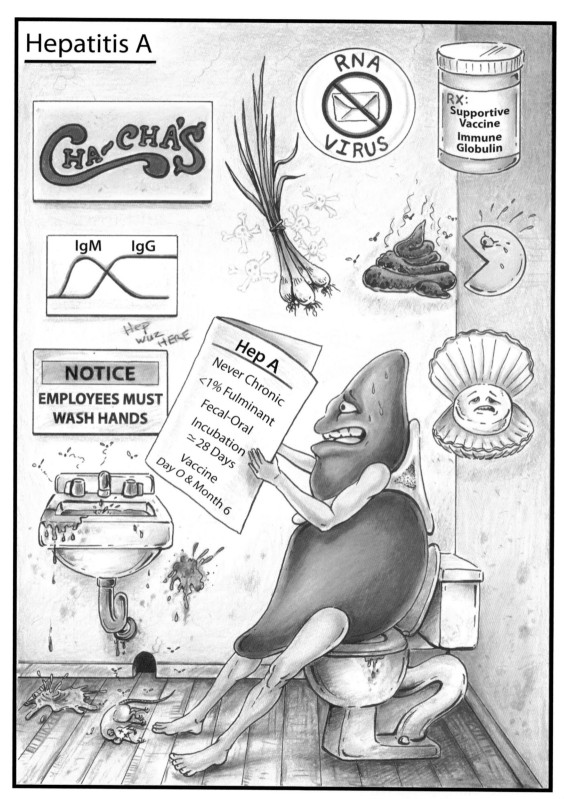

Disease Name: **Hepatitis B**

Synonyms:	Serum Hepatitis
Causative Agent:	Hepatitis B Virus (HBV)
Incubation:	60–150 days; Average: 90 days
Geographic Regions Affected:	Worldwide, Higher Incidence in Asia
Reservoir:	Humans

Description: HBV is a double-stranded DNA virus that causes acute and chronic hepatitis. The disease can be transmitted vertically at birth or through contact with infected bodily fluids, such as blood, semen, and vaginal secretions. Hepatitis B can be transmitted sexually and through IV drug use. Healthcare workers are at risk of infection from needlestick injuries.

Signs and Symptoms: *Acute*: Most infants and young children with acute infections are asymptomatic. Older patients are more likely to show symptoms, which include fever, malaise, anorexia, nausea, vomiting, abdominal pain, and jaundice. Approximately 70% of acutely infected adults will have symptoms. Symptoms can last for several weeks. The incidence of fulminant hepatic failure is <1%. *Chronic*: Chronic hepatitis B is often asymptomatic but patients can have symptomatic flairs. If untreated, the disease can be spread to others, cause cirrhosis, and predispose patients to hepatocellular carcinoma. The likelihood of developing chronic hepatitis B is inversely proportional to age at time of infection. The risk of vertical transmission is very high and is dependent on the mother's HBeAg/HBeAb status. Those women who are HBeAg+ and HBeAb− are more likely to pass on the infection. The Centers for Disease Control and Prevention report that infected newborns develop chronic hepatitis B approximately 90% of the time, whereas children infected between the ages of 1 and 5 years have a 25%–50% chance of developing chronic disease. Older children and adults are more likely to clear the disease and have a 5%–10% chance of chronicity.

Diagnostic Testing: Acute and chronic hepatitis B are diagnosed by specific serum markers and HBV viral load testing using PCR. Chronic hepatitis B is defined as the presence of HBsAg detectable in serum for 6 months or longer after symptom onset. Please see our summary of hepatitis B markers for more information.

Treatments: Treatment of acute disease is supportive, except in cases of fulminant hepatic failure, wherein nucleoside/nucleotide analog medications are indicated. In chronic hepatitis B infections, treatment options and the decision to treat are highly dependent on individual patient factors, such as viral load, presence/absence of cirrhosis or hepatocellular cancer, HBeAg/HBeAb status, pregnancy status, patient age, and biochemical markers. Treatment options for chronic hepatitis B include PEGylated interferon or nucleoside/nucleotide analogs. Nucleoside/nucleotide analogs include lamivudine, adefovir, entecavir, telbivudine, and tenofovir. The authors recommend referencing current American Association for the Study of Liver Diseases (AASLD) and/or European Association for the Study of the Liver (EASL) guidelines prior to initiating treatment. Hepatitis B is vaccine preventable, and infection after acute exposure can be prevented with vaccination and immune globulin.

Hepatitis B

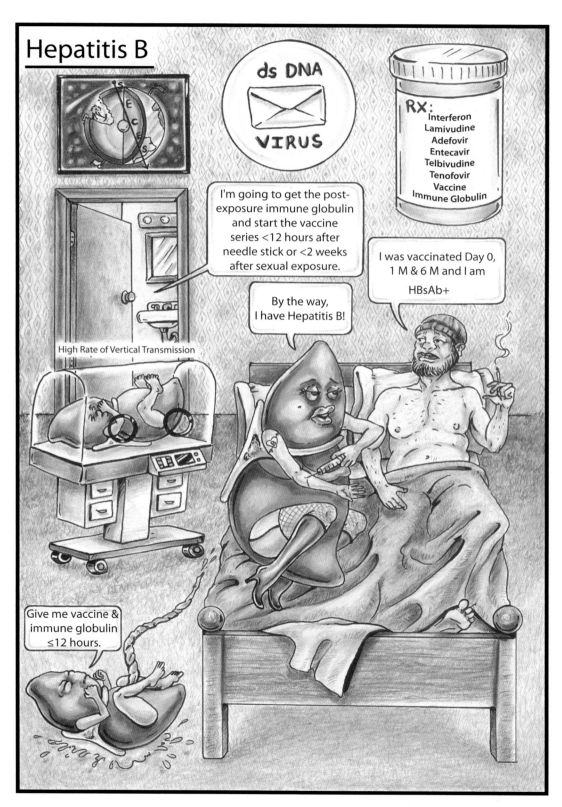

Disease Name: **Hepatitis B Serum Markers**

Hepatitis B Surface Antigen (HBsAg):

HBsAg is the first serum marker to appear and is detectable prior to the onset of clinical symptoms. It peaks approximately 12 weeks after exposure and should become undetectable within 24 weeks (6 months). The elimination of HBsAg and seroconversion to hepatitis B surface antibody (HBsAb) indicates that the infection has resolved. If HBsAg persists in the serum for >6 months, the patient has a chronic infection.

Hepatitis B e Antigen (HBeAg):

HBeAg is associated with viral replication and is detectable within 6–14 weeks after exposure. In chronic hepatitis B, HBeAg serves as a marker of both disease activity and infectivity. Patients who are HBeAg+ (HBeAb−) have higher viral loads and greater disease activity and are more infectious. In pregnancy, HBsAg+ women are more likely to pass the infection on to their infants. Any infant born to a mother with chronic HBV should be vaccinated and given immune globulin, ideally within 12 hours.

Hepatitis B Virus Core Antibody (HBcAb):

HBcAb is the first antibody to be detected via serum. Although there is a core antigen, it is intracellular and cannot be detected in serum. HBcAb exists as both IgM (signifying acute infection or significant reactivation of chronic disease) and IgG (indicating a past exposure to the hepatitis B disease). Because HBcAb can only exist in those exposed to the disease, it is used when screening donated blood and/or distinguishing whether a person is immune from disease exposure or vaccination. Because the HBV vaccine consists only of HBsAg, those patients who have been successfully vaccinated will test HBsAb+ and HBcAb−. This indicates that they have antibodies to the hepatitis B surface antigen but have never been exposed to the full virus. Patients who are HBsAb+ and HBcAb+ have been exposed to the full hepatitis B virus, had the disease to some extent, and are now immune.

Hepatitis B e Antibody (HBeAb):

Antibodies to the e antigen are associated with decreased viral loads and herald convalescence. Seroconversion to HBeAb occurs early in acute disease but can be delayed for years in chronic infection. Those patients with chronic hepatitis B that are HBeAb− seroconvert to HBeAb+ at a rate of approximately 0.5% per year.

HBsAb:

HBsAb confirms immunity, either via vaccination or resolved infection. HBsAb begins to elevate after HBsAg levels taper off. Again, presence of HBsAg and absence of HBsAb at 6 months indicates chronic infection. In some cases, there is a window when neither HBsAg nor HBsAb can be detected. In this case an HBcAb IgM level can be obtained to evaluate for acute infection.

Hepatitis B Serum DNA:

PCR can be used in either a qualitative (yes or no) or quantitative (How much?) fashion when determining the presence or absence of HBV DNA in serum samples. In patients who contract HBV infection and seroconvert to an HBsAb+ state, HBV DNA should be 100% cleared from their serum. Those patients with chronic hepatitis B will have detectable HBV DNA in their serum, the amount highly dependent on their HBeAg/HBeAb status. HBV DNA quantitative studies, HBeAg/HBeAb status, and liver biopsy results (to grade liver damage) are important in determining treatment eligibility and options.

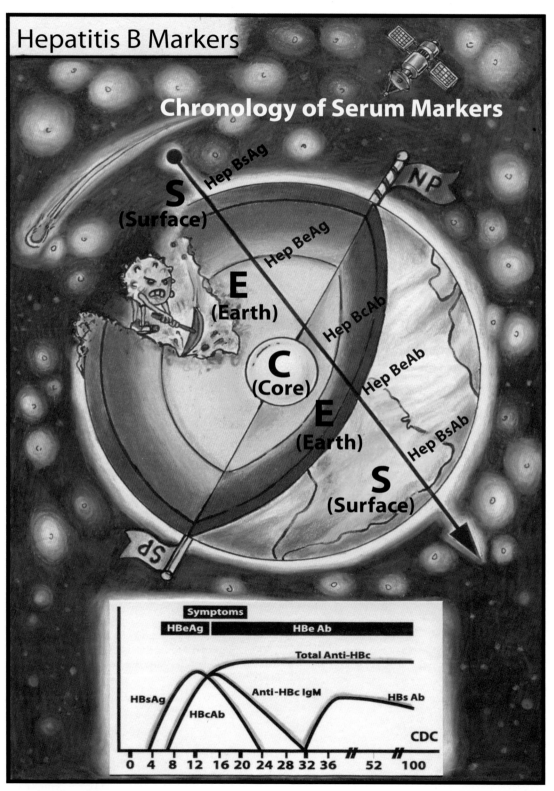

Hepatitis B Markers

Chronology of Serum Markers

S (Surface)

Hep BsAg

NP

Hep BeAg

E (Earth)

Hep BcAb

C (Core)

Hep BeAb

E (Earth)

Hep BsAb

S (Surface)

SP

Symptoms

HBeAg   HBe Ab

Total Anti-HBc

HBsAg   Anti-HBc IgM   HBs Ab

HBcAb

CDC

0 4 8 12 16 20 24 28 32 36   52   100

Disease Name: Hepatitis C

Causative Agent: Hepatitis C Virus, HCV

Incubation: 14–180 days; Average: 45 days

Geographic Regions Affected: Worldwide

Reservoir: Humans

Description: HCV is a single-stranded RNA virus responsible for both acute and chronic viral hepatitis, with up to 85% of infections becoming chronic. Risk factors for HCV transmission include IV drug use, blood transfusions and organ transplantation before July 1992, receiving clotting factors before 1987, intranasal drug use (cocaine), long-term hemodialysis, unsterile tattoos (e.g., prison), and vertical transmission. Sexual and household transmission can occur but is low.

Signs and Symptoms: *Acute*: Approximately 85% of acute infections are asymptomatic, and about 85% of hepatitis C infections become chronic. Acute symptoms can include malaise, fatigue, nausea, vomiting, abdominal pain, and jaundice. *Chronic*: Often asymptomatic but can cause malaise and fatigue. People with chronic HCV infections can develop cirrhosis and are predisposed to developing primary hepatocellular carcinoma. Extrahepatic manifestations of chronic HCV can include diabetes, cryoglobulinemia, and glomuleronephritis.

Diagnostic Testing: People with chronic hepatitis C may have normal liver enzymes. Hepatitis C antibody testing screens for the disease, and positive results should be followed by PCR testing for viral load and genotype. Positive HCV antibody tests with negative viral load may indicate a false-positive antibody test or identify a patient who previously had hepatitis C and cleared the virus either spontaneously or via treatment.

Treatments: Since the treatment for hepatitis C is continuously evolving, the authors recommend consulting the American Association for the Study of Liver Disease (AASLD) and/or the Infectious Disease Society of America (IDSA) for current guidelines. Initially, PEGylated interferon combined with oral ribavirin provided about 50% sustained virologic response (SVR) or "cure" rate. Direct-acting antivirals (DAAs) are now the preferred treatment and include oral agents: elbasvir/grazoprevir, ledipasvir/sofosbuvir, simeprevir/sofosbuvir, and sofosbuvir/velpatasvir.

Treatment is often based on genotype, viral load, presence/absence of cirrhosis, previous treatment failures, and insurance formularies. New drugs are constantly entering the development pipeline, and many patients may be offered enrollment in clinical trials. All patients with chronic hepatitis C should be vaccinated against hepatitis A virus and hepatitis B virus to prevent additional liver disease from these infections.

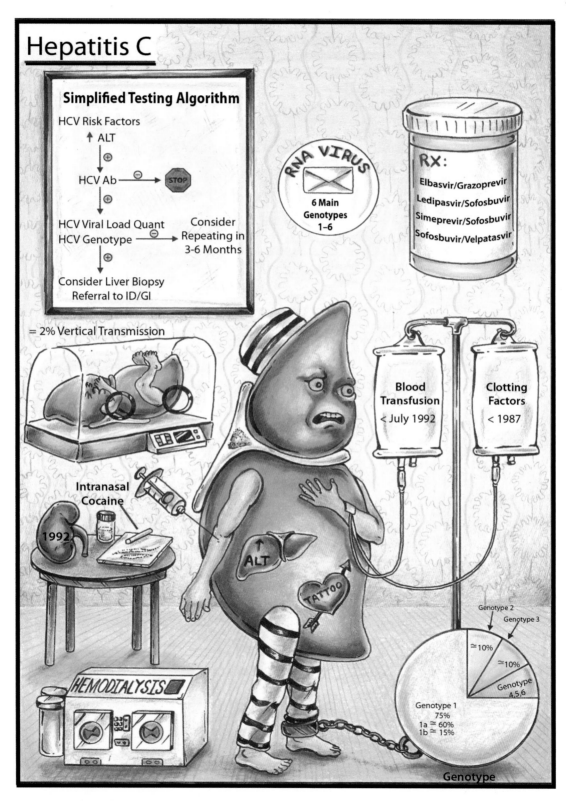

Hepatitis C

Simplified Testing Algorithm

HCV Risk Factors

↑ ALT

⊕

HCV Ab ⟶ ⊖ ⟶ STOP

⊕

HCV Viral Load Quant
HCV Genotype ⊖ ⟶ Consider Repeating in 3-6 Months

⊕

Consider Liver Biopsy
Referral to ID/GI

RNA VIRUS
6 Main Genotypes 1–6

RX:
Elbasvir/Grazoprevir
Ledipasvir/Sofosbuvir
Simeprevir/Sofosbuvir
Sofosbuvir/Velpatasvir

= 2% Vertical Transmission

Intranasal Cocaine

1992

ALT

TATTOO

Blood Transfusion
< July 1992

Clotting Factors
< 1987

HEMODIALYSIS

Genotype 2
Genotype 3
≈ 10%
≈ 10%
Genotype 4,5,6
Genotype 1
75%
1a ≈ 60%
1b ≈ 15%

Genotype

Disease Name: **Hepatitis D**

Causative Agent: Hepatitis D Virus (HDV), Delta Virus

Incubation: *Coinfection*: 45–160 days; Average: 90
Superinfection: 2–8 weeks

Geographic Regions Affected: Worldwide; Higher incidences where hepatitis B is endemic. Hepatitis D is rare in the United States.

Reservoir: Humans with hepatitis B virus (HBV)/HDV coinfections.

Description: Hepatitis D is a "defective" single-stranded RNA virus that requires the machinery and assistance of hepatitis B to replicate. HDV is acquired as either a coinfection (simultaneously acquired with hepatitis B) or as a superinfection (acquired by a person who already has chronic hepatitis B).

Signs and Symptoms: When acquired as a coinfection, HDV can increase the likelihood of severe illness and fulminant hepatic failure. Coinfections are less likely to result in chronic hepatitis D. Superinfections are more likely to cause chronic hepatitis D and can worsen preexisting liver disease.

Diagnostic Testing: Since patients cannot have hepatitis D without hepatitis B, patients will test positive for hepatitis B serum markers. IgM and IgG anti-HDV antibody testing is available in the United States, and an elevated anti-HDV IgG titer can be seen in chronic hepatitis D infections. Patients testing positive for HDV antibodies can be followed up with HDV viral levels via PCR technology.

Treatments: Vaccination against hepatitis B is also preventative against hepatitis D. PEGylated interferon is the only treatment that is effective for chronic hepatitis D, but successful clearance of the virus with treatment is low (approximately 20%–25%).

Pearls: HDV infections cannot exist without hepatitis B. The incubation period for hepatitis D coinfection is identical to that of acute hepatitis B (the HDV infection occurs concurrently with HBV). The presence of HBsAg and IgM anti-HBc is essential for the diagnosis of HDV infections.

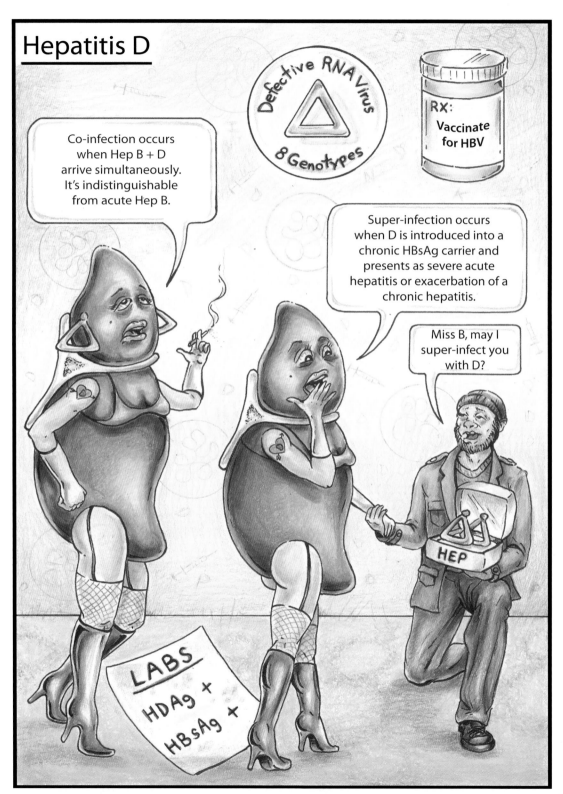

Disease Name: **Hepatitis E**

Causative Agent:	Hepatitis E Virus, HEV
Incubation:	15–60 days; Average: 40 days
Geographic Regions Affected:	Central America, Africa, Middle East, India, and Asia
Reservoir:	Swine and small rodents may serve as an animal reservoir.
Description:	HEV is a fecal-oral (genotype 1 and 2) and foodborne (genotype 3 and 4) single-stranded RNA virus responsible for acute viral hepatitis. There are four major viral genotypes, each associated with specific regions and unique clinical presentations. Genotype 3 is found in developed countries, tends to affect those patients >40 years old or immunocompromised, and can cause chronic infections. Genotypes 1, 2, and 4 more commonly affect younger adults. HEV infections can occur as sporadic outbreaks affecting many people or as isolated cases affecting isolated individuals.
Signs and Symptoms:	Most cases are asymptomatic, with fewer than 5% of patients showing signs of acute infection. When symptomatic, patients may exhibit malaise, fever, nausea, vomiting, abdominal pain, arthralgia, and jaundice. Fulminant hepatic failure can occur in up to 3% of infections and is more common in pregnant females and in those with preexisting liver disease.
Diagnostic Testing:	There are no commercially approved tests for HEV in the United States. Some countries have access to IgM, IgG, and HEV PCR testing capabilities. Acute infection would be determined by a positive IgM and HEV PCR viral load. IgM is elevated in the acute setting and indicates recent exposure to the HEV virus, whereas IgG increases during convalescence and confirms past exposure. In chronic HEV infections, HEV RNA will be detectable via PCR in serum or stool more than 6 months after initial infection.
Treatments:	Supportive. Ribavirin may be beneficial in the treatment of chronic HEV infection. There is an HEV vaccine that is licensed in China.
Pearls:	Acute hepatitis E infection during pregnancy has a high mortality rate (up to 25%).

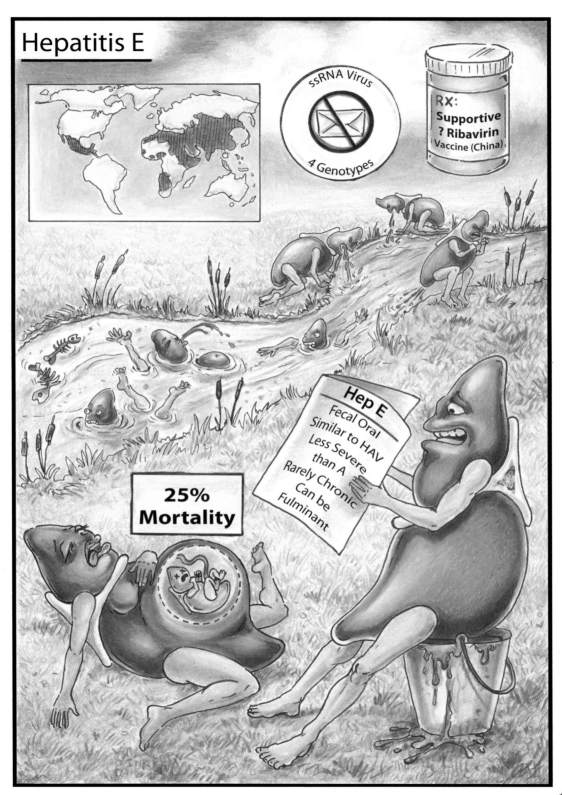

PART 2

INFECTIOUS DIARRHEA

Section 1

BACTERIAL

Disease Name: # Shigellosis

Synonyms:	Bacillary Dysentery
Causative Agent:	Four serogroups of *Shigella*, broken down into group A: *S. dysenteriae*; group B: *S. flexneri*; group C: *S. boydii*; and group D: *S. sonnei*.
Transmission:	Transmission is fecal-oral. Because a very small inoculum of bacteria (10–100 organisms) is required for transmission, infected food handlers can easily spread the disease. Person-to-person transmission is common. Consumption of contaminated water, food, or produce grown where sewage is used as fertilizer often results in illness. Given the low inoculum required for transmission, there can be rapid spread in closed quarters such as military campaigns, refugee camps, day care centers, and households.
Incubation:	1–7 days; Average: 3 days
Geographic Regions Affected:	Worldwide—more common in developing nations.
Description:	An acute bacterial hemorrhagic diarrheal illness caused by any one of four *Shigella* serogroups. Key symptoms include bloody diarrhea, abdominal pain, and fever. Severe dehydration is uncommon.
Signs and Symptoms:	Diarrhea, fever, abdominal pain and cramps, tenesmus, malaise, nausea, and vomiting. Diarrhea is initially watery and nonbloody then becomes mucoid and bloody as the infection transitions into the large bowel. Symptoms typically last 5–7 days without treatment. Complications can include hemolytic uremic syndrome (HUS), seizures in children, and reactive arthritis.
Diagnostic Testing:	Shigella should be suspected in patients presenting with bloody diarrhea, abdominal pain, fever, and small, frequent stool volumes. Stool can be cultured or tested using PCR.
Treatments:	Antibiotics can reduce the duration of symptoms in infected patients. Because antibiotic resistance to TMP/SMX and ampicillin is commonplace, current recommendations call for either azithromycin or ciprofloxacin. However, providers should be aware of emerging resistance to these antibiotics as well. Antispasmodics should be avoided.
Pearls:	*Shigella* is the most infectious bacterial diarrheal disease, commonly passed via person-to-person transmission. *S. dysenteriae* serotype 1 (formerly *Shigella shigae*) tends to be a more aggressive pathogen, whereas *S. sonnei* tends to cause milder disease. *S. sonnei* is more common in developed nations, and *S. flexneri* is more common in less-developed nations.

BACTERIAL

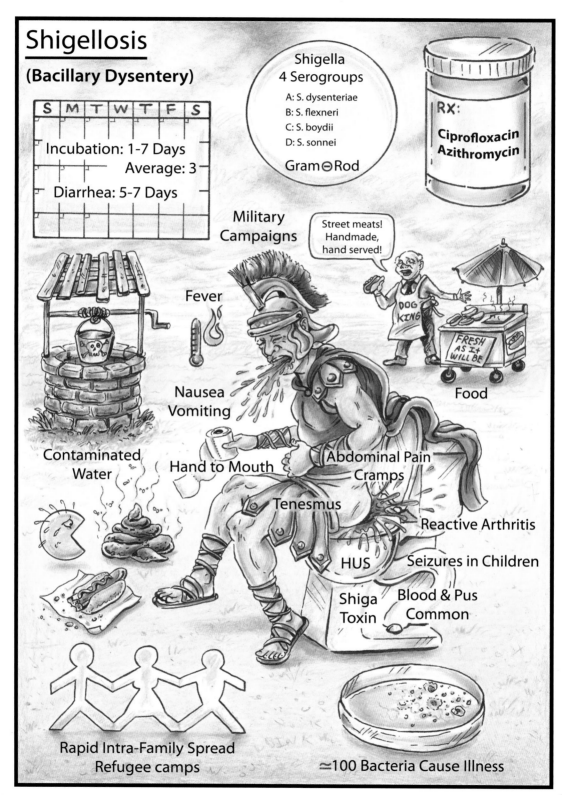

Shigellosis
(Bacillary Dysentery)

Incubation: 1-7 Days
Average: 3
Diarrhea: 5-7 Days

Shigella
4 Serogroups

A: S. dysenteriae
B: S. flexneri
C: S. boydii
D: S. sonnei

Gram ⊖ Rod

RX:
Ciprofloxacin
Azithromycin

Military Campaigns

Street meats! Handmade, hand served!

DOG KING

FRESH AS IT WILL BE

Fever

Food

Nausea Vomiting

Contaminated Water

Hand to Mouth

Abdominal Pain
Cramps

Tenesmus

Reactive Arthritis

HUS

Seizures in Children

Shiga Toxin

Blood & Pus Common

Rapid Intra-Family Spread
Refugee camps

≃100 Bacteria Cause Illness

BACTERIAL

Disease Name: **Salmonellosis**

Synonym: Nontyphoidal Salmonella

Causative Agents: *Salmonella bongori, Salmonella enterica*

Reservoir: Poultry is the most common. Some reptiles.

Transmission: Typically foodborne via consumption of undercooked poultry, foodstuffs in contact with raw/undercooked poultry (contaminated cutting board), raw eggs, and raw/unpasteurized milk. There have been several major U.S. foodborne outbreaks traced back to commercially packaged chicken, peanut butter (Peanut Corporation of America in 2008), and ice cream (Schwan's in 1994). Reptiles such as turtles, lizards, and snakes may be carriers of salmonella *(S. bongori).*

Incubation: 12–48 hours

Geographic Regions Affected: Worldwide

Description: An acute, febrile, bacterial diarrheal illness often transmitted by undercooked poultry (chicken/raw eggs) and characterized by watery and/or bloody diarrhea.

Signs and Symptoms: Typical symptoms include fever, malaise, nausea, vomiting, abdominal pain/cramps, tenesmus, and diarrhea. Bloody diarrhea can also occur and is more common in children. The illness is often self-limiting, and symptoms typically resolve within 3–7 days. More severe infections are seen with larger bacterial inoculums, in young children and older adults, and the immunocompromised. Salmonella may become invasive and can cause bacteremia, meningitis, septic arthritis, and osteomyelitis (sickle cell patients are at increased risk). Postinfectious irritable bowel syndrome and reactive arthritis may occur in some patients.

Diagnostic Testing: Stool culture is the gold standard for diagnosis.

Treatments: The mainstay of treatment is often supportive and consists of fluids and a gentle diet. Antibiotics are indicated in cases of severe illness, persistent fever, high-risk patients (extremes of age, weakened immune systems), and those with invasive disease. Treatment options may include fluoroquinolones (ciprofloxacin or levofloxacin), macrolides (azithromycin), or cephalosporins (ceftriaxone or cefotaxime). Resistance to TMP/SMX and other antibiotics is on the rise.

Pearls: The Food and Drug Administration has banned the sale of pet turtles less than 4 inches in length since 1975 to reduce the incidence of salmonellosis in children. The Centers for Disease Control and Prevention estimates that 100,000 cases of the disease have been prevented as a result of this ban.

Salmonellosis
(Non-typhoidal Salmonella)

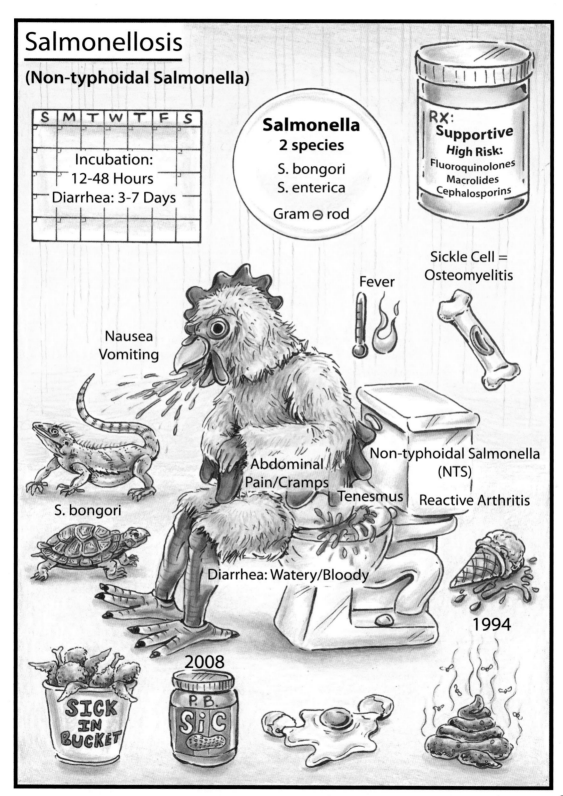

Incubation:
12-48 Hours
Diarrhea: 3-7 Days

Salmonella
2 species
S. bongori
S. enterica

Gram ⊖ rod

RX:
Supportive
High Risk:
Fluoroquinolones
Macrolides
Cephalosporins

Sickle Cell =
Osteomyelitis

Fever

Nausea
Vomiting

Abdominal
Pain/Cramps

Tenesmus

Non-typhoidal Salmonella
(NTS)
Reactive Arthritis

S. bongori

Diarrhea: Watery/Bloody

1994

2008

SICK IN BUCKET

P.B. SiC

BACTERIAL

| Disease Name: | **Cholera** |

| Synonym: | Blue Death |

| Causative Agent: | *Vibrio cholerae* |

| Transmission: | Fecal-oral transmission can occur through consumption of contaminated water, foodstuffs, or naturally contaminated shellfish. |

| Incubation: | 1–5 days; Average: 2–3 days |

| Geographic Regions Affected: | Resource-poor countries, mostly in Africa, Asia, the Caribbean, and Central and South America. Peaks are seen before and after rainy seasons. |

| Description: | An acute, afebrile, painless, bacterial diarrheal illness characterized by profound fluid loss and the passage of "rice water stools." Severe cases can cause severe electrolyte abnormalities, renal failure, acidosis, hypovolemic shock, circulatory collapse, and death. |

| Signs and Symptoms: | Cholera is a spectrum disease with diarrheal symptoms ranging from asymptomatic or mild to severe. Severe illness causes hypovolemic shock and death. After a brief incubation period, patients develop nausea, vomiting, painless diarrhea, and lethargy. Fever is uncommon. Diarrhea is nonbloody, may contain flecks of mucus (rice water stools), and has a fishy odor. Volume losses of 10–20 liters per day can occur in adults, resulting in hypovolemic shock, sunken eyes, and loss of skin turgor and elasticity (washerwoman hands). Severe acidosis secondary to bicarbonate loss can trigger Kussmaul respirations. |

| Diagnostic Testing: | Clinical signs and symptoms, specifically in the setting of an outbreak of watery diarrhea, should raise suspicions to the diagnosis. Darkfield microscopy may show motile *Vibrio* bacteria. Rapid diagnostic tests can identify the O1 and/or O139 antigens in stool samples. Labs from severely ill patients will reflect the electrolyte, pH, and renal abnormalities associated with severe dehydration and acidosis. Ultimately, a positive stool culture is considered the gold standard for diagnosis. |

| Treatments: | The mainstay of treatment consists of IV fluid resuscitation with lactated Ringer's solution followed by transition to oral rehydration salts once tolerated. Antibiotics can shorten the duration of illness in severe disease and include doxycycline, azithromycin, tetracycline, or erythromycin. Vaccines are available in endemic areas of the world and for those U.S. travelers headed to endemic regions (relief workers, extended medical missions, etc.). |

| Pearls: | There was a significant outbreak of cholera in Haiti after a major earthquake in 2010. Patients with blood group O may have worse disease. Cholera epidemics are associated with O1 and O139 serogroups; O139 is only found in Asia. |

Cholera

(Blue Death)

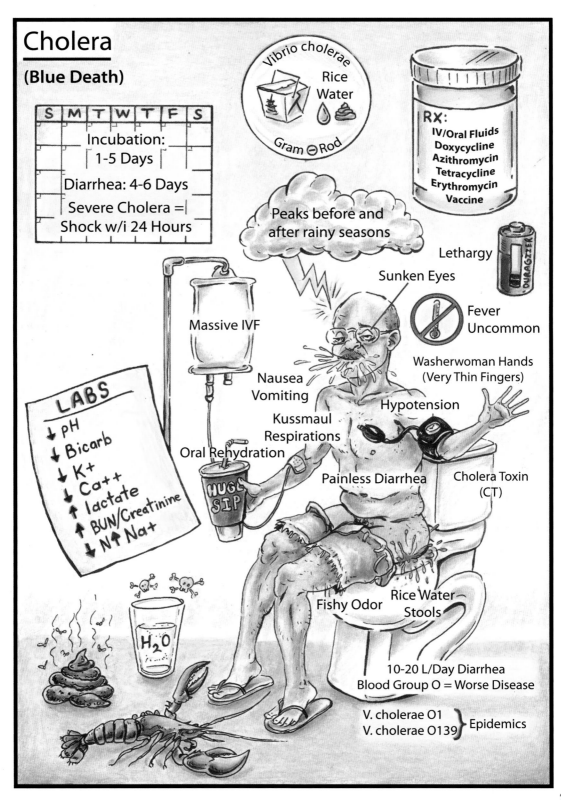

Vibrio cholerae
Rice Water
Gram ⊖ Rod

Incubation:
1-5 Days

Diarrhea: 4-6 Days

Severe Cholera =
Shock w/i 24 Hours

RX:
IV/Oral Fluids
Doxycycline
Azithromycin
Tetracycline
Erythromycin
Vaccine

Peaks before and after rainy seasons

Lethargy

Sunken Eyes

Fever Uncommon

Massive IVF

Washerwoman Hands (Very Thin Fingers)

Nausea Vomiting

Hypotension

Kussmaul Respirations

Oral Rehydration

LABS
↓ pH
↓ Bicarb
↓ K+
↓ Ca++
↓ lactate
↑ BUN/Creatinine
↓ N ↑ Na+

Painless Diarrhea

Cholera Toxin (CT)

HUGE SIP

H_2O

Fishy Odor

Rice Water Stools

10-20 L/Day Diarrhea
Blood Group O = Worse Disease

V. cholerae O1
V. cholerae O139 } Epidemics

BACTERIAL

Disease Name:	**Campylobacteriosis**

Causative Agents: *Campylobacter jejuni, Campylobacter coli*

Reservoir: Gastrointestinal tract of animals and livestock; poultry is the most common. Domestic dogs and cats may also be colonized.

Transmission: Typically foodborne via consumption of undercooked poultry, foodstuffs in contact with raw/undercooked poultry, raw/unpasteurized milk, chicken paté, or fecal-oral transmission from symptomatic individuals.

Incubation: 1–7 days; Average: 3 days

Geographic Regions Affected: Worldwide

Description: An acute, febrile, bacterial diarrheal illness characterized by watery diarrhea that frequently becomes bloody after a few days.

Signs and Symptoms: Patients may have a febrile prodrome before the diarrhea occurs. Typical symptoms include fever, malaise, abdominal pain/cramps, tenesmus, and watery diarrhea that often becomes bloody. Nausea and vomiting may occur in some patients. The illness is often self-limiting and symptoms typically resolve within 7 days. In the acute setting, some patients may develop right lower quadrant abdominal pain prior to the onset of diarrhea (pseudoappendicitis). Postinfectious complications can include Guillain-Barré syndrome and reactive arthritis.

Diagnostic Testing: Stool culture is the gold standard for diagnosis. Darkfield or phase-contrast microscopy may reveal the motile, gram-negative, curved/helical-shaped rods. There are some stool antigen and PCR tests available as well.

Treatments: The mainstay of treatment is often supportive and consists of fluids and a gentle diet. Antibiotics will decrease the duration of illness and options include azithromycin 500 mg daily × 3 days or erythromycin 500 mg four times daily × 5 days. There is worldwide emerging campylobacter resistance to fluoroquinolones, specifically in Southeast Asia.

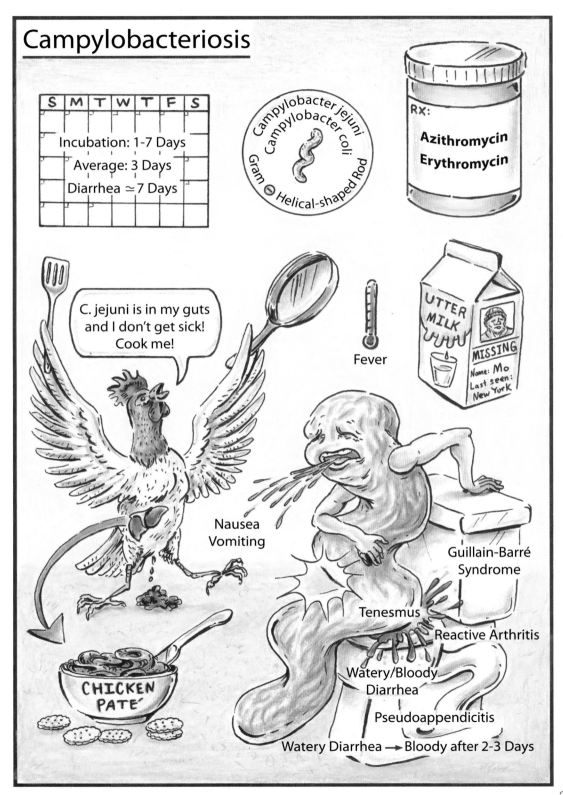

BACTERIAL

Disease Name: Enterohemorrhagic *Escherichia coli*

Causative Agent: *Escherichia coli* bacteria strains capable of producing Shiga toxin, known as "Shiga toxin–producing *E. coli*" (STEC). Strains identified in significant outbreaks have included *E. coli* O157:H7 (most common in North America, Jack in the Box in 1993), O104:H4 (Germany and Europe in 2011), and O26 (Chipotle in 2015).

Reservoir: Ruminant animals: Cattle, goats, sheep, deer, and elk. Cattle are the main reservoir.

Transmission: Transmission is fecal-oral, most commonly from the consumption of foodstuffs like leafy green vegetables, undercooked meat, and raw milk

Incubation: 3–8 days; Average: 3–4 days

Geographic Regions Affected: Worldwide

Description: An acute bacterial hemorrhagic diarrheal illness caused by STEC. Key symptoms include bloody diarrhea, abdominal pain, cramps, leukocytosis, and absence of fever.

Signs and Symptoms: Bloody diarrhea, abdominal pain, cramps, tenesmus, malaise, and anorexia. Fever is notably absent. Symptoms typically resolve over 5–7 days without intervention. Hemolytic uremic syndrome (HUS), a triad of hemolytic anemia, renal failure, and thrombocytopenia, occurs in 5%–10% of cases. HUS is more common in children under 10 years old (affecting about 15%) and those treated with antibiotics (up to 25% of children). HUS typically occurs 5–10 days after the onset of diarrhea, just as the diarrhea is becoming less frequent.

Diagnostic Testing: STEC should be suspected in patients presenting with bloody diarrhea, abdominal pain, and absence of fever. Stool can be cultured using sorbitol-MacConkey agar. Enzyme-linked immunosorbent assays for Shiga toxin 1 and 2. PCR for Shiga toxin gene, anti-LPS (anti-lipopolysaccharide) IgM and IgG antibodies can also be obtained.

Treatments: The mainstay of treatment is supportive and consists of fluids. Antispasmodics should be avoided, as they increase the likelihood of systemic complications like HUS and seizure. Ciprofloxacin and TMP/SMX have been shown to increase the release of Shiga toxin from bacteria, thus increasing the likelihood of HUS. If an antibiotic is used, azithromycin is probably the safest choice.

Pearls: There have been several infamous outbreaks of STEC in the United States associated with fast food restaurants, including Jack in the Box in 1993 and Chipotle in 2015.

BACTERIAL

Enterotohemorrhagic E. coli

(EHEC)

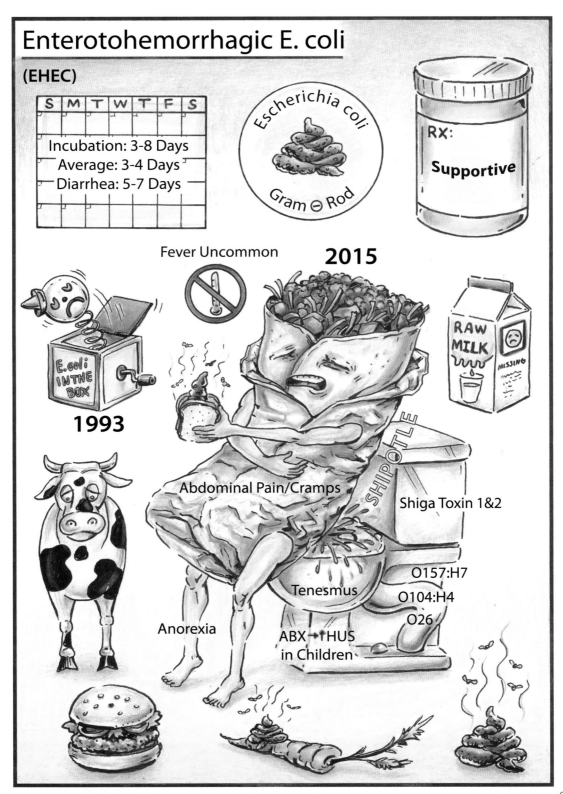

Incubation: 3-8 Days
Average: 3-4 Days
Diarrhea: 5-7 Days

Escherichia coli
Gram ⊖ Rod

RX: Supportive

Fever Uncommon

2015

E.coli IN THE BOX

1993

RAW MILK
MISSING

Abdominal Pain/Cramps

SHIPOTLE

Shiga Toxin 1&2

Tenesmus

O157:H7
O104:H4
O26

Anorexia

ABX→↑HUS
in Children

27

BACTERIAL

Disease Name: Enterotoxigenic *Escherichia coli*

Synonyms: Traveler's Diarrhea, Montezuma's Revenge, Delhi Belly, Turista

Causative Agent: *Escherichia coli* bacteria strains capable of producing one of two toxins: heat-stable (ST) enterotoxin, which increases intracellular cGMP, and heat-labile (LT) enterotoxin, which increases intracellular cAMP. These toxins stimulate the intestines to increase fluid secretion, causing non-bloody diarrhea. Enterotoxigenic *Escherichia coli* (ETEC) bacteria may produce either or both toxins.

Transmission: Transmission is fecal-oral, through the consumption of contaminated foodstuffs, drinking water, or ice. Following the "Boil it, cook it, peel it, or forget it" mantra reduces the odds of getting ill.

Incubation: 8 hours–3 days

Geographic Regions Affected: Worldwide. Most common cause of "traveler's diarrhea."

Description: An acute, profuse watery diarrheal illness caused by ST or LT toxin producing strains of *E. coli* (ETEC) bacteria. Key symptoms include watery diarrhea, abdominal pain, cramps, malaise, anorexia, and absence of fever.

Signs and Symptoms: Profuse watery diarrhea, abdominal pain and cramps, tenesmus, malaise, and anorexia. Fever is notably absent. Symptoms typically resolve over 3–4 days without intervention.

Diagnostic Testing: ETEC or "traveler's diarrhea" is often diagnosed based on patient's symptoms and history of recent travel. Often, by the time the patient comes to a healthcare provider's attention, symptoms have begun to resolve. Since both bacterial and viral causes of "traveler's diarrhea" have very short incubation periods, giardia or other parasites should strongly be considered in those patients who develop diarrhea 1–2 weeks after returning from travel.

Treatments: The mainstay of treatment is supportive and consists of fluids and a gentle diet. Handwashing, drinking bottled water, and avoiding street meats/street vendors, iced drinks, salads (uncooked vegetables), and fruits may reduce risk of transmission. Bismuth subsalicylate taken prophylactically may reduce likelihood of infection. Azithromycin 1000 mg as a single dose or 500 mg daily × 3 days, ciprofloxacin 750 mg twice daily for 1–3 days, or levofloxacin 500 mg daily for 1–3 days can be prescribed to travelers to take if they develop diarrhea while abroad. Since the actual cause of "traveler's diarrhea" cannot be determined in the field, while the traveler is abroad, azithromycin is the preferred antibiotic—it covers campylobacter, a bacterium with emerging resistance to fluoroquinolones, specifically in Southeast Asia.

Enterotoxigenic E. coli

(ETEC/Traveler's Diarrhea/Montezuma's Revenge)

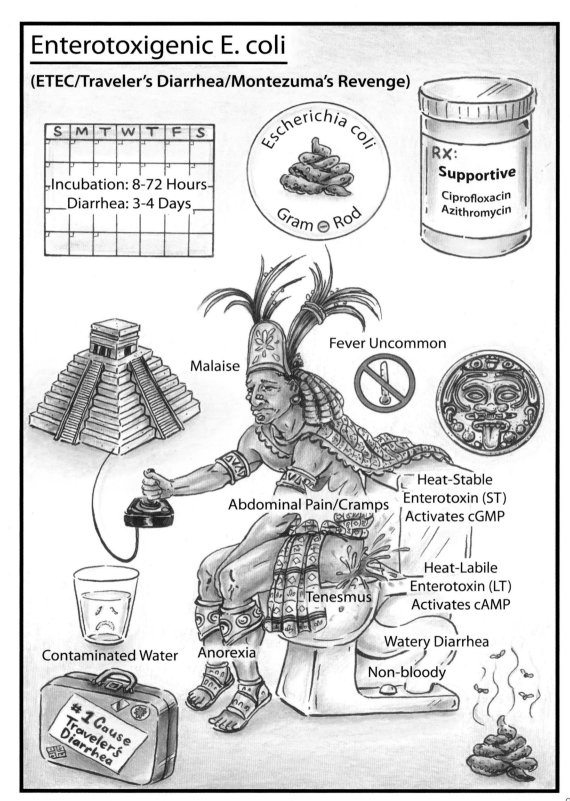

S M T W T F S

Incubation: 8-72 Hours
Diarrhea: 3-4 Days

Escherichia coli
Gram ⊖ Rod

RX:
Supportive
Ciprofloxacin
Azithromycin

Malaise

Fever Uncommon

Abdominal Pain/Cramps

Heat-Stable
Enterotoxin (ST)
Activates cGMP

Tenesmus

Heat-Labile
Enterotoxin (LT)
Activates cAMP

Watery Diarrhea

Non-bloody

Contaminated Water

Anorexia

#1 Cause
Traveler's
Diarrhea

BACTERIAL

Disease Name: **Yersiniosis**

Causative Agents: *Yersinia enterocolitica, Yersinia pseudotuberculosis*

Reservoir: Pigs, rodents, rabbits, sheep, horses, dogs, and cats. Pigs are the most important.

Transmission: Fecal-oral or foodborne transmission via the handling or consumption of undercooked pork (especially chitterlings), raw/unpasteurized milk, or contaminated water.

Incubation: 1–14 days; Average: 4–6 days

Geographic Regions Affected: Worldwide

Description: Yersiniosis may have a variety of presentations. *Y. enterocolitica* often causes an acute, febrile, bacterial diarrheal illness characterized by nausea, vomiting, abdominal pain, and bloody diarrhea. *Y. pseudotuberculosis* often presents as pseudoappendicitis, occasionally without diarrhea.

Signs and Symptoms: Infants and children often have worse disease than adults. Infants may develop necrotizing enterocolitis. Typical symptoms in children and adults include fever, malaise, abdominal pain, cramps, tenesmus, nausea, vomiting, and bloody diarrhea. The illness is often self-limiting, and symptoms typically resolve within 1–3 weeks. *Y. enterocolitica* may present as pharyngitis without diarrhea. Some patients may develop right lower quadrant abdominal pain secondary to mesenteric lymphadenitis and present as pseudoappendicitis. Bacteremia and hematogenous spread can occur and is more common in infants and the immunocompromised. Postinfectious complications include erythema nodosum and reactive arthritis.

Diagnostic Testing: Culture from the source of infection (stool, pharynx, blood, etc.) is the gold standard for diagnosis. Serologic testing is used in Europe and Japan, but it is not widely available in the U.S.

Treatments: For diarrheal illness, the mainstay of treatment is often supportive and consists of fluids. Antibiotics are indicated for severe infections and include doxycycline combined with an aminoglycoside, TMP/SMX, or fluoroquinolones.

Pearls: Hemochromatosis and iron overload states predispose patients to yersinia infections. Desferrioxamine therapy increases disease severity and should be discontinued in infected patients.

Yersiniosis

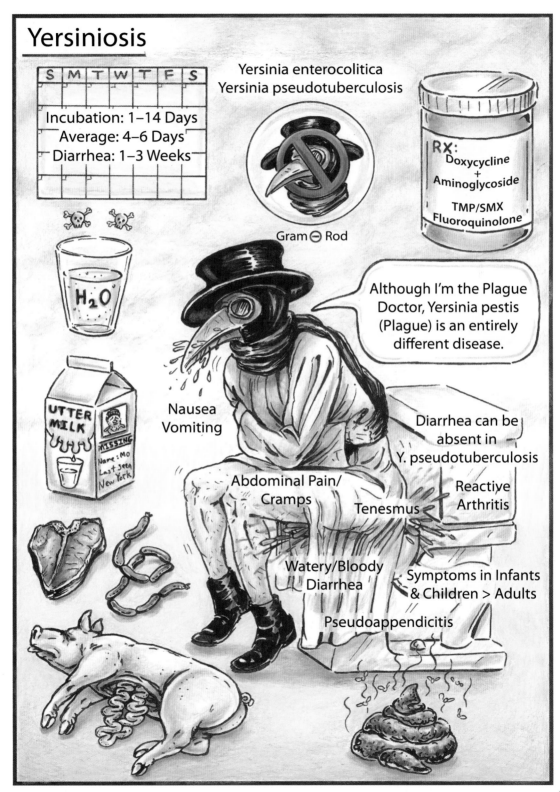

Incubation: 1–14 Days
Average: 4–6 Days
Diarrhea: 1–3 Weeks

Yersinia enterocolitica
Yersinia pseudotuberculosis

Gram ⊖ Rod

RX:
Doxycycline
+
Aminoglycoside

TMP/SMX
Fluoroquinolone

H₂O

UTTER MILK
MISSING
Name: Mo
Last Seen
New York

Although I'm the Plague Doctor, Yersinia pestis (Plague) is an entirely different disease.

Nausea
Vomiting

Abdominal Pain/
Cramps

Diarrhea can be absent in
Y. pseudotuberculosis

Tenesmus

Reactive
Arthritis

Watery/Bloody
Diarrhea

Symptoms in Infants
& Children > Adults

Pseudoappendicitis

BACTERIAL

Disease Name: *Clostridium difficile* Infection

Synonyms: Pseudomembranous Colitis, *C. diff*

Causative Agent: *Clostridium difficile*

Incubation: Varied

Geographic Regions Affected: Worldwide

Description: *Clostridium difficile* is a gram-positive spore and toxin-forming bacteria that can colonize the human gastrointestinal tract and causes antibiotic-associated diarrhea. The infection is a spectrum disorder, with symptoms ranging from asymptomatic colonization to severe colitis. The disease is more common in elderly patients and is associated with antibiotic use. Antibiotics decrease normal colonic flora and can allow for *C. diff* overgrowth and symptom manifestation. The antibiotics most associated with *C. diff* include clindamycin, fluoroquinolones, and second-generation (and above) cephalosporins.

Signs and Symptoms: Watery diarrhea beginning during or after recent antibiotic use is the classic disease manifestation. Other symptoms include fever, malaise, abdominal pain, cramps, and tenesmus. Severe disease can cause profound dehydration, hypotension, shock, acidosis, abdominal distension, and toxic megacolon (which may lead to perforation).

Diagnostic Testing: Leukocytosis is common. Leukocytosis, elevated creatinine, decreased albumin, and elevated lactate are markers for disease severity. Fecal leukocytes will be positive. Stool can be cultured and/or sent for PCR analysis and/or EIA testing for Toxin A and B. Since only Toxin B is associated with diarrheal illness, PCR and EIA testing may be limited to that toxin in some institutions.

Treatments: Discontinue the offending antibiotics if possible. Treatment of *C. diff* can be with oral metronidazole, vancomycin, or fidaxomicin. Severe disease requires intravenous (IV) metronidazole. IV vancomycin is not effective for *C. diff*. Fecal microbial transplant is being investigated as another treatment option.

Pearls: Proton-pump inhibitors (PPIs) and H2 acid blockers are associated with increased risk of *C. diff*. If colonoscopy is performed, mucosal friability, edema, inflammation, and pseudomembranes will be visualized. Only liquid stool is sent for culture/PCR testing, as diarrhea with solid/semi-solid stool is not consistent with *C. diff* infection.

Clostridium difficile Infection

(Pseudomembranous Colitis)

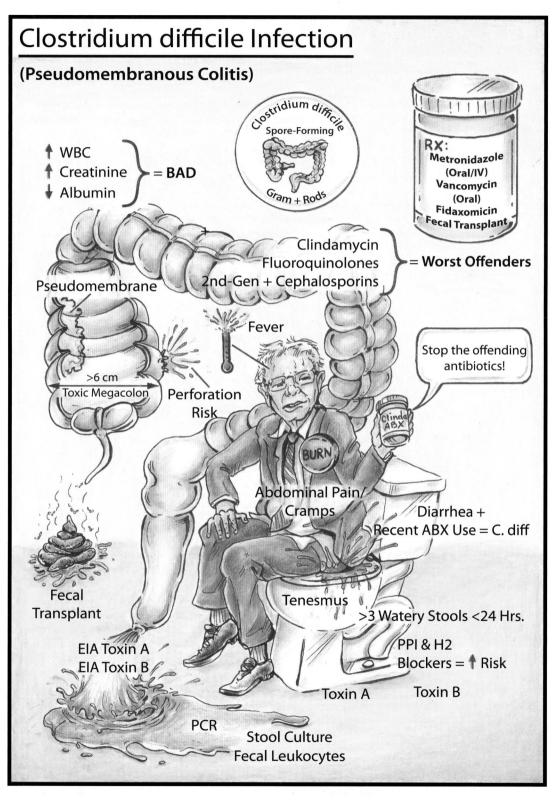

↑ WBC
↑ Creatinine } = **BAD**
↓ Albumin

Clostridium difficile
Spore-Forming
Gram + Rods

RX:
Metronidazole
(Oral/IV)
Vancomycin
(Oral)
Fidaxomicin
Fecal Transplant

Clindamycin
Fluoroquinolones
2nd-Gen + Cephalosporins } = **Worst Offenders**

Pseudomembrane

>6 cm
Toxic Megacolon

Fever

Stop the offending antibiotics!

Clinda ABX

BURN

Perforation Risk

Abdominal Pain/ Cramps

Diarrhea +
Recent ABX Use = C. diff

Fecal Transplant

Tenesmus

>3 Watery Stools <24 Hrs.

EIA Toxin A
EIA Toxin B

PPI & H2
Blockers = ↑ Risk

Toxin A   Toxin B

PCR

Stool Culture
Fecal Leukocytes

Disease Name:	**Vibriosis**

Causative Agents: *Vibrio parahaemolyticus, Vibrio vulnificus*

Incubation: 24–72 hours

Geographic Regions Affected: Worldwide

Description: Vibrio bacteria are common to marine and brackish waters (estuaries, saltwater marshlands), and shellfish living in these waters concentrate the bacteria, making vibrio a common cause of shellfish-associated diarrhea. Since bacterial concentration increases as water temperatures rise, highest disease incidence is noted in the United States between April and September. In addition to causing gastrointestinal illness, vibrio can also cause significant wound infections and/or septicemia. Vibrio infection tends to be worse in the immunocompromised, those with chronic liver disease, and alcoholics.

Signs and Symptoms: *Gastroenteritis:* Vibriosis should be suspected when watery diarrhea begins shortly after recent raw or undercooked shellfish consumption (oysters and clams are most common). Other symptoms include abdominal pain, cramps, nausea, and vomiting. Diarrhea may become bloody. *Soft Tissue Infection:* Wound exposure to vibrio can occur if cut while swimming in marine or brackish waters or when handling infected shellfish. In severe cases, cellulitis can expand rapidly, cause hemorrhagic bullae and/or necrotizing fasciitis. *Septicemia:* High-risk patients exposed to vibrio may develop bacteremia and sepsis after consumption of infected shellfish or secondary from a wound infection. Shock rapidly follows the onset of sepsis and patients have an extremely high mortality. This pathologic process is most common in those with compromised immune systems and/or chronic liver disease.

Diagnostic Testing: Stool, wound, or blood cultures confirm the diagnosis.

Treatments: *Gastroenteritis:* Mild to moderate disease can be treated with intravenous or oral hydration. Antibiotics may shorten the duration of illness in more-severe cases. *Soft Tissue Infections and/or Septicemia:* Doxycycline or minocycline 100 mg twice daily + ceftriaxone 2 grams IV daily is the suggested regimen for severe infections. Intravenous cefotaxime + ciprofloxacin and fluoroquinolone monotherapy are alternatives. Aggressive treatment is necessary in soft tissue infections and sepsis.

Pearls: While either species can present in any of the above scenarios, *V. parahaemolyticus* is more commonly associated with gastroenteritis and *V. vulnificus* is more commonly implicated in severe soft tissue infections and septicemia. Most restaurant menus warn consumers with chronic liver disease and/or immunodeficiency to avoid raw shellfish for this reason.

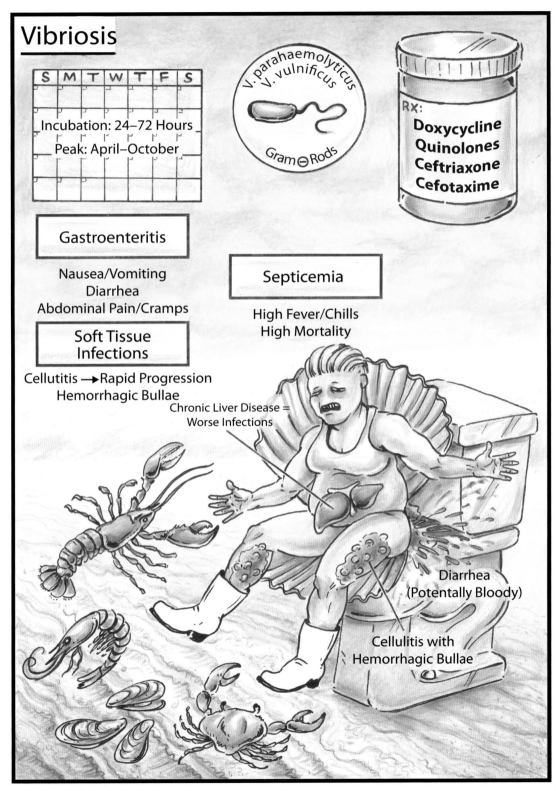

Vibriosis

Incubation: 24–72 Hours

Peak: April–October

V. parahaemolyticus
V. vulnificus

Gram ⊖ Rods

RX:
Doxycycline
Quinolones
Ceftriaxone
Cefotaxime

Gastroenteritis

Nausea/Vomiting
Diarrhea
Abdominal Pain/Cramps

Septicemia

High Fever/Chills
High Mortality

Soft Tissue Infections

Cellutitis ➞ Rapid Progression
Hemorrhagic Bullae

Chronic Liver Disease =
Worse Infections

Diarrhea
(Potentally Bloody)

Cellulitis with
Hemorrhagic Bullae

Section **2**

2

VIRAL

Disease Name: **Norovirus**

Synonyms:	Norwalk Virus, Winter Vomiting Bug, "Stomach Flu"
Causative Agent:	Norovirus (NoV)
Transmission:	Fecal-oral transition, typically spread via contact with contaminated surfaces, the consumption of contaminated food or water, or aerosolized virus from vomitus. The virus can live outside the body for long periods of time and can be shed for weeks after symptoms have resolved.
Incubation:	12–48 hours. Peaks in the winter months.
Geographic Regions Affected:	Worldwide
Description:	Norovirus is an extremely contagious virus responsible for up to 1/5 of all cases of gastroenteritis worldwide. It is known for causing outbreaks on cruise ships and in daycare centers, nursing homes, and schools.
Signs and Symptoms:	Norovirus infections typically present acutely with generalized malaise, headache, myalgia, nausea, vomiting, watery diarrhea, abdominal cramping, and low-grade fever. The disease is self-limiting, and symptoms tend to resolve over 1–3 days.
Diagnostic Testing:	Norovirus infections are often diagnosed based on clinical presentation alone. PCR testing of stool samples is not routinely done or recommended since asymptomatic shedding is common. However, if PCR testing is pursued, stool samples should be obtained within 48–72 hours of symptom onset.
Treatments:	Supportive.
Pearls:	The Centers for Disease Control (CDC) investigates and tracks outbreaks of gastroenteritis on cruise ships, and, not surprisingly, most are caused by NoV.

VIRAL

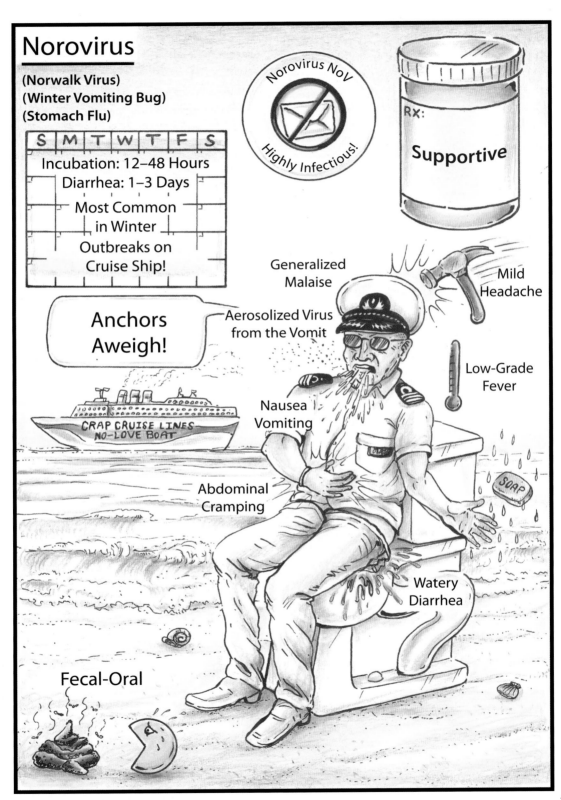

VIRAL

VIRAL

Disease Name: **Rotavirus**

Causative Agent: Rotavirus

Transmission: Fecal-oral transmission, typically spread via contact with contaminated surfaces, the consumption of contaminated food or water, or aerosolized virus. The virus can live outside the body in water for several days.

Incubation: Typically <48 hours

Geographic Regions Affected: Worldwide. Greater morbidity and mortality is noted in less-developed nations.

Description: Rotavirus causes viral gastroenteritis and is the common cause of diarrhea in infants and young children.

Signs and Symptoms: Rotavirus is a spectrum diarrheal illness, with symptoms ranging from mild to severe. The disease has the most profound impact on children 6–24 months old and rarely affects adults. Symptoms include malaise, nausea, vomiting, watery diarrhea, and low-grade fever. With significant fluid loss, severe dehydration and even death can occur. Signs of dehydration in infants include decreased tears, decreased urine output, decreased skin turgor, and irritability or lassitude. When profound dehydration is not an issue, the disease is self-limiting, and symptoms tend to resolve over 4–8 days. Most people have been infected by rotavirus at least once before the age of 5 years. Reinfection can occur throughout life; subsequent illnesses are less severe.

Diagnostic Testing: Diagnosis is often based on clinical suspicion. ELISA testing can be used to detect viral antigens in stool samples. PCR can also be performed on stool samples and is the most sensitive technique for rotavirus detection.

Treatments: Supportive. There are two licensed vaccines available in the United States.

Pearls: After the introduction of safe and effective vaccines, the number and severity of cases and subsequent hospitalizations in the United States and other developed nations has trended down dramatically. Diarrheal illness is still a leading cause of death in children under the age of 5 worldwide.

Rotavirus

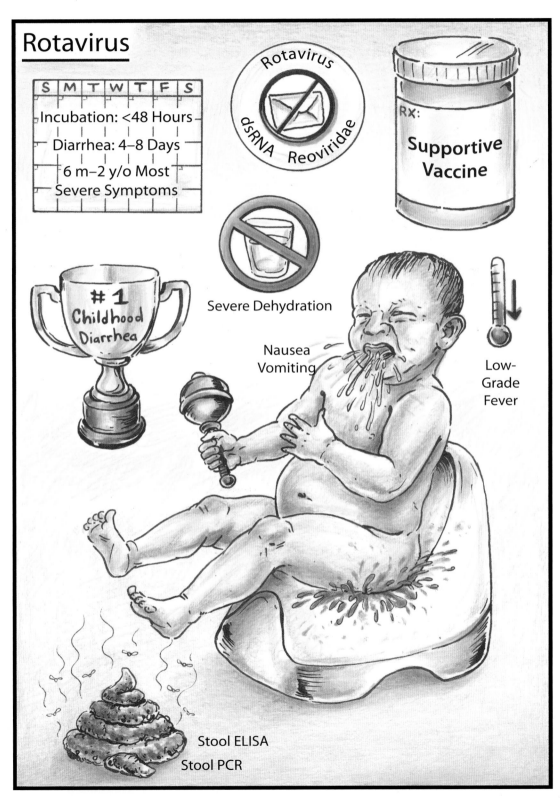

S M T W T F S

Incubation: <48 Hours

Diarrhea: 4–8 Days

6 m–2 y/o Most Severe Symptoms

Rotavirus
dsRNA   Reoviridae

RX:

Supportive Vaccine

Severe Dehydration

#1 Childhood Diarrhea

Nausea Vomiting

Low-Grade Fever

Stool ELISA

Stool PCR

VIRAL

Section  **3**

PROTOZOAN

Disease Name: Giardiasis

Synonym: Beaver fever

Causative Agent: *Giardia lamblia*, AKA: *Giardia intestinalis*

Reservoir: Humans. Beavers and dogs may be potential reservoirs.

Incubation: 1–3 weeks

Geographic Regions Affected: Worldwide—It is the number 1 intestinal parasite disease in the United States.

Description: *Giardia* is a flagellated intestinal protozoan responsible for acute and chronic outbreaks of gastrointestinal (GI) and diarrheal illnesses worldwide. It is contracted via the ingestion of infectious cysts through the fecal-oral route, often from consuming contaminated food or water.

Signs and Symptoms: The disease may be asymptomatic, acute and self-limiting, or chronic. Acutely, patients may have abdominal pain and cramping, malaise, upper GI upset, and diarrhea. The diarrhea is often described as green, frothy, foul smelling, and often floats, indicating malabsorption. Chronically, patients may develop anorexia, weight loss, malabsorption, B12 deficiency, postinfectious irritable bowel syndrome, and lactose intolerance.

Diagnostic Testing: Ovum and parasite stool studies ×3 can be obtained. Stool antigen and nucleic acid amplification testing (NAAT) are also available.

Treatments: Tinidazole 2 grams by mouth once, nitazoxanide 500 mg twice a day × 3 days, or metronidazole 250 mg three times a day × 5 days.

Prevention: Proper sanitation and handwashing limits spread. Water can be boiled, filtered, or halogenated (chlorine or iodine) to eliminate and/or decrease the number of cysts.

Pearls: The disease is more common in children and middle-aged adults. Backpackers, campers, international travelers, people in child care centers, and men who have sex with men (MSM) are at higher risk of acquiring giardiasis. Giardia, given its incubation period, delayed onset, and potential for chronicity, should be considered in the returned traveler presenting with diarrheal illness. This is in contrast to acute-onset "traveler's diarrhea," which is often self-limiting and bacterial or viral in nature.

PROTOZOAN

Giardiasis

(Beaver Fever)

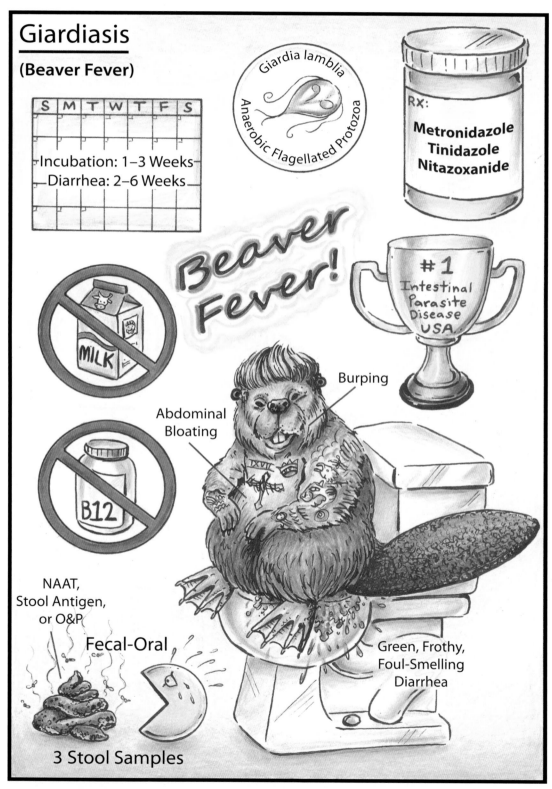

S M T W T F S

Incubation: 1–3 Weeks
Diarrhea: 2–6 Weeks

Giardia lamblia
Anaerobic Flagellated Protozoa

RX:
Metronidazole
Tinidazole
Nitazoxanide

MILK

B12

Beaver Fever!

#1 Intestinal Parasite Disease USA

Burping

Abdominal Bloating

NAAT, Stool Antigen, or O&P

Fecal-Oral

Green, Frothy, Foul-Smelling Diarrhea

3 Stool Samples

PROTOZOAN

45

Disease Name: **Cryptosporidiosis**

Causative Agents: *Cryptosporidium parvum, Cryptosporidium hominis*

Transmission: Transmission is fecal-oral secondary to ingestion of infectious oocysts from animals (cattle, calves) or humans. Since oocytes are resilient to chlorine, and filtration and can survive for months outside of a host, contaminated water (swimming holes, drinking water, and community swimming pools) plays an important role in transmission.

Incubation: 2–28 days; Average: 5–10 days

Geographic Regions Affected: Worldwide

Description: Cryptosporidiosis is a spectrum illness caused by intracellular protozoa; symptoms can range from an asymptomatic carrier state to profound diarrhea with significant fluid loss. The illness affects both immunocompetent and immunocompromised individuals, with more significant disease seen in the latter. Diarrhea can be acute, intermittent, or chronic.

Signs and Symptoms: Symptoms of intestinal disease include malaise, fatigue, low-grade fever, abdominal pain, cramps, and watery diarrhea. Diarrhea in immunocompetent patients often resolves within 2 weeks. Immunocompromised (HIV/AIDS) patients have more significant disease and biliary tree involvement (cholecystitis, cholangitis) and are more likely to have chronic diarrhea and associated weight loss. Respiratory cryptosporidiosis can occur, is rare, and is more common in immunocompromised patients.

Diagnostic Testing: Up to three stool samples may be required to make the diagnosis via microscopy. PCR is the diagnostic method of choice. Serologic antigen tests are also available.

Treatments: Oral nitazoxanide 500 mg twice a day orally for 3 days is effective for immunocompetent patients. For those with HIV/AIDS, the best means of treatment is to maximize the HAART antiretroviral therapy.

Pearls: Exposure to fecal matter, such as work in child care centers or sexual activity, increases risk of infection. Outbreaks in community pools are not uncommon in the United States and have been linked to infants swimming while wearing diapers.

PROTOZOAN

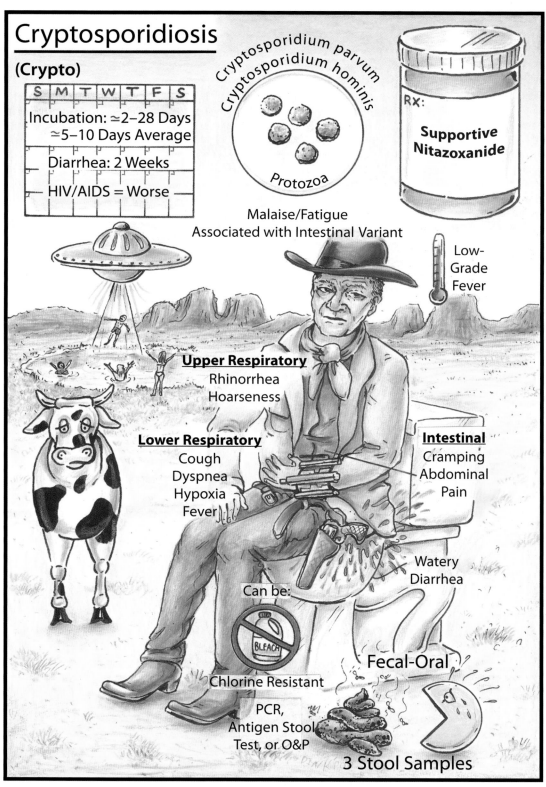

Cryptosporidiosis
(Crypto)

S	M	T	W	T	F	S

Incubation: ≈2–28 Days
≈5–10 Days Average

Diarrhea: 2 Weeks

HIV/AIDS = Worse

Cryptosporidium parvum
Cryptosporidium hominis

Protozoa

RX:
Supportive Nitazoxanide

Malaise/Fatigue
Associated with Intestinal Variant

Low-Grade Fever

Upper Respiratory
Rhinorrhea
Hoarseness

Lower Respiratory
Cough
Dyspnea
Hypoxia
Fever

Intestinal
Cramping
Abdominal
Pain

Watery
Diarrhea

Can be:

BLEACH

Chlorine Resistant

Fecal-Oral

PCR,
Antigen Stool
Test, or O&P

3 Stool Samples

PROTOZOAN

Disease Name: **Amebiasis**

Causative Agent:	*Entamoeba histolytica*
Transmission:	Fecal-oral transmission of infectious cysts. Cysts can survive outside the human body for weeks to months and are transmitted via person-to-person contact or the ingestion of contaminated food or water. Once ingested, cysts mature into trophozoites and typically invade the colonic mucosa.
Incubation:	2–4 weeks
Geographic Regions Affected:	Worldwide, more common in tropics and developing nations with poor sanitation.
Description:	Amebiasis is a spectrum diarrheal illness ranging from asymptomatic carrier states to hemorrhagic colitis and dysentery. Hematogenous spread may cause extraintestinal disease.
Signs and Symptoms:	Symptom onset tends to be gradual and includes fever, malaise, abdominal pain, weight loss, and bloody diarrhea. These invasive amebas can cause characteristic flask-shaped ulcers in the colonic mucosa and rarely, large granulomatous masses (amebomas) resembling cancerous tumors may form. Toxic megacolon and perforation are potential complications of severe acute disease. There is also a potential for invasive, extraintestinal disease secondary to hematogenous spread to the liver, brain, or lungs. Amebic liver abscesses are the most common extraintestinal manifestation and cause fever, chills, weight loss, and right upper quadrant pain. Abscesses may enlarge to the point of rupture.
Diagnostic Testing:	Microscopy may identify cysts and/or trophozoites of amebas, but it cannot differentiate between pathologic and nonpathologic species. Stool antigen and PCR testing confirm the diagnosis. Serology is helpful in the diagnosis of amebic liver abscess and extraintestinal disease. Imaging for liver abscess includes CT, US, and/or MRI. Abscesses may be aspirated by interventional radiology and sent for microscopy, antigen, and/or PRC testing.
Treatments:	Asymptomatic patients should be treated to prevent disease progression and transmission to others. Luminal agents, such as paromomycin, iodoquinol, and diloxanide, are poorly absorbed from the GI tract and are effective at cyst eradication. Mild to moderate disease can be treated with oral metronidazole or tinidazole, followed by paromomycin or iodoquinol to kill luminal-dwelling cysts. More-severe diarrheal disease and extraintestinal disease should be treated with intravenous metronidazole or tinidazole and followed by paromomycin or iodoquinol to kill luminal-dwelling cysts.

PROTOZOAN

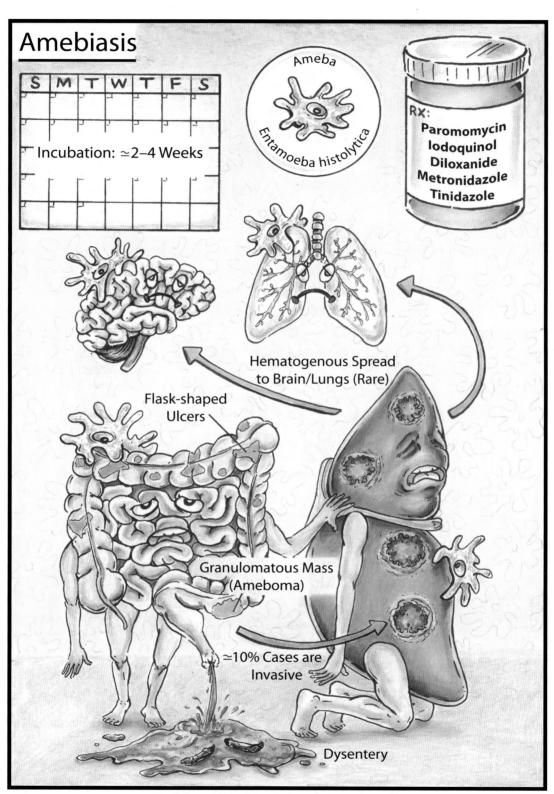

Amebiasis

Incubation: ≃2–4 Weeks

Ameba

Entamoeba histolytica

RX:
Paromomycin
Iodoquinol
Diloxanide
Metronidazole
Tinidazole

Hematogenous Spread
to Brain/Lungs (Rare)

Flask-shaped
Ulcers

Granulomatous Mass
(Ameboma)

≃10% Cases are
Invasive

Dysentery

PART 3

CHILDHOOD ILLNESSES

Disease Name: **Measles**

Synonym:	Rubeola
Causative Agent:	Measles Virus (MV)
Incubation:	7–21 Days; Average: 10–14 days
Geographic Regions Affected:	Worldwide

Description: Measles is a highly contagious, vaccine-preventable, viral illness characterized by a high fever, cough, coryza, and conjunctivitis followed by a maculopapular rash.

Signs and Symptoms: Following a 7- to 21-day incubation period, patients develop prodromal symptoms, including high fever (up to 40°C), malaise, conjunctivitis, coryza (runny nose), and cough. Koplik spots, small white to gray spots on the buccal mucosa opposite the lower molars, are pathognomonic and may appear 2–3 days before the viral exanthem. Koplik spots have been described as "grains of salt on a red background." After 3–4 days (range 1–7 days) of prodromal symptoms, patients enter the exanthem phase of the disease, characterized by the development of a red, maculopapular rash that starts at the head and proceeds in a cephalocaudal (head to toe) and outward progression. The rash persists for up to 7 days and fades in the same order it appeared. As the rash resolves, patients enter the recovery phase and may continue to have a mild cough for 1–2 weeks. Complications of measles include diarrhea, otitis media, pneumonia, encephalitis, seizures, and death. Infection with measles confirms lifelong immunity.

Diagnostic Testing: Serum IgM and IgG levels can be checked. IgM will become elevated in the acute phase of the illness and remain elevated for 1–2 months. Polymerase chain reaction can be used to detect the MV in serum, urine, and oropharyngeal and nasopharyngeal secretions.

Treatments: Supportive. Measles is preventable by vaccine.

Pearls: Koplik spots are a temporary viral enanthem and are pathognomonic for measles. Fever is high grade and tends to last for about 4 days and occurs concurrently with conjunctivitis, coryza, and cough. Subacute sclerosing panencephalitis is a rare and fatal degenerative disease of the central nervous system that occurs in some patients 7–10 years after initial infection.

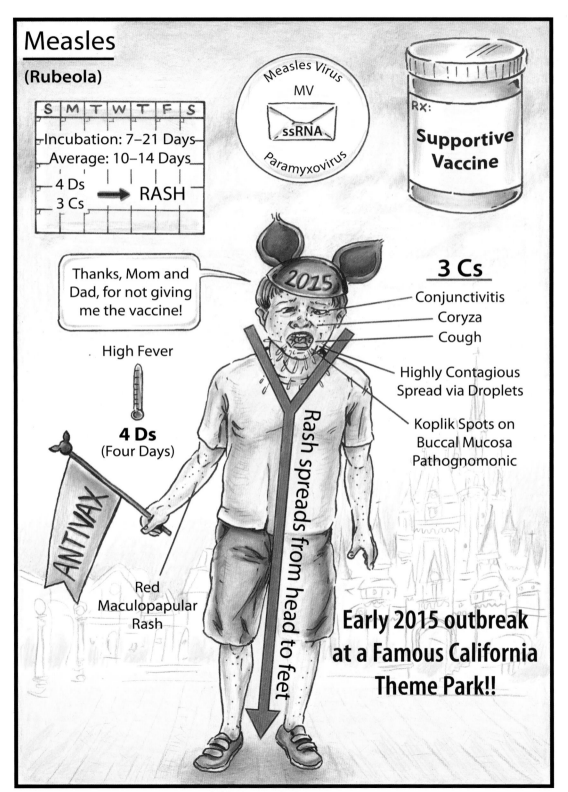

Disease Name: **Mumps**

Synonym:	Epidemic Parotitis
Causative Agent:	Mumps Virus
Incubation:	12–25 days; Average: 16–18 days
Geographic Regions Affected:	Worldwide
Peak Incidence:	Late Winter—Early Spring, Sporadic outbreaks
Description:	Mumps is a vaccine-preventable, viral illness known to cause parotitis. The virus reproduces in the upper respiratory tract and is spread via saliva, oropharyngeal secretions, and respiratory droplets. Patients with mumps are considered contagious and should be isolated, with droplet precautions for at least 5 days after the onset of parotitis.
Signs and Symptoms:	After a 12- to 25-day incubation period, patients develop prodromal symptoms, including low-grade fever, headache, malaise, fatigue, and myalgia, followed by parotitis. Parotid swelling is often bilateral (75%) and progresses over the next 72 hours. Glands remain swollen for about 1 week. While most cases of mumps are self-limiting, complications, including orchitis, oophoritis (ovarian inflammation), infertility, pancreatitis, meningitis, and/or deafness, can occur.
Diagnostic Testing:	Diagnosis is often based on history and clinical presentation. Serology can reveal an acute rise of IgM or a fourfold rise of IgG in the convalescence phase. IgG is of no value in previously vaccinated patients. Serum and buccal/oral swabs can be tested for mumps using PCR.
Treatments:	Treatment is mostly supportive. Vaccination is the best way to prevent mumps.

Mumps
(Epidemic Parotitis)

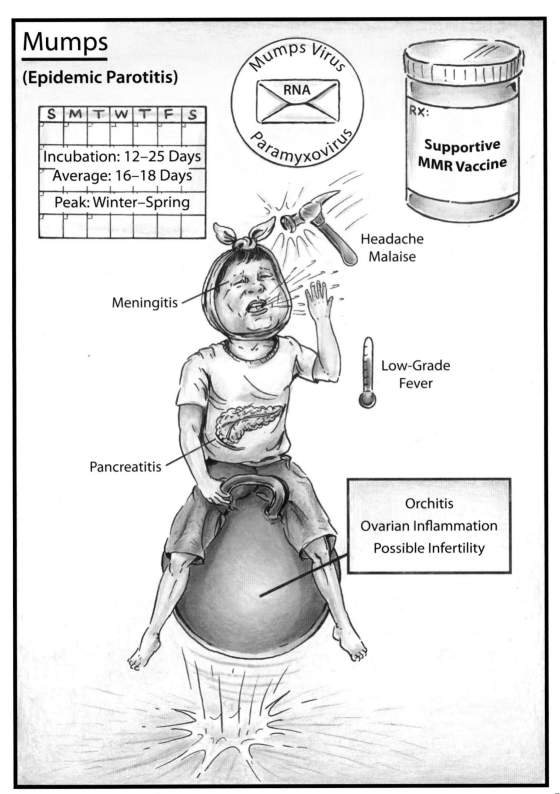

S	M	T	W	T	F	S
Incubation: 12–25 Days						
Average: 16–18 Days						
Peak: Winter–Spring						

Mumps Virus
RNA
Paramyxovirus

RX:
Supportive
MMR Vaccine

Headache
Malaise

Meningitis

Low-Grade
Fever

Pancreatitis

Orchitis
Ovarian Inflammation
Possible Infertility

Disease Name: **Rubella**

Synonyms: German Measles, 3-Day Measles

Causative Agent: Rubella Virus

Incubation: 12–23 Days; Average: 14 days

Geographic Regions Affected: Worldwide

Description: Rubella is a contagious, vaccine-preventable, viral illness characterized by low-grade fever, lymphadenopathy, and a mild 3-day maculopapular rash.

Signs and Symptoms: Many cases are asymptomatic, and children exhibit milder disease than adults. Following a 12- to 23-day incubation period, patients develop a low-grade fever, lymphadenopathy, and a mild maculopapular rash that proceeds in a cephalocaudal (head to toe) and outward progression. Lymphadenopathy tends to affect the posterior auricular, suboccipital, and posterior lymph nodes. Fever and lymphadenopathy may precede the rash by a few days or occur concurrently. The rash is fainter than in measles and lasts about 3 days; hence, the term "3-day measles." Headache, malaise, conjunctivitis, coryza, and cough may occur as part of the prodrome, more commonly in older patients. Up to 70% of adolescents and adult females develop arthralgia and arthritis that may persist for several months. Complications are more common in older patients and may include thrombocytopenic purpura and encephalitis. Rubella during pregnancy—specifically the first trimester—can cause stillbirth or birth defects. Congenital rubella syndrome causes cataracts, heart defects, and deafness.

Diagnostic Testing: Serum IgM and IgG levels can be obtained. IgM will be elevated in the acute phase of the illness, and a fourfold rise in IgG in convalescence will confirm recent infection. PCR testing can be performed on oropharyngeal or nasopharyngeal swabs and urine. Obtaining samples from both sources will increase the likelihood of detecting the virus.

Treatments: Supportive. Rubella is preventable by vaccine.

Pearls: Rubella and measles are similar but have some distinct differences. Rubella is characterized by low-grade fever, lymphadenopathy, and rash. Measles is characterized by high-grade fever, cough, coryza, conjunctivitis, and rash. The rash in rubella is fainter (pink vs. red) and lasts for a shorter duration (3 days vs. 7 days). Rubella is a milder disease but can cause congenital defects in pregnancy. Forchheimer spots are transient erythematous petechiae seen as enanthem on the hard palate in about 20% of patients with rubella. Since these spots can also be seen in measles and scarlet fever, they are not pathognomonic for rubella. Koplik spots, however, small white to gray spots on the buccal surface opposite the lower molars, are a pathognomonic enanthem for measles.

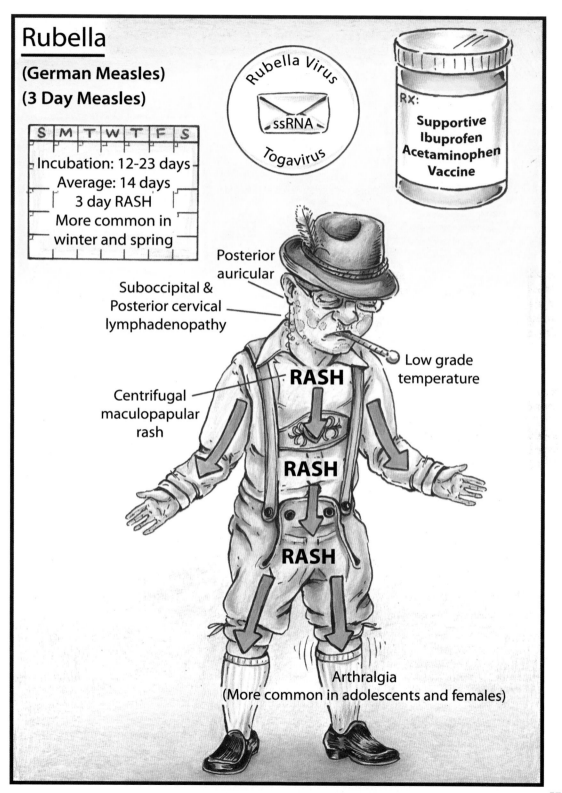

Rubella

(German Measles)

(3 Day Measles)

Rubella Virus

ssRNA

Togavirus

RX:
Supportive
Ibuprofen
Acetaminophen
Vaccine

S	M	T	W	T	F	S

Incubation: 12-23 days
Average: 14 days
3 day RASH
More common in
winter and spring

Posterior
auricular

Suboccipital &
Posterior cervical
lymphadenopathy

Low grade
temperature

RASH

Centrifugal
maculopapular
rash

RASH

RASH

Arthralgia
(More common in adolescents and females)

Disease Name: **Erythema Infectiosum**

Synonyms:	Fifth Disease, Slap Face, Slapped Cheek Syndrome
Causative Agent:	Parvovirus B19
Incubation:	4–14 days
Geographic Regions Affected:	Worldwide
Peak Incidence:	Late Winter—Early Spring. Peak incidence is in children 5–15 years old.
Description:	Erythema infectiosum (EI) is a self-limiting febrile viral illness that produces a characteristic "slapped cheek" facial rash followed by a lace-like reticular rash of the trunk and extremities. Patients are most infectious prior to the development of the rash.
Signs and Symptoms:	After a 4- to 14-day incubation period, most patients experience a prodrome of low-grade fever, malaise, headache, and rhinorrhea. After 2–5 days, a "slapped cheek" facial rash develops followed 1–4 days later by a lacelike reticular rash on the trunk and extremities. The rash can be pruritic, worsens with sunlight, and spares the palms and soles. The rash typically lasts for 5–10 days and may periodically return with exposure to sunlight, heat, exertion, or stress. Older children, adolescents, and adults, particularly females, may develop a mild polyarthritis of the hands, wrists, ankles, and knees that can last for several weeks or become chronic in some patients.
Diagnostic Testing:	EI is typically diagnosed based on history and clinical presentation. IgM/IgG serology and nucleic acid detection can be performed, but they should be reserved for pregnant women with known exposure (risk of congenital defects) and immunocompromised patients.
Treatments:	Supportive. Ibuprofen or acetaminophen as needed for fever, myalgia, and arthralgia.

Erythema Infectiosum

(Fifth Disease)

(Slap Face)

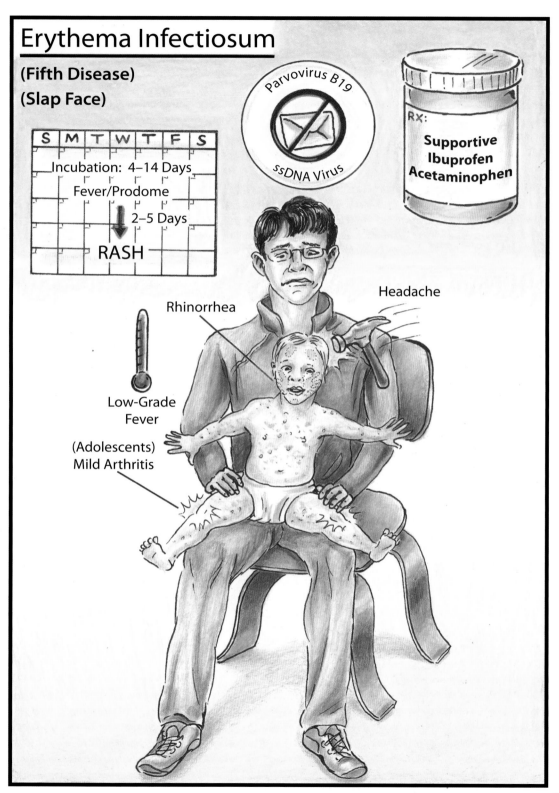

Parvovirus B19
ssDNA Virus

RX:
Supportive Ibuprofen Acetaminophen

S	M	T	W	T	F	S

Incubation: 4–14 Days

Fever/Prodome

2–5 Days

RASH

Rhinorrhea

Headache

Low-Grade Fever

(Adolescents) Mild Arthritis

Disease Name: **Exanthem Subitum**

Synonyms: Sixth Disease, Roseola

Causative Agent: Human Herpes Virus 6 (HHV 6) is the most frequent cause, but can also be caused by Human Herpes Virus 7 (HHV 7), enteroviruses, or adenoviruses.

Incubation: 5–15 days

Geographic Regions Affected: Worldwide

Peak Incidence: Occurs year round, mostly affecting children less than 2 years old.

Description: Exanthem subitum is an acute viral illness characterized by 3–5 days of high fever followed by defervescence and the appearance of a blanching macular or maculopapular centrifugal rash.

Signs and Symptoms: After an incubation period, children develop a high fever (up to 40°C) lasting for 3–5 days. During the febrile phase, children may have some irritability, malaise, and anorexia; however, most children are unphased. Within 24 hours of defervescence a blanching, nonpruritic, macular or maculopapular rash appears on the trunk and later spreads to the face and extremities. The disease is self-limiting and results in few complications. Occasionally, infants may experience febrile seizures.

Diagnostic Testing: Diagnosis is often based on history and clinical presentation.

Treatments: Treatment is supportive.

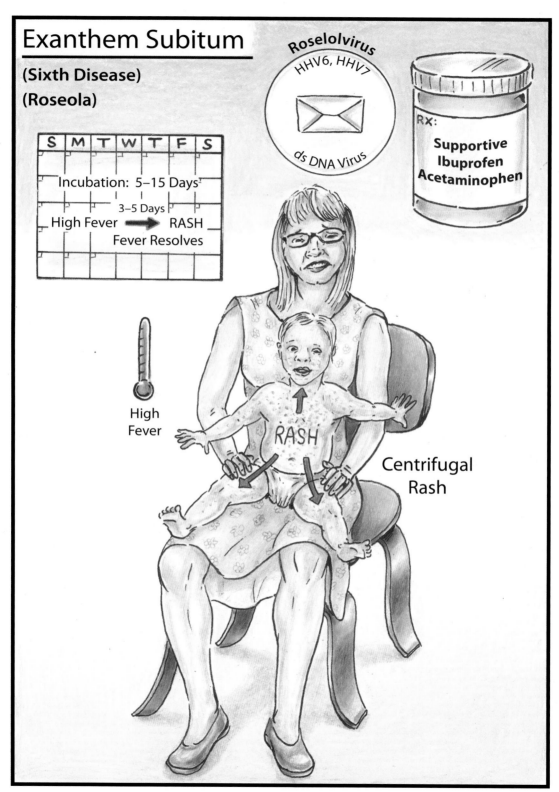

Exanthem Subitum

(Sixth Disease)

(Roseola)

Roselolvirus
HHV6, HHV7

ds DNA Virus

RX:
**Supportive
Ibuprofen
Acetaminophen**

S	M	T	W	T	F	S

Incubation: 5–15 Days

3–5 Days

High Fever ➞ RASH

Fever Resolves

High Fever

RASH

Centrifugal Rash

Disease Name: **Chickenpox**

Synonym:	Varicella
Causative Agent:	Varicella-zoster Virus (VZV)
Incubation:	10–21 Days; Average: 14–16 days
Geographic Regions Affected:	Worldwide
Description:	Chickenpox is a highly contagious, vaccine-preventable, viral illness characterized by a rash that spreads in a cephalocaudal (head to toe) progression and rapidly progresses from macules and papules to vesicles and then scabs.
Signs and Symptoms:	Primary infection occurs after an incubation period averaging 14–16 days. Initial symptoms include a prodrome of fever and malaise (more common in adults) 1–2 days before the onset of a characteristic rash. The rash is pruritic and first appears on the head, chest, and back before spreading to the extremities. Lesions rapidly progress from macules and papules to vesicles before scabbing over. New crops of lesions occur over the next 3–4 days, and most lesions crust over within a week. Scabs remain for about 2 weeks before falling off. It is typical to have crops of lesions at various stages; this is how the disease is diagnosed clinically. Chickenpox tends to be a mild illness in young children and causes more severe presentations and complications in adolescents, adults, and the immunocompromised. Complications can include secondary bacterial skin infections, pneumonia, and encephalitis. Pregnant women who develop chickenpox can pass the infection on to the fetus or neonate, causing congenital varicella syndrome or neonatal varicella, respectively.
Diagnostic Testing:	Chickenpox is often a clinical diagnosis. Polymerase chain reaction (PCR) testing of blister fluid can be done in pregnant females to diagnose acute infections.
Treatments:	Supportive. Calamine lotion can be applied to soothe the lesions and make them less itchy. Acyclovir may have some benefit in the treatment of varicella pneumonia and encephalitis. There are vaccines to prevent both primary infection (chickenpox) and the reactivation of VZV (shingles).
Pearls:	After a single dose of vaccine, some patients exposed to a wild strain of VZV may develop a mild form of chickenpox referred to as "breakthrough disease." These patients will have a lower-grade fever, atypical rash pattern, and fewer lesions and are less likely to develop complications. Although "breakthrough disease" could potentially occur after the second dose of vaccine, it would be rare.

Chickenpox

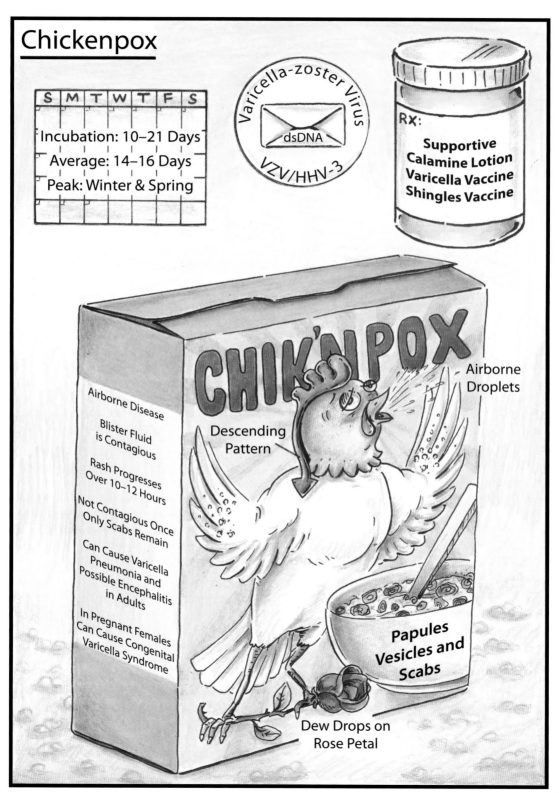

S	M	T	W	T	F	S

Incubation: 10–21 Days
Average: 14–16 Days
Peak: Winter & Spring

Varicella-zoster Virus
dsDNA
VZV/HHV-3

RX:
**Supportive
Calamine Lotion
Varicella Vaccine
Shingles Vaccine**

CHIK'N'POX

Airborne Disease

Blister Fluid is Contagious

Rash Progresses Over 10–12 Hours

Not Contagious Once Only Scabs Remain

Can Cause Varicella Pneumonia and Possible Encephalitis in Adults

In Pregnant Females Can Cause Congenital Varicella Syndrome

Descending Pattern

Airborne Droplets

Papules Vesicles and Scabs

Dew Drops on Rose Petal

Disease Name: Congenital and Perinatal Infections

Below is the CHEAP TORCHES mnemonic for congenital and perinatal infections proposed by Ford-Jones and Kellner in the *Pediatric Infectious Diseases Journal* in 1995.

C—Chickenpox: Varicella can be passed on to the child in utero, during the perinatal period, or just after birth. In utero transmission, particularly early in pregnancy (<20 weeks), can cause congenital varicella syndrome (CVS). This syndrome is characterized by one or more abnormalities, including low birth weight, hypoplastic limbs, ocular defects, neurologic defects (mental retardation, microcephaly, hydrocephalus), and/or cutaneous scars that follow dermatomal patterns. Neonatal varicella, an early infection not associated with birth defects, can occur via placental transmission in late pregnancy or via exposure to maternal respiratory droplets shortly after birth.

H—Hepatitis: Both hepatitis B and C are concerns during pregnancy and can be transmitted whether the child is born vaginally or via C-section. Hepatitis B is more likely to be transmitted if the mother has an acute infection or a chronic infection and is HBeAg+ (lacks antibodies to the e antigen). Infants born to mothers infected with hepatitis B should receive hepatitis B immunoglobulin and the first dose of the hepatitis B vaccine within hours of birth to decrease the likelihood of infection. Those infants infected with hepatitis B during childbirth have a higher likelihood (about 90%) of becoming chronically infected themselves. Women with chronic hepatitis C have about a 4% chance of passing the infection on to their children.

E—Enterovirus: Non-polio enteroviruses are very common, specifically in the summer and fall. Mothers infected shortly before delivery can potentially pass the infection on to the infant. Infected infants will most likely have mild disease. According to the Centers for Disease Control and Prevention (CDC), there is no clear evidence that infection during pregnancy increases the risk of miscarriage, stillbirth, or congenital defects.

A—AIDS: HIV transmission can occur anytime during pregnancy, labor and delivery, or during breastfeeding. Prior to the use of antiretroviral therapy (ART) in pregnancy, risk of transmission to the infant was >90%. Risk of transmission is determined by several factors, including the mother's HIV viral load and use of or lack of antepartum or intrapartum antiretroviral drugs. The CDC recommends that maternal ART should be initiated as early in pregnancy as possible and continued by the infant for at least 4–6 weeks. Those infants born to HIV-positive mothers who did not receive intrapartum ART should be initiated on ART prophylaxis within hours after birth. With proper HIV treatment during pregnancy and after, risk of transmission can be reduced to <1%.

P—Parvovirus B-19: Parvovirus B-19 causes erythema infectiosum (slap face); fortunately, most women are immune prior to pregnancy. Infection during pregnancy can cause a severe fetal aplastic anemia and resultant complications (hydrops fetalis) leading to miscarriage.

T—Toxoplasmosis:	Toxoplasmosis is a parasitic protozoan infection caused by *Toxoplasma gondii* and causes asymptomatic or mild flulike illness in immunocompetent patients. The parasite can remain in the host in an inactive state and become reactivated if the immune system becomes compromised. Toxoplasmosis can be passed to the fetus if the mother contracts the infection just before or during pregnancy.

Maternal infection with toxoplasmosis can cause spontaneous abortion, stillbirth, or congenital infection. Congenital infections can range in severity from mild to severe and may not manifest until much later in the child's life. The classic triad of congenital toxoplasmosis includes chorioretinitis, hydrocephalus, and intracranial calcifications. Congenital infections that manifest later in life include chorioretinitis (potentially leading to blindness), mental retardation, and/or seizures.

To prevent toxoplasmosis infection during pregnancy, women are encouraged not to clean the litter box, to feed the cat only dry or canned cat food, to keep the cat indoors, and to refrain from getting any new cats or kittens prior to or during the pregnancy. Litter boxes should be cleaned daily, as it takes 1–5 days for the toxoplasma parasite in the cat feces to become infectious. Proper handwashing with soap and water after exposure to uncooked meats, sand, and soil is encouraged.

O—Other: This is the catch-all for the mnemonic and includes: Group B Strep (GBS), Listeria, Lyme, and Zika. Others may be added over time.

Group B Strep: GBS is a bacteria that can be passed to the infant during childbirth. Since 25% of women carry GBS in their reproductive tract (are carriers/are colonized), the CDC recommends routine screening of pregnant women for GBS between 35 and 37 weeks of pregnancy. Those women who test positive or have an unknown GBS status are treated with intravenous (IV) antibiotics during delivery to decrease the risk of transmission to the infant. Infants that contract GBS during childbirth may become ill and develop pneumonia, sepsis, and/or meningitis.

Listeria: Pregnant women are at a greater risk than the general population at contracting an infection with *Listeria monocytogenes*, specifically during the third trimester. Infection can manifest as flulike symptoms and can cause miscarriage or premature delivery. About 20% of perinatal listeria infections will result in stillbirth or neonatal death. Neonatal infections can cause sepsis, meningitis, and/or granulomatous infantisepticemia. Foods to avoid during pregnancy include pate, young cheeses, raw milk, and unwashed fruits and vegetables.

Lyme Disease: The CDC reports that untreated Lyme disease during pregnancy may potentially cause brain, nerve, spinal cord, and cardiac defects. Avoidance of tick exposure during pregnancy and early treatment of pregnant females is highly recommended. Since doxycycline is contraindicated in pregnancy, treatment would consist of either amoxicillin or cefuroxime in penicillin-allergic patients.

Zika: The CDC reports that Zika infection during pregnancy may cause congenital Zika syndrome, a pattern of birth defects that includes microcephaly, decreased brain development and mental retardation, ocular abnormalities, club foot, and/or increased muscle tone at birth.

R—Rubella:

Congenital rubella syndrome (CRS) is characterized by a triad of deafness, cataracts, and congenital heart disease (pulmonary artery stenosis and/or patent ductus arteriosus). Infants may also have a "blueberry muffin" rash indicating extramedullary hematopoiesis. Risk of CRS is greatest if the mother contracts rubella during the first two trimesters.

C—Cytomegalovirus:

Cytomegalovirus (CMV) can be passed to the fetus via the placenta if the mother has an active infection. The CDC has recognized that most congenital CMV infections are asymptomatic and/or never cause any long-term consequences. However, CMV may cause spontaneous abortion or stillbirth. Signs of congenital CMV infection include premature birth, low birth weight, microcephaly, seizures, mental retardation, or hearing and/or vision loss. Hearing loss may be present at birth or may manifest later in life.

H—Herpes:

Congenital HSV infection can result in microcephaly, hydrocephaly, chorioretinitis, and skin lesions. Neonatal herpes is often contracted at birth via asymptomatic shedding of the virus at the cervix and can cause localized skin infection, encephalitis, or disseminated disease. Infected neonates should be treated with IV acyclovir.

E—Everything Sexually Transmitted:

Another catch-all for the mnemonic. Both gonorrhea and chlamydia can be contracted by the infant via vaginal delivery or in C-section if there has been premature rupture of membranes. Both infections typically present as conjunctivitis (ophthalmia neonatorum). A purulent conjunctival discharge 2–5 days after birth is classic for gonorrhea, while a more watery (eventually progressing to purulent) discharge occurring 5–14 days after birth is classic for chlamydia. Erythromycin ophthalmic ointment can be used as prophylaxis in the infant against gonorrheal conjunctivitis, but it has no effect on chlamydial conjunctivitis. Gonorrhea contracted at birth can also cause infection in an infant's pharynx, urethra, anus, and/or vagina, as well as disseminated infections presenting as sepsis, meningitis, and/or arthritis. Chlamydial infections contracted at birth can cause neonatal pneumonia.

S—Syphilis:

Congenital syphilis occurs when the spirochete *Treponema pallidum* is passed to the fetus via the placenta during pregnancy and may result in prematurity, LBW, miscarriage, congenital infection, stillbirth, or neonatal death. The likelihood of the mother passing the infection on to the fetus is highest in primary and secondary syphilis and lowest in the tertiary stage. The CDC reports the risk of stillbirth or neonatal death is near 40% for pregnant women with untreated syphilis. Of those born with congenital infection, the disease is characterized as either early (diagnosed before 2 years of age) or late (diagnosed after 2 years of age).

Early congenital syphilis presents with jaundice, hepatosplenomegaly, lymphadenopathy, rhinitis (snuffles), a characteristic maculopapular rash, and radiographic long bone abnormalities. Late congenital syphilis can present with notched upper incisors (Hutchinson teeth), perioral fissures (rhagades), interstitial keratitis, deafness, frontal bossing, saddle nose deformity, short maxilla and protruding mandible, anterior bowing of the lower legs (saber shins), and arthritis of the knees (Clutton joints). Hutchinson triad consists of deafness, Hutchinson teeth, and interstitial keratitis. Children with congenital syphilis should be treated with penicillin.

Congenital & Perinatal Infections

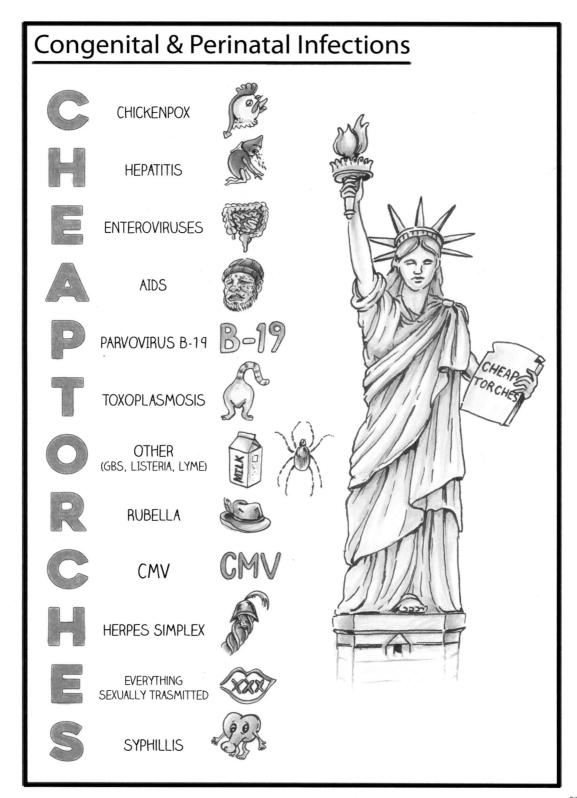

C CHICKENPOX

H HEPATITIS

E ENTEROVIRUSES

A AIDS

P PARVOVIRUS B-19

T TOXOPLASMOSIS

O OTHER
(GBS, LISTERIA, LYME)

R RUBELLA

C CMV

H HERPES SIMPLEX

E EVERYTHING
SEXUALLY TRASMITTED

S SYPHILLIS

Disease Name: **Pertussis**

Synonyms: Whooping Cough, 100-Day Cough

Causative Agent: *Bordetella pertussis*

Incubation: 4–21 days; Average: 5–10 days

Geographic Regions Affected: Worldwide

Description: Pertussis is a highly contagious, vaccine-preventable, bacterial illness that causes a characteristic triad of prolonged cough syndrome, inspiratory whoop, and posttussive vomiting.

Signs and Symptoms: Pertussis is divided into three stages. The *Catarrhal Stage* presents like most upper respiratory infections with rhinorrhea, sneezing, low-grade temperature, and a mild cough. These symptoms persist for about 7–10 days until the cough becomes progressively worse. The *Paroxysmal Stage* is characterized by coughing spells or paroxysms, the classic inspiratory whoop, and posttussive vomiting. Paroxysms occur more frequently at night, increase in frequency for the first few weeks, remain at a constant frequency for several weeks, and then gradually decrease in frequency. Complications can include exhaustion, rib fractures, subconjunctival hemorrhages, pneumonia, cyanosis, and apnea in children. The paroxysmal phase lasts 1–6 weeks, but sometimes as long as 10. The *Convalescent Stage* is a gradual recovery associated with less frequent and less persistent paroxysms. This stage lasts about 7–10 days but can persist for as long as 21 days. Subsequent upper respiratory infections may trigger paroxysmal coughing spells months after pertussis has resolved.

Diagnostic Testing: A nasopharyngeal swab should be used to obtain patient samples for both culture and polymerase chain reaction (PCR) testing. Culture and PCR specimens can be obtained immediately at the onset of cough and provide accurate results if obtained in the first 2 weeks (culture) or 4 weeks (PCR) of symptoms. Serology can be obtained between 2 to 8 weeks after cough onset and are of greater value later in disease presentation.

Treatments: Azithromycin, clarithromycin, erythromycin, or TMP/SMX are effective for eradicating nasal carriage of the bacteria (lessening likelihood of transmitting infection) and can decrease the duration of symptoms if initiated during the catarrhal stage. The disease is preventable by vaccination, but, as a result of decreasing immunity with age, the United States Committee on Immunization Practices recommends a booster with Tdap (tetanus, diphtheria, acellular pertussis) at least once for those patients between 15 to 65 years of age. Postexposure antibiotics may be indicated to prevent illness in certain populations.

Pertussis

(Whooping Cough)
(100-Day Cough)

S	M	T	W	T	F	S
		Incubation: 4–21 Days				
	Average Incubation: 5–10 Days					
	Catarrhal Stage: 1–2 Weeks					
Paroxysmal Cough Stage: 1–6 Weeks						
	Convalescence: Weeks to Months					

Bordetella pertussis
Gram ⊖ Aerobic Coccobacillus

RX:
Azithromycin
Erythromycin
TMP/SMX
Vaccine

Catarrhal Stage

Runny Nose

Sneezing

Low-grade Temperature

Mild Cough

↓

Cough Becomes Worse

> Cough, cough WHOOP!

Paroxysmal Stage

Coughing Spells/Paroxysms

↓

Inspiratory Whoop

Posttussive Vomiting

Cyanosis

Apnea in Infants

Subconjunctival Hemorrhage

Rib Fractures/PTX

Pneumonia

> Paroxysms are worse at night!

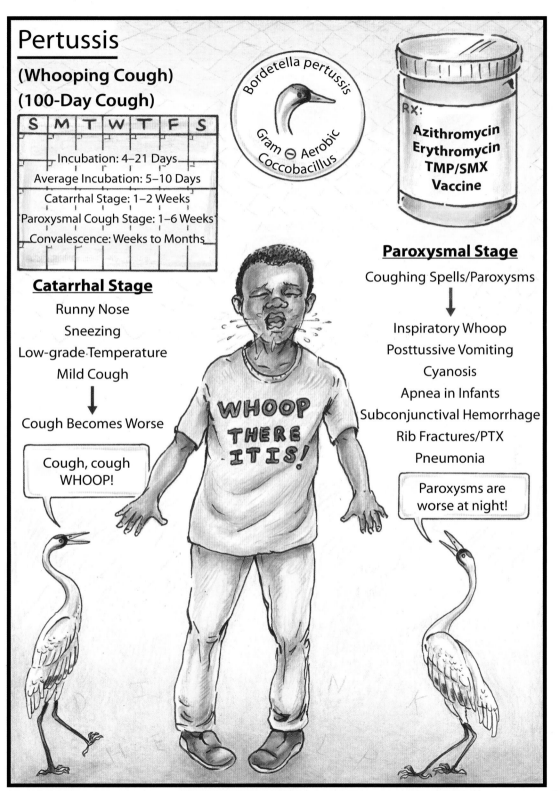

WHOOP THERE IT IS!

Disease Name: Hand, Foot, and Mouth Disease

Causative Agents:	ssRNA Enteroviruses: Coxsackievirus A16 and Enterovirus A71
Incubation:	3–6 days
Geographic Regions Affected:	Worldwide
Peak Incidence:	Spring–Fall, Occasional outbreaks in day care centers and elementary schools
Brief Description:	Hand, foot, and mouth disease (HFMD) is a self-limiting febrile viral enanthem of the mouth with associated papular, maculopapular, or vesicular rash of the hands and feet. The disease is most common in children under the age of 10, with most cases occurring in children younger than 5 years of age.
Signs and Symptoms:	HFMD classically presents as a low-grade fever, headache, and malaise for 1–3 days, followed by an oral enanthem with a papular, maculopapular, or vesicular rash of the hands and feet. The rash may occasionally involve the legs and buttocks. The sores in the mouth may cause poor feeding and irritability. The disease is self-limiting and tends to resolve after 7–10 days. Fingernail and toenail loss can occur in some children 4–8 weeks after infection with HFMD.
Diagnostic Testing:	HFMD tends to be a clinical diagnosis based on history, symptoms, and characteristic exam findings.
Treatments:	Supportive. "Magic Mouthwash" made of equal parts of liquid magnesium hydroxide and liquid diphenhydramine as a swish and spit may help control oral pain. Weight-based ibuprofen is helpful for pain and fever control. Ice pops can help improve oral intake and decrease oral pain.
Prevention:	Handwashing. Enteroviruses tend to be transmitted via the fecal-oral route. HFMD can be transmitted via oral and nasal secretions, as well as via the fecal-oral route.

Hand, Foot, and Mouth Disease

(HFMD)

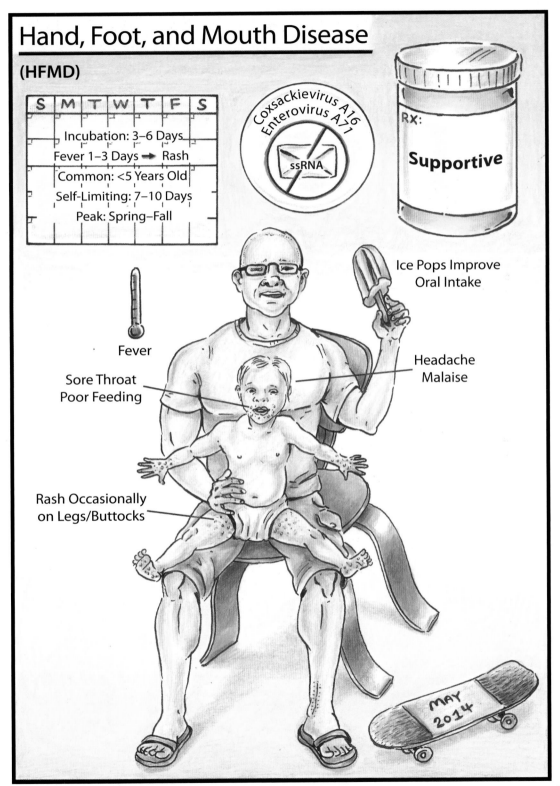

S	M	T	W	T	F	S

Incubation: 3–6 Days

Fever 1–3 Days ➡ Rash

Common: <5 Years Old

Self-Limiting: 7–10 Days

Peak: Spring–Fall

Coxsackievirus A16
Enterovirus A71

ssRNA

RX:

Supportive

Ice Pops Improve
Oral Intake

Fever

Headache
Malaise

Sore Throat
Poor Feeding

Rash Occasionally
on Legs/Buttocks

MAY 2014

Disease Name: **Bronchiolitis**

Causative Agents: Respiratory syncytial virus (RSV) is the most common cause. Other viruses include metapneumovirus, influenza, parainfluenza, adenovirus, coronavirus, and rhinovirus.

Incubation: 3–5 days

Geographic Regions Affected: Worldwide

Peak Incidence: Winter

Description: Bronchiolitis is an acute viral lower respiratory tract infection most commonly caused by RSV in children less than 2 years old. Bronchiolitis peaks in infants 3–6 months old and is the most common cause for hospitalization in children younger than 1 year old. Infants with higher risk for severe disease include preemies, low–birth weight infants, and those born with congenital heart defects.

Signs and Symptoms: RSV affects both children and adults, often presenting as a typical viral upper respiratory infection with possible wheezing in the latter. In young children, bronchiolitis initially presents with rhinorrhea and then progresses to the lower respiratory tract after a few days. Inflammation of the smaller airways (bronchioles) causes cough, wheezing, and rhonchi. Severe disease is characterized by lethargy, poor feeding, tachypnea, nasal flaring, retractions, hypoxia, cyanosis, apnea, and respiratory failure. Infants younger than 4 weeks of age and smaller, low birth–weight, premature infants (preemies) are at higher risk of central apnea. Symptoms tend to resolve after 7–10 days.

Diagnostic Testing: Diagnosis is often based on history and clinical presentation. Chest x-ray may show hyperinflation and peribronchial cuffing. Nasopharyngeal swabs can be used to obtain samples for polymerase chain reaction (PCR) testing in the acute setting. IgM/IgG serology exists but is of limited value in the acutely ill patient.

Treatment: Treatment is mostly supportive. Management and disposition is based on patient age, past medical history, risk factors for apnea, and severity of illness. Nasal suctioning helps clear secretions. Supplemental oxygen and a trial of bronchodilators are beneficial. Steroids, antibiotics, and/or ribavirin have no proven benefits. Intravenous fluids may be necessary given insensible losses and decreased oral intake.

Bronchiolitis

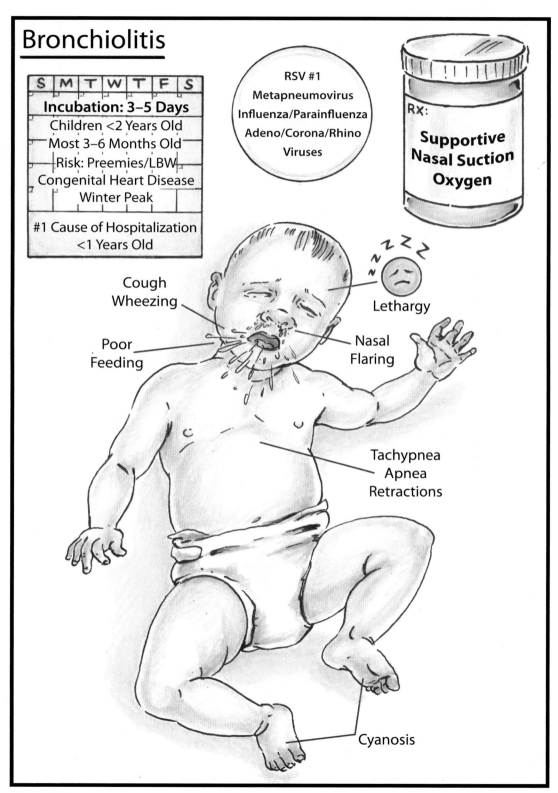

S	M	T	W	T	F	S

Incubation: 3–5 Days

Children <2 Years Old

Most 3–6 Months Old

Risk: Preemies/LBW

Congenital Heart Disease

Winter Peak

#1 Cause of Hospitalization <1 Years Old

RSV #1
Metapneumovirus
Influenza/Parainfluenza
Adeno/Corona/Rhino
Viruses

RX:
**Supportive
Nasal Suction
Oxygen**

Cough
Wheezing

Poor
Feeding

Lethargy

Nasal
Flaring

Tachypnea
Apnea
Retractions

Cyanosis

Disease Name: **Kawasaki Disease**

Synonyms: KD, Mucocutaneous lymph node syndrome

Causative Agent: Unknown—Possibly viral and/or autoimmune

Incubation: Unknown

Geographic Regions Affected: Worldwide, with greatest incidence in Japan and East Asian countries. Children of East Asian and Pacific Island descent living worldwide are affected to a greater degree than Caucasians.

Description: KD is a febrile childhood illness characterized by vasculitis of medium-sized arteries, inflammation of mucocutaneous tissues, and lymphadenopathy.

Signs and Symptoms: The disease begins with irritability and a high fever that tends to be unresponsive to traditional antipyretics. Children will likely next develop bilateral conjunctivitis and inflammation of the oral mucosa, including cracked red lips, inflamed "strawberry tongue," and/or oropharyngeal erythema. Rash, typically occurring 1–2 days after fever onset, is polymorphic and can be erythematous, macular, maculopapular, desquamating, or target-like and involves the trunk and extremities. Hand and foot erythema and edema are the last symptoms to appear. Periungal desquamation can occur in the convalescent phase of the disease. Lymphadenopathy, when it occurs, is limited to the anterior cervical chain. Without treatment, the disease resolves within 10–12 days. Coronary artery aneurysms can develop in untreated patients as the disease resolves, thus early diagnosis and treatment with intravenous immunoglobulin (IVIG) is paramount.

Diagnostic Testing: Labs will reveal elevated CRP and SED rates, leukocytosis with a left shift (increased neutrophils), increased platelets, and normocytic anemia.

Diagnostic criteria established by Tomisaku Kawasaki require the presence of a fever >5 days' duration and four of the five following criteria: (1) bilateral conjunctival injection, (2) polymorphous rash, (3) cervical lymphadenopathy with one node at least >15 mm, (4) strawberry tongue, cracked lips, or injected pharynx, (5) hand or foot erythema, edema, or periungal desquamation.

Treatments: IVIG is the standard treatment and is ideally initiated within 7–10 days to decrease the likelihood of coronary artery aneurysms. High-dose aspirin tapered down over time is still a part of some treatment protocols.

Pearls: Diagnostic criteria for KD can be remembered by the mnemonic: **Fever >5 Days** and **CRASH: C**onjunctivitis, **R**ash, **A**denopathy, **S**trawberry tongue, **H**ands and Feet.

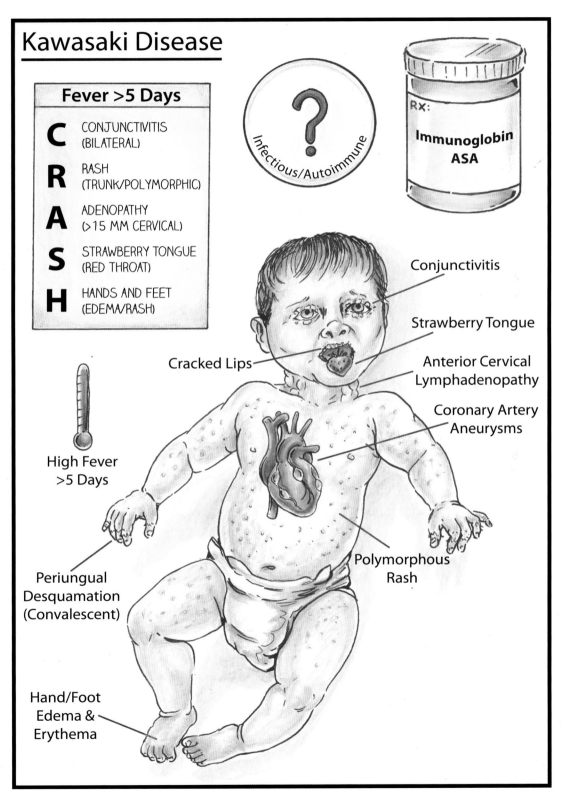

Kawasaki Disease

Fever >5 Days

C CONJUNCTIVITIS
(BILATERAL)

R RASH
(TRUNK/POLYMORPHIC)

A ADENOPATHY
(>15 MM CERVICAL)

S STRAWBERRY TONGUE
(RED THROAT)

H HANDS AND FEET
(EDEMA/RASH)

Infectious/Autoimmune

?

RX:

**Immunoglobin
ASA**

Conjunctivitis

Strawberry Tongue

Anterior Cervical
Lymphadenopathy

Coronary Artery
Aneurysms

Cracked Lips

High Fever
>5 Days

Periungual
Desquamation
(Convalescent)

Polymorphous
Rash

Hand/Foot
Edema &
Erythema

Disease Name: **Croup**

Synonym: Laryngotracheobronchitis

Causative Agents: ssRNA Parainfluenza virus is the most common cause. Other viral causes can include influenza virus, respiratory syncytial virus, human metapneumovirus, adenovirus, and rhinovirus.

Incubation: 2–6 days

Geographic Regions Affected: Worldwide

Peak Incidence: Fall–Winter. Most common in children 6 months to 3 years old, with a peak incidence at age 2.

Description: Croup is a viral infection of the upper airway that causes stridor, hoarseness, and a characteristic bark-like cough, often worse at night.

Signs and Symptoms: Croup is often preceded by a prodrome of several days of malaise, rhinorrhea, and a low-grade fever before the onset of hoarseness, stridor, and the characteristic seal-like barking cough. The Westley Croup Score categorizes the severity of illness on the basis of five criteria: chest wall retractions, stridor, cyanosis, level of consciousness, and air entry. Fortunately, most cases are mild and can be managed as an outpatient or with overnight observation. Symptoms often resolve in most patients within 3–7 days.

Diagnostic Testing: Croup tends to be a clinical diagnosis based on history, symptoms, and characteristic exam findings. An anterior-posterior (AP) soft tissue neck x-ray will likely reveal the "steeple sign," a tapering of the upper trachea resembling a church steeple. Astute clinicians need to consider epiglottitis (drooling and high fever) and bacterial tracheitis (toxic appearance and high fever) in their differential.

Treatments: Supportive. Steam or humidified mist may be of some benefit in providing calm for both the infant and family. Nebulized epinephrine can be given every 20 minutes and decrease upper airway edema and stridor. Oral corticosteroids (dexamethasone) take effect within 6 hours of administration, decrease the frequency of nebulized epinephrine treatments, and shorten the emergency department/hospital lengths of stay.

Croup
(Laryngotracheobronchitis)

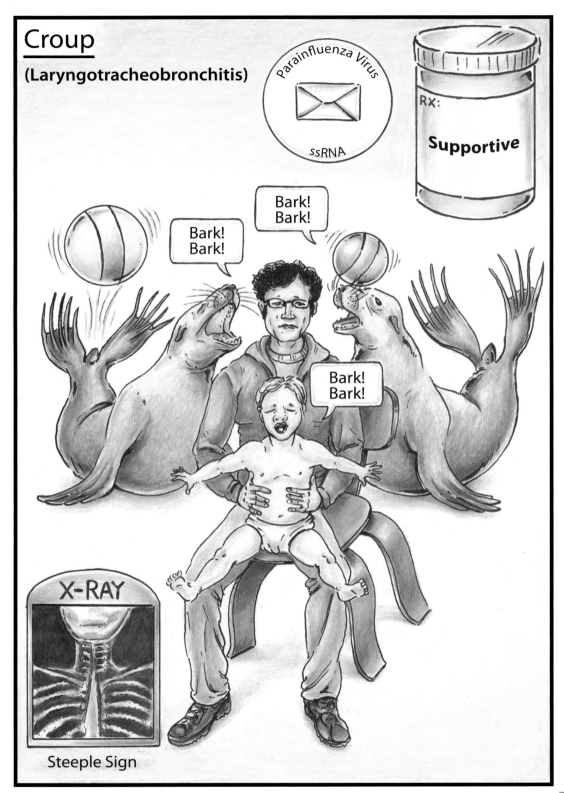

Steeple Sign

PART 4

TICK-BORNE ILLNESSES

Disease Name: Tick-Borne Illness and Ticks as Vectors

Lyme Disease:
- Causative Agent: *Borrelia burgdorferi*
- Vector: *Ixodes scapularis* (deer tick), *Ixodes pacificus* (western black-legged tick), *Ixodes ricinus* (sheep tick), *Ixodes persulcatus* (taiga tick)
- Region: North America, Eurasia
- Symptoms: fever, malaise, myalgia, erythema migrans rash, neurologic, cardiac, arthritis
- Treatment: doxycycline, amoxicillin, ceftriaxone

Relapsing Fever:
- Causative Agent: *Borrelia hermsii, Borrelia parkeri, Borrelia duttoni, Borrelia miyamotoi*
- Vector: Ornithodoros species (soft body ticks)
- Region: Africa, Spain, Middle East, Western United States, and Canada
- Symptoms: relapsing fevers, headaches, myalgia, cough, rash
- Treatment: doxycycline, tetracycline, erythromycin

Rocky Mountain Spotted Fever:
- Causative Agent: *Rickettsia rickettsii*
- Vector: *Dermacentor variabilis* (dog tick), *Dermacentor andersoni* (Rocky Mountain wood tick)
- Region: United States
- Symptoms: headache, fever, myalgia, rash
- Treatment: doxycycline, tetracycline

Ehrlichiosis—HME:
- Causative Agent: *Ehrlichia chaffeensis*
- Vector: *Amblyomma americanum* (lone star tick), *Dermacentor variabilis* (dog tick)
- Region: South Central and Eastern North America
- Symptoms: headache, myalgia, fatigue, rash (uncommon)
- Treatment: doxycycline, minocycline, rifampin

Anaplasmosis—HGA:
- Causative Agent: *Anaplasma phagocytophilum*
- Vector: *Ixodes scapularis* (deer tick), *Ixodes pacificus* (black-legged tick), *Ixodes ricinus* (sheep tick) *Ixodes persulcatus* (taiga tick), *Haemaphysalis longicornis* (Cattle Tick)
- Region: Northern latitudes of North America, Europe, and Asia
- Symptoms: headache, myalgia, fatigue, rash (rare)
- Treatment: doxycycline, minocycline, rifampin

Tularemia:
- Causative Agent: *Francisella tularensis*
- Host: rabbits, beavers, muskrats
- Vector: *Dermacentor variabilis* (dog tick), *Dermacentor andersoni* (Rocky Mountain wood tick)
- Region: United States, Eurasia
- Symptoms: fever, malaise, lymphadenopathy, skin ulceration
- Treatment: doxycycline, ciprofloxacin, streptomycin, gentamicin, chloramphenicol

Tick-borne Meningoencephalitis:	• Causative Agent: tick-borne encephalitis virus (TBEV) • Vector: *Ixodes scapularis* (deer tick), *Ixodes ricinus* (sheep tick), *Ixodes persulcatus* (taiga tick) • Region: Europe, North Asia • Symptoms: meningitis, encephalitis, meningoencephalitis • Treatment: supportive, TBEV vaccine
Colorado Tick Fever:	• Causative Agent: Colorado tick fever virus (CTFV) • Vector: *Dermacentor andersoni* (Rocky Mountain wood tick) • Region: Western U.S. • Symptoms: Two phases of disease. Initially fever, chills, headache, malaise, myalgia, nausea, vomiting, splenomegaly, rash. In the second phase, symptoms intensify. • Treatment: supportive
Crimean-Congo Hemorrhagic Fever:	• Causative Agent: Crimean-Congo hemorrhagic fever virus (CCHFV) • Vector: *Hyalomma marginatum*, *Rhipicephalus sanguineus* • Region: Africa, Southern Europe, Southern Asia • Symptoms: flulike symptoms, altered mental status (AMS), petechiae, epistaxis, nausea, vomiting, melena, shock, and disseminated intravascular coagulation (DIC). 75% of patients will hemorrhage and the disease has a 30% mortality. • Treatment: supportive, vaccine, ribavirin
Babesiosis:	• Causative Agent: *Babesia microti*, *Babesia duncani* • Vector: *Ixodes scapularis* (deer tick), *Ixodes pacificus* (black-legged tick), *Ixodes ricinus* (sheep tick) • Region: North-Eastern states, Upper Midwest, Pacific Northwest, and parts of Europe • Symptoms: flulike symptoms, malaise, headache, fatigue, and fever. Hemolytic anemia and thrombocytopenia can occur. • Treatment: Atovaquone and azithromycin or clindamycin and quinine
Tick paralysis:	• Causative Agent: neurotoxin • Vector: *Dermacentor variabilis* (dog tick), *Dermacentor andersoni* (Rocky Mountain wood tick) • Region: United States • Symptoms: ascending paralysis, beginning in legs and spreading to trunk and extremities, decreased deep tendon reflexes, and ataxia. Respiratory failure can occur if left untreated. • Treatment: Tick removal causes rapid abatement of symptoms

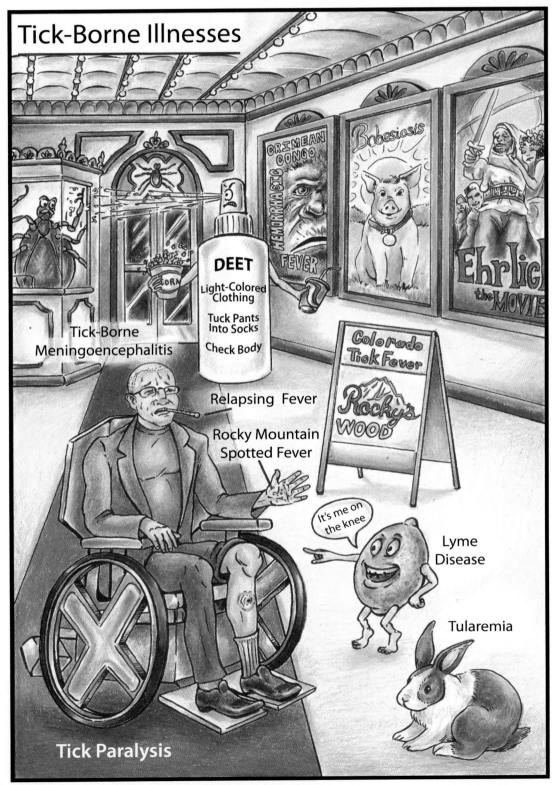

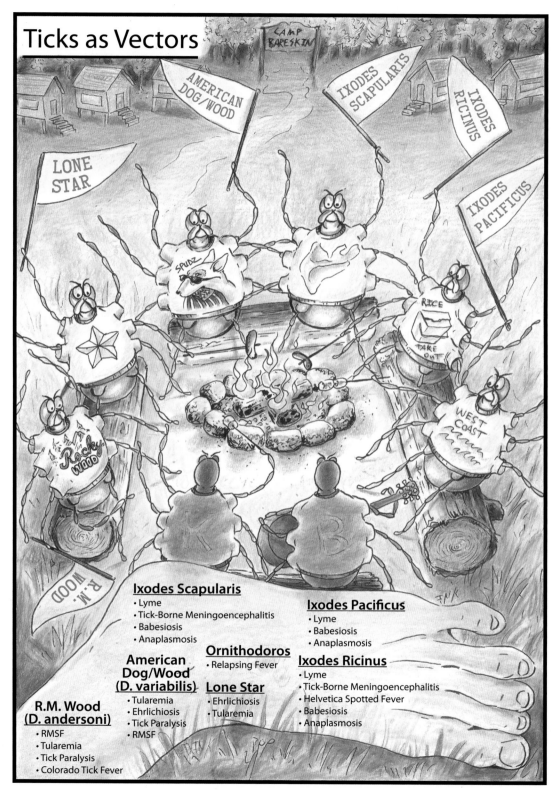

Ticks as Vectors

Ixodes Scapularis
- Lyme
- Tick-Borne Meningoencephalitis
- Babesiosis
- Anaplasmosis

Ixodes Pacificus
- Lyme
- Babesiosis
- Anaplasmosis

Ornithodoros
- Relapsing Fever

Ixodes Ricinus
- Lyme
- Tick-Borne Meningoencephalitis
- Helvetica Spotted Fever
- Babesiosis
- Anaplasmosis

American Dog/Wood (D. variabilis)
- Tularemia
- Ehrlichiosis
- Tick Paralysis
- RMSF

Lone Star
- Ehrlichiosis
- Tularemia

R.M. Wood (D. andersoni)
- RMSF
- Tularemia
- Tick Paralysis
- Colorado Tick Fever

Disease Name: Rocky Mountain Spotted Fever

Synonyms: RMSF, Blue Disease, Black Measles

Causative Agent: *Rickettsia rickettsii* in America

Vector: United States: American dog tick *(Dermacentor variabilis)*, Rocky Mountain wood tick *(D. andersoni)*, brown dog tick *(Rhipicephalus sanguineus)*. Central and South America: Cayenne tick *(Amblyomma cajennense)*. Female ticks pass the infection to their eggs in a process called transovarial transmission.

Reservoir: Small woodland animals, domestic dogs and cats, deer.

Incubation Period: 2–14 days

Geographic Regions Affected: North Atlantic and South Central regions of the United States, North America, Central America, and South America.

Peak Incidence: Late spring and early summer

Description: RMSF is a tick-borne rickettsial zoonotic disease caused by *Rickettsia rickettsii*, a gram-negative obligate intracellular bacteria. The transmission of the infectious agent occurs within 6–10 hours of tick attachment.

Signs and Symptoms: Patients with mild disease have fever, malaise, myalgia, nausea, vomiting, headache, arthralgia, and rash. The characteristic rash of RMSF is a centripetal "inward" spreading macular rash, beginning on the wrist, forearm, and ankles and spreading inward toward the trunk. The palms and soles are involved in up to 80% of patients. Patients with severe disease may have skin necrosis, digit gangrene, acute respiratory distress syndrome, pulmonary edema, nausea, vomiting, abdominal pain, diarrhea, confusion, acute renal failure, meningoencephalitis, ataxia, blindness, retinal hemorrhages, papilledema, disseminated intravascular coagulation, jaundice, rhabdomyolysis, hepatomegaly, stupor, circulatory shock, and death.

Diagnostic Testing: The disease should be considered in patients presenting with fever, rash, and history of tick exposure/bite. Labs will reveal hyponatremia, thrombocytopenia, elevated liver enzymes, increased bilirubin, and increased BUN. Serologic detection of a fourfold rise in IgG antibodies against *R. rickettsii* by indirect immunofluorescence assay; Western blot with cross-absorption; detection of rickettsial nucleic acids by PCR in blood, skin biopsy, and eschar biopsy or swab; immunohistochemical detection of *R. rickettsia* in skin biopsy.

Treatments: Doxycycline 100 mg twice a day for 7–10 days. Chloramphenicol can be used as an alternative in pregnancy, but has a wide range of side effects and requires blood monitoring.

Pearls: Prevention by avoidance of tick exposures and early removal of attached ticks. Early therapy improves outcomes and prevents severe complications or sequelae. More-severe infections are seen in males, alcoholics, the elderly, African Americans, the immunocompromised, and patients with G6PD deficiency. Fever without rash can occur in the elderly and African Americans.

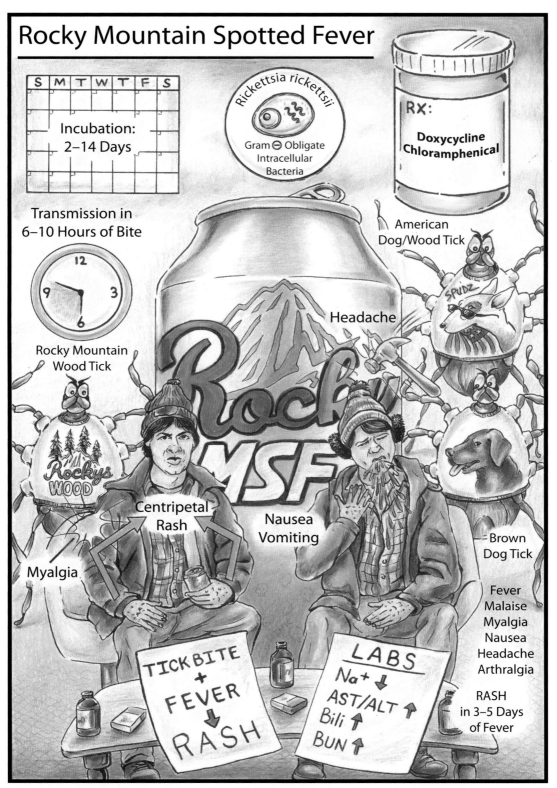

Rocky Mountain Spotted Fever

Incubation: 2–14 Days

Rickettsia rickettsii

Gram ⊖ Obligate Intracellular Bacteria

RX: Doxycycline Chloramphenical

Transmission in 6–10 Hours of Bite

American Dog/Wood Tick

Rocky Mountain Wood Tick

Headache

Centripetal Rash

Nausea Vomiting

Myalgia

Brown Dog Tick

Fever Malaise Myalgia Nausea Headache Arthralgia

RASH in 3–5 Days of Fever

TICK BITE + FEVER → RASH

LABS
Na+ ↓
AST/ALT ↑
Bili ↑
BUN ↑

Disease Name: Lyme Disease

Synonym:	Lyme borreliosis
Causative Agents:	*Borrelia burgdorferi* in North America; *B. afzelii* and *B. garinii* in Europe
Vector:	Deer tick *(Ixodes scapularis)* in Eastern U.S., black-legged tick *(Ixodes pacificus)* in Western U.S., sheep tick *(Ixodes ricinus)* in Europe, taiga tick *(Ixodes persulcatus)* in parts of Asia
Reservoir:	White-footed mouse *(Peromyscus leucopus)*
Incubation Period:	3–30 days
Geographic Regions Affected:	Northern latitudes of North America, Europe, and Asia
Peak Incidence:	Spring through fall, with peaks in summer months, in accordance with the activity of nymph stage of *Ixodes spp.* ticks. Nymphs are more likely than adult ticks to transmit Lyme disease.
Description:	Lyme disease is a tick-borne spirochetal zoonosis that may affect the skin, joints, nervous system, and heart. The disease is broken down into three stages of infection: early localized, early disseminated, and late disseminated.
Signs and Symptoms:	Early localized infection is characterized by a circular, outwardly-expanding bull's-eye rash known as *erythema migrans* (EM), occurring in 70%–80% of patients. Flulike symptoms, including fatigue, malaise, headache, myalgia, and fever, may be present or delayed. Early disseminated infection occurs within several days to weeks of the initial EM lesion and can present as multiple areas of EM. Within months, patients may develop neurologic symptoms, including facial palsy (can be bilateral), photosensitivity, polyneuropathy, vertigo, ataxia, insomnia, memory loss, psychosis, meningitis, and encephalitis. Cardiac symptoms can also present that include myopericarditis and heart block. Late disseminated infection is characterized by chronic arthritis and joint effusions, usually involving the knee.
Diagnostic Testing:	Culture of *B. burgdorferi* in Barbour-Stoenner-Kelly medium of biopsies of EM skin lesions; IgM and IgG serologic antibody testing can be obtained but is of limited use early in the disease course.
Treatments:	For early infection: doxycycline 100 mg orally twice a day, amoxicillin 500 mg orally three times a day, or cefuroxime 500 mg orally twice a day for 14–21 days. Treatment for cardiac, nervous system, or joint involvement: ceftriaxone 2 g intravenously once a day for 28 days can be used. Treatment regiments may vary based on severity of disease.
Pearls:	Prevention by avoidance of tick exposure and early removal of attached tick. Transmission rarely occurs unless the tick has been attached for >24 to 36 hours. Early therapy improves outcomes and prevents severe complications or sequelae. When an engorged nymph is found attached, a single dose of 200 mg of oral doxycycline given within 72 hours of the tick bite can prevent Lyme disease. Multiple EM indicates spirochetemia and not multiple tick bites. Coinfection with *Babesia microti* can occur. Lyme disease is the most common vector-borne infection in the United States and is very common in the Northeast and upper Midwest U.S.

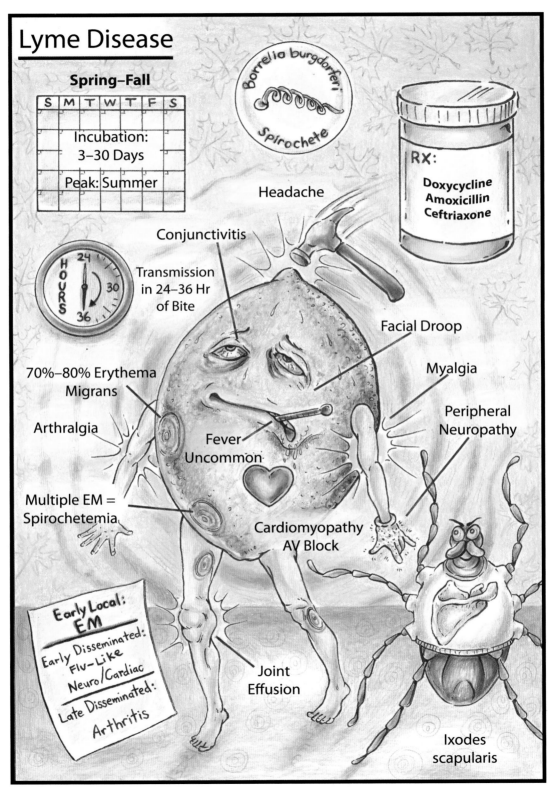

Lyme Disease

Spring–Fall

Incubation:
3–30 Days

Peak: Summer

Borrelia burgdorferi
Spirochete

RX:
Doxycycline
Amoxicillin
Ceftriaxone

Headache

Conjunctivitis

HOURS 24 30 36

Transmission
in 24–36 Hr
of Bite

Facial Droop

Myalgia

70%–80% Erythema
Migrans

Peripheral
Neuropathy

Arthralgia

Fever
Uncommon

Multiple EM =
Spirochetemia

Cardiomyopathy
AV Block

Early Local:
EM
Early Disseminated:
Flu–Like
Neuro/Cardiac
Late Disseminated:
Arthritis

Joint
Effusion

Ixodes
scapularis

Disease Name: **Ehrlichiosis**

Synonym:	Human monocytic ehrlichiosis (HME)
Causative Agents:	*Ehrlichia chaffeensis*, *Ehrlichia ewingii* (less common)
Vector:	Lone star tick *(Amblyomma americanum)*, dog tick/wood tick *(Dermacentor variabilis)*
Reservoir:	White-tail deer *(Odocoileus virginianus)*
Incubation Period:	7–14 days
Geographic Regions Affected:	South Central and Eastern North America
Peak Incidence:	Spring and summer
Description:	Ehrlichiosis (HME) is a tick-borne rickettsial zoonosis caused by an obligate intracellular bacteria that affects monocytes.
Signs and Symptoms:	Many cases are thought to be asymptomatic. In mild disease, fever, chills, headache, malaise, myalgia, nausea, vomiting, diarrhea, conjunctivitis, and rash can occur. Unlike HGA, rash occurs in about 30% of adults and up to 60% of children with HME. In severe disease, septic shock-like syndrome, respiratory distress, meningoencephalitis, renal failure, and death can occur. Severe disease is more common in immunosuppressed, HIV-positive, elderly, or asplenic patients.
Diagnostic Testing:	Labs will reveal leukopenia, thrombocytopenia, anemia, elevated liver enzymes, increased LDH. Serologic detection of a fourfold rise in antibodies against *Ehrlichia chaffeensis* by immunofluorescence assay; detection of bacterial DNA in blood or cerebrospinal fluid by PCR; and peripheral blood smear examination for morulae in monocytes.
Treatment:	Doxycycline 100 mg twice a day for up to 10 days.
Pearls:	Prevention by avoidance of tick exposure and early removal of attached ticks. Diagnosis is often based on history and clinical suspicion. Consider the diagnosis in patients presenting with fever, leukocytosis, thrombocytopenia, abnormal liver enzymes, elevated LDH, and a history of tick bite. Early therapy improves outcomes and prevents severe complications or sequelae. Treatment response is expected within 48 hours and failure to respond within 3 days suggests infection with a different agent. Doxycycline is indicated for use in children of any age, according to the CDC and American Academy of Pediatrics. There can be coinfection with *Rickettsia rickettsii*.

Ehrlichiosis - HME

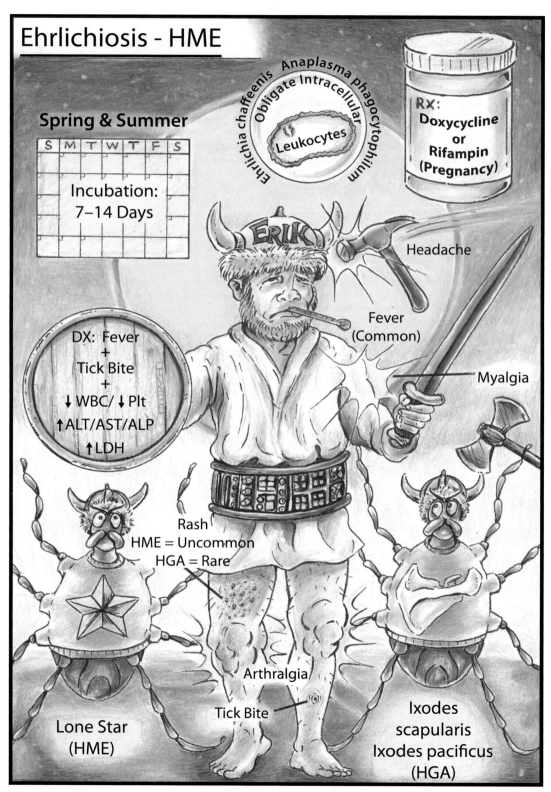

Spring & Summer

Incubation: 7–14 Days

Ehrlichia chaffeensis *Anaplasma phagocytophilum*
Obligate Intracellular
Leukocytes

RX:
Doxycycline
or
Rifampin
(Pregnancy)

ERIK

Headache

Fever
(Common)

Myalgia

DX: Fever
+
Tick Bite
+
↓WBC/↓Plt
↑ALT/AST/ALP
↑LDH

Rash
HME = Uncommon
HGA = Rare

Arthralgia

Tick Bite

Lone Star
(HME)

Ixodes
scapularis
Ixodes pacificus
(HGA)

Disease Name: **Anaplasmosis**

Synonym:	Human granulocytic anaplasmosis (HGA)
Causative Agent:	*Anaplasma phagocytophilum*
Vector:	Deer tick *(Ixodes scapularis)* in Eastern United States; black-legged tick *(Ixodes pacificus)* in Western United States; sheep tick *(Ixodes ricinus)* in Europe; taiga tick *(Ixodes persulcatus)* in parts of Asia; cattle tick *(Haemaphysalis longicornis)* in China
Reservoir:	White-footed mouse *(Peromyscus leucopus)*, white-tail deer *(Odocoileus virginianus)* red deer, roe deer, and multiple small mammals such as squirrels, voles, and wood rats.
Incubation Period:	7–14 days
Geographic Regions Affected:	Northern latitudes of North America, Europe, and Asia
Peak Incidence:	Spring and summer
Description:	Anaplasmosis (HGA) is a tick-borne rickettsial zoonosis caused by an obligate intracellular bacteria that affects granulocytes, specifically neutrophils.
Signs and Symptoms:	Many cases are thought to be asymptomatic. When symptomatic, about two thirds of patients develop fever, chills, malaise, headache, nausea, vomiting, diarrhea, cough, arthralgia, stiff neck, and myalgia. Rash is a rare finding in HGA. One third of patients can have severe disease with respiratory insufficiency, septic shock-like illness, rhabdomyolysis, renal failure, meningoencephalitis, hemorrhage, and opportunistic viral and fungal infections that can lead to death. Severe disease is more common in immunosuppressed, HIV, elderly, or asplenic patients.
Diagnostic Testing:	Labs will reveal leukopenia, thrombocytopenia, anemia, elevated liver enzymes, and elevated LDH. Peripheral blood smear examination for morulae in circulating neutrophils; detection of bacterial DNA in blood by PCR; serologic detection of a fourfold rise in IgG antibodies against *Anaplasm phagocytophilum*.
Treatments:	Doxycycline 100 mg twice a day for 10 days; rifampin has been successfully used in children and during pregnancy.
Pearls:	Prevention by avoidance of tick exposure and early removal of attached ticks. Diagnosis is often based on history and clinical suspicion. Consider the diagnosis in patients presenting with fever, leukocytosis, thrombocytopenia, abnormal liver enzymes, elevated LDH, and a history of tick bite. Early therapy improves outcomes and prevents severe complications or sequelae. There can be coinfection with *Borrelia burgdorferi* or *Babesia microti*.

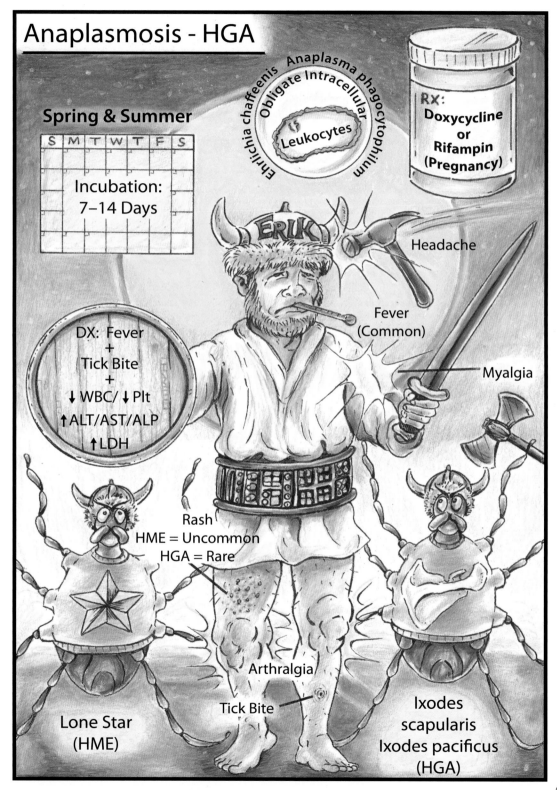

Anaplasmosis - HGA

Ehrlichia chaffeenis Anaplasma phagocytophilum
Obligate Intracellular
Leukocytes

Spring & Summer

S M T W T F S

Incubation:
7–14 Days

RX:
**Doxycycline
or
Rifampin
(Pregnancy)**

ERIK

Headache

Fever
(Common)

DX: Fever
+
Tick Bite
+
↓WBC/ ↓Plt
↑ALT/AST/ALP
↑LDH

Myalgia

Rash
HME = Uncommon
HGA = Rare

Arthralgia

Tick Bite

Lone Star
(HME)

Ixodes
scapularis
Ixodes pacificus
(HGA)

Disease Name: **Babesiosis**

Synonyms:	Nantucket fever, Texas cattle fever, red water fever, tick fever
Causative Agents:	*Babesia microti, Babesia duncani, Babesia divergens*
Vector:	Deer tick *(Ixodes scapularis)*; black-legged tick *(Ixodes pacificus)*, sheep tick *(Ixodes ricinus)* in Europe
Reservoir:	White-footed mouse *(Peromyscus leucopus)*, shrews, chipmunks, raccoons, white tailed deer, and rabbits
Incubation Period:	1–6 weeks
Geographic Regions Affected:	Northeastern United States and Upper Midwest *(Babesia microti)*, Pacific Northwest *(Babesia duncani)*, and parts of Europe *(Babesia divergens)*
Peak Incidence:	May through September. The initial infection occurs in late spring to early summer, in accordance with the activity of nymph stage of *Ixodes spp.* ticks. Since there is a 1- to 6-week incubation period, 50% of the cases are seen in July and 25% in August. Adult ticks may cause infection in late summer or early fall.
Description:	Babesiosis is a tick-borne protozoan zoonosis that causes the lysis of host erythrocytes. The disease can range from mild to severe and has symptoms resembling malaria.
Signs and Symptoms:	*Mild Disease*: weakness, fatigue, malaise, fever, chills, night sweats, headache, myalgia, anorexia, cough, arthralgia, nausea, vomiting, diarrhea, neck stiffness, and hemolytic anemia. *Severe Disease*: ARDS, CHF, DIC, liver failure, splenic infarct and rupture, and kidney injury. Coma and death can ensue.
Diagnostic Testing:	Labs will reveal hemolytic anemia, elevated liver enzymes, increased bilirubin, thrombocytopenia, and leukopenia. Giemsa-stained peripheral blood smear examination for ring trophozoites or Maltese cross-shaped tetrads of merozoites in erythrocytes; detection of parasitic 18S rRNA gene by PCR serologic detection of IgM and IgG antibodies.
Treatments:	*Mild Disease*: Atovaquone plus azithromycin for 7–10 days. *Severe Disease*: Clindamycin plus quinine for 7–10 days, but up to 6 weeks for relapsing disease. Exchange transfusion should be considered for patients with severe anemia and high parasite load.
Pearls:	Prevention by avoidance of tick exposures and early removal of attached ticks. Early therapy improves outcomes and prevents severe complications or sequelae. There can be coinfection with *Borrelia burgdorferi* or *Anaplasm phagocytophilum*. It can be transmitted by blood transfusion and via the placenta. Immunosuppressed, asplenic, and patients older than 50 years of age are at increased risk for severe disease. While *B. divergens, B. odocoilei, B. venatori,* and *B. bigemina* are more commonly associated with various animals, human infection can occur but is rare.

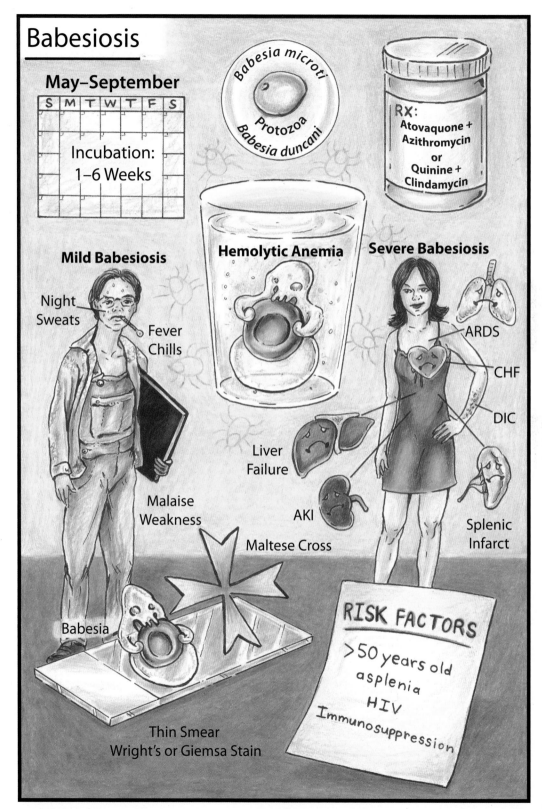

Babesiosis

May–September

Incubation: 1–6 Weeks

Babesia microti

Protozoa

Babesia duncani

RX: Atovaquone + Azithromycin or Quinine + Clindamycin

Mild Babesiosis

Hemolytic Anemia

Severe Babesiosis

Night Sweats

Fever Chills

ARDS

CHF

DIC

Liver Failure

AKI

Malaise Weakness

Maltese Cross

Splenic Infarct

Babesia

Thin Smear
Wright's or Giemsa Stain

RISK FACTORS
>50 years old
asplenia
HIV
Immunosuppression

Disease Name: Tularemia

Synonyms:	Rabbit fever, deer fly fever
Causative Agent:	*Francisella tularensis*
Vector:	American dog/wood tick *(Dermacentor variabilis)*, Rocky Mountain wood tick *(Dermacentor andersoni)*, lone star tick *(Amblyomma americanum)*, and deer flies *(Chrysops callidus)*. Mosquitoes in Europe.
Reservoir:	Lagomorphs: rabbits, hares, and pikas; aquatic rodents: beavers and muskrats
Incubation Period:	1–14 days; Average: 3–5 days
Geographic Regions Affected:	Worldwide—primarily in the Northern hemisphere
Peak Incidence:	April through October, with a peak in June and July due to ticks
Description:	Tularemia is a gram-negative zoonotic bacterial disease associated with rabbits that presents as one of six clinical variants. It is transmitted by tick or deerfly bites or from contact with infected host animals.
Signs and Symptoms:	*Ulceroglandular*: Painful skin ulcer at the site of insect bite or animal exposure with associated regional tender lymphadenopathy. The lymph nodes may become suppurative.
	Glandular: Regional lymphadenopathy without evidence or recall of skin ulceration.
	Oropharyngeal: Fever and sore throat predominate, with cervical, preparotid, and retropharyngeal lymphadenopathy. Nausea, vomiting, and diarrhea can occur. The source of infection is associated with the ingestion of contaminated water or undercooked contaminated animal meat.
	Pneumonic: Fever, dyspnea, and pneumonia predominate and are caused by the direct inhalation of aerosolized bacteria or from hematogenous spread.
	Oculoglandular: Often unilateral and caused by conjunctival exposure to the bacteria. Presenting symptoms include conjunctivitis and preauricular lymphadenopathy.
	Typhoidal: Febrile illness without lymphadenopathy. Symptoms can include fever, chills, malaise, anorexia, headache, myalgia, nausea, vomiting, diarrhea, and abdominal pain. Illness can progress to cause meningoencephalitis, hepatosplenomegaly, cholangitis, hepatitis, liver abscess, necrotic bowel, shock, kidney failure, rhabdomyolysis, pneumonia, and death.
Diagnostic Testing:	Specimens from swabs or scraping of skin lesions, lymph node aspirates or biopsies, pharyngeal washings, sputum, or gastric aspirates can be used for culture, immunostaining, and PCR. Acute and convalescent serologic titers can be followed.
Treatments:	Mild disease can be treated with oral doxycycline 100 mg or ciprofloxacin 500 mg twice a day for 14 days. Moderate to severe disease requires streptomycin or gentamicin, with the addition of doxycycline or chloramphenicol when meningitis is present.

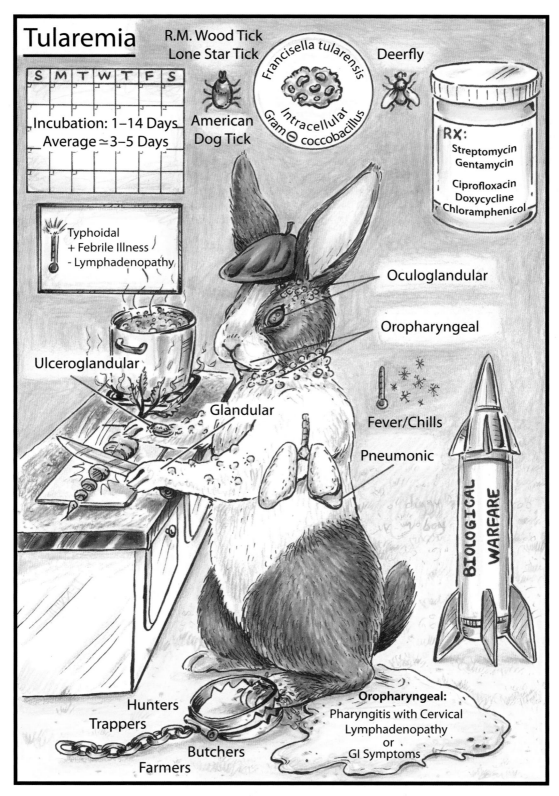

Tularemia

R.M. Wood Tick
Lone Star Tick

Francisella tularensis
Intracellular
Gram ⊖ coccobacillus

Deerfly

S M T W T F S

Incubation: 1–14 Days
Average ≃ 3–5 Days

American
Dog Tick

RX:
Streptomycin
Gentamycin

Ciprofloxacin
Doxycycline
Chloramphenicol

Typhoidal
+ Febrile Illness
– Lymphadenopathy

Oculoglandular

Oropharyngeal

Ulceroglandular

Glandular

Fever/Chills

Pneumonic

BIOLOGICAL WARFARE

Hunters
Trappers

Butchers
Farmers

Oropharyngeal:
Pharyngitis with Cervical
Lymphadenopathy
or
GI Symptoms

Disease Name: Crimean-Congo Hemorrhagic Fever

Causative Agent: Crimean-Congo hemorrhagic fever virus (CCHFV)

Vector: Ticks: *Hyalomma spp.*; infected animal blood during slaughter/butchering

Reservoir: Many wild and domestic animals including cattle, goats, sheep, hares, and ostriches.

Incubation Period: Tick bite: 1–3 days; exposure to infected blood: 5–6 days

Geographic Regions Affected: Africa, the Balkans, Eastern Europe, Middle East, and Asia

Peak Incidence: Between March and May and a second peak between August and October.

Description: CCHF is a tick-borne zoonotic viral hemorrhagic fever spread via the *Hyalomma* spp. ticks and/or exposure to infected blood via the slaughter and butchering of domestic livestock. Human-to-human transmission is possible via contact with infected blood or surgical instruments.

Signs and Symptoms: After the incubation period, there is a 3-day–long prehemorrhagic phase characterized by the sudden onset of facial flushing, malaise, myalgia, dizziness, diarrhea, nausea, vomiting, headache, high fever, back pain, arthralgia, stomach pain, conjunctivitis, pharyngitis, and petechiae on the palate. The hemorrhagic phase occurs next, between days 3 and 5 and lasts for up to 2 weeks. The hemorrhagic phase is characterized by gingival bleeding, ecchymosis, epistaxis, mucosal bleeding, hematemesis, melena, hematuria, hemoptysis, and abdominal muscle hematomas. Females can have vaginal and uterine bleeding. There may be hepatosplenomegaly, massive liver necrosis, hemorrhagic pneumonia, cardiovascular disturbances, changes in mood and sensory perception, multisystem organ failure, cerebral hemorrhage, shock, and death between the days 5 and 14 of illness. Fatality rate averages 30% and ranges between 5% and 80%.

Diagnostic Testing: Polymerase chain reaction (PCR), serology for IgM and IgG antibodies, and viral recovery in cell cultures.

Treatments: Supportive care. Ribavirin and platelet transfusion may be useful. Recovery is slow.

Pearls: Ticks can serve as both vectors and reservoirs. Livestock serve as amplifying hosts of the disease and, if infected, put herders and butchers at risk of infection, specifically through exposure to infected animal blood.

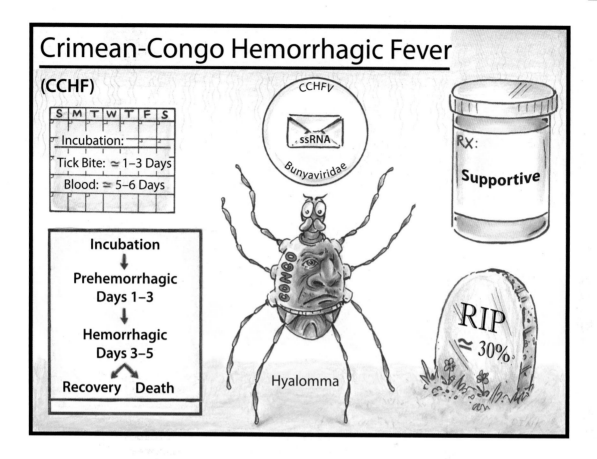

Crimean-Congo Hemorrhagic Fever

(CCHF)

S	M	T	W	T	F	S

Incubation:

Tick Bite: ≃ 1–3 Days

Blood: ≃ 5–6 Days

Incubation
↓
Prehemorrhagic
Days 1–3
↓
Hemorrhagic
Days 3–5
↗ ↖
Recovery   Death

CCHFV

ssRNA

Bunyaviridae

Hyalomma

RX:

Supportive

RIP

≃ 30%

Disease Name: Colorado Tick Fever

Synonyms: Mountain tick fever, American tick fever

Causative Agents: Colorado tick fever virus, Coltivirus (**Colo**rado **ti**ck virus)

Vector: Rocky Mountain wood tick (*Dermacentor andersoni*)

Reservoir: Small mammals, porcupine, ground squirrels, chipmunks

Incubation Period: 1–14 days; Average: 3–5 days

Geographic Regions Affected: Rocky Mountain region of the United States at altitudes from 4000 to 10,000 feet with rocky outcroppings. Also found in Europe and China.

Peak Incidence: March to September, with a peak in June

Description: Colorado tick fever is a tick-borne viral zoonosis that infects erythrocytes and is characterized by flu-like symptoms and a saddleback fever pattern.

Signs and Symptoms: Saddleback (biphasic) fever pattern with an initial 3-day phase with abrupt onset of fever, chills, headaches, pharyngitis, retro-orbital pain, photophobia, conjunctivitis, myalgia, generalized malaise, abdominal pain, splenomegaly, nausea, vomiting, diarrhea, and rash; remittance of symptoms for 1–3 days followed by a second 2-day phase with high fever, worsening of symptoms, generalized weakness, lethargy, aseptic meningitis, encephalitis, and hemorrhagic fever. It may rarely cause myocarditis, pericarditis, pneumonitis, and hepatitis. Children are at risk of death from hemorrhagic shock, meningoencephalitis, or disseminated intravascular coagulation. Full resolution of symptoms typically occurs within 1 week.

Diagnostic Testing: Labs will reveal leukopenia, thrombocytopenia, and elevated liver enzymes. PCR testing of blood or CSF is diagnostic in the first few days of infection, while serology is often negative in the first 2 weeks after symptom onset.

Treatments: Supportive. Avoid aspirin in children due to increased risk of Reye syndrome, and avoid nonsteroidal antiinflammatory drugs due to risk of bleeding secondary to thrombocytopenia.

Pearls: Prevention by avoidance of tick exposures and early removal of attached ticks. Must use gloves and tweezers close to the head of the tick for removal and wash the wound with soap and water. Infection can occur even with brief tick attachment. It can be transmitted by blood transfusion. Intrauterine transmission can lead to miscarriage and congenital anomalies. Viremia may persist for up to 4 months.

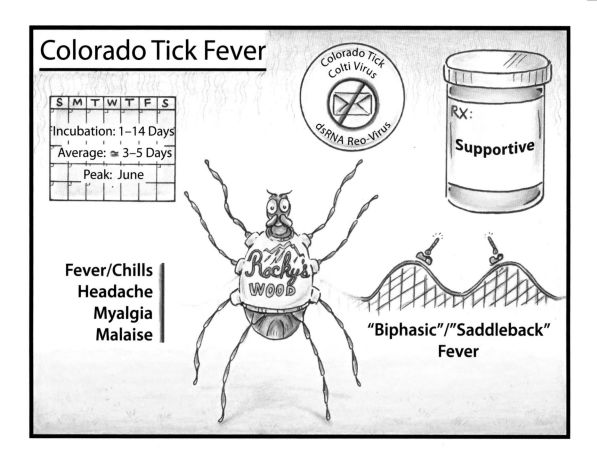

Colorado Tick Fever

S	M	T	W	T	F	S

Incubation: 1–14 Days

Average: ≃ 3–5 Days

Peak: June

Colorado Tick
Colti Virus

dsRNA Reo-Virus

RX:

Supportive

Fever/Chills
Headache
Myalgia
Malaise

Rocky's
WOOD

"Biphasic"/"Saddleback"
Fever

PART 5

WORMS

Section **1**

ROUNDWORMS

ROUNDWORMS

Disease Name:	# Ascariasis

Causative Agent: *Ascaris lumbricoides*

Lifecycle: Immature eggs are passed in the feces to soil where they embryonate for 2–4 weeks before becoming infectious. Infectious eggs can be consumed through poor handwashing and sanitation or through ingestion of unwashed vegetables, particularly where human waste is used as fertilizer. Once ingested, eggs hatch in the small intestine, they invade intestinal mucosa, and are carried through the portal and systemic circulatory systems to the lungs. Once in the lungs, the larvae mature over 2 weeks and penetrate the alveolar walls. Mature larvae are coughed up the bronchial tree and are swallowed. Once swallowed, they migrate to the small intestine where they mature into adult worms. The entire cycle takes 2–3 months and once mature, worms live 1–2 years. Adult females produce about 200,000 eggs per day.

Geographic Regions Affected: Worldwide. There is a higher prevalence in underdeveloped, tropical nations with poor sanitation, including parts of Asia, the Western Pacific, South America, and Africa.

Description: Ascariasis is a human nematode infection caused by the ingestion of infectious embryonated eggs from fecal contaminated soil, water, or vegetables. Ascariasis is the largest human roundworm parasitizing the human intestine and is more common in children.

Signs and Symptoms: Most infections are asymptomatic unless there is significant worm burden. Shortness of breath, cough, and fever may be present in the early phase of the disease followed by abdominal pain, nausea, and diarrhea. Loffler syndrome can occur in early infections with significant worm burden. Children with chronic infection can have malabsorption of protein, fats, vitamin A, and iodine leading to malnutrition, and growth and developmental delays. Individual worms may migrate to and potentially obstruct the common bile duct, gallbladder, pancreatic duct, and appendix, causing organ-specific symptoms. Significant worm burden may cause small bowel obstruction requiring surgical removal.

Diagnostic Testing: Eosinophilia may be present on labs. Stool samples ×3 to identify eggs.

Treatments: Mebendazole, albendazole, or ivermectin are effective treatment options.

Prevention: Sanitation and proper hygiene.

Pearls: Ascariasis eggs are quite hardy and can survive up to 5–6 years, specifically in moist, warm, shady soil. The hardiness of the eggs and large numbers released daily by females leads to a high prevalence of the disease.

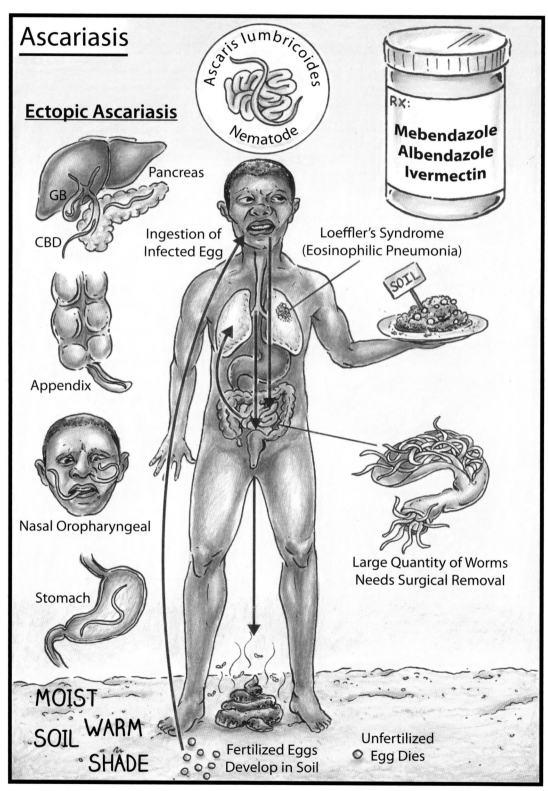

Ascariasis

Ascaris lumbricoides
Nematode

RX:
Mebendazole
Albendazole
Ivermectin

Ectopic Ascariasis

Pancreas

GB

CBD

Appendix

Nasal Oropharyngeal

Stomach

Ingestion of Infected Egg

Loeffler's Syndrome
(Eosinophilic Pneumonia)

SOIL

Large Quantity of Worms
Needs Surgical Removal

MOIST
SOIL WARM
SHADE

Fertilized Eggs
Develop in Soil

Unfertilized
Egg Dies

Disease Name: **Filariasis**

Filariasis is a complex of parasitic diseases caused by threadlike nematodes transmitted by the bites of mosquitos and black flies. Filarial infections can be broken down into three main categories, based on the body cavities they occupy.

Lymphatic Filariasis:

Elephantiasis, a severe manifestation of lymphatic filariasis, is caused by one of several nematodes including: *Wucheria bancrofti*, *Brugia malayi*, and *Brugia timori*. These nematode worms can be transmitted by the bites of several major mosquito species including: *Anopheles*, *Culex*, and *Aedes*. Numerous mosquito bites from vector mosquitos are required for full-blown disease to manifest. Characteristic findings are secondary to lymph channel blockage and include lymphedema of the upper and lower extremities as well as male genital regions. *Treatment*: Diethylcarbamazine (DEC) and doxycycline.

Subcutaneous Filariasis:

Loiasis is caused by *Loa loa* (the eye worm) and is transmitted by female day-feeding horse or deer flies of the genus *Chrysops*. The disease is common in West Africa and is often asymptomatic unless there is a large worm burden. Calabar swellings are localized patches of pruritic angioedema that correlate to worm migration. The *Loa loa* worm can migrate to the conjunctiva of the eye and be visualized, giving rise to its name. *Treatment*: DEC, which can also be given weekly as chemoprophylaxis to travelers to endemic areas. Albendazole can also be used. The *Loa loa* worm is unique among filarial worms as it does not harbor the *Wolbachia* symbiotic bacteria.

Onchocerciasis or **River Blindness** is caused by *Onchocerca volvulus* and is transmitted by the female day-feeding black fly. The disease is common in West Africa, East Africa, Arabian Peninsula, and South America. It is characterized by specific acute and chronic cutaneous manifestations and is the second most common cause of infectious blindness. *Treatment*: Ivermectin and doxycycline.

Streptocerciasis is caused by *Mansonella streptocerca* and is transmitted by the midge. It is common in Central African rain forests and is often asymptomatic. Pruritus and dermatitis are the predominant symptoms, and a cultured skin biopsy will reveal microfilaria. *Treatment*: DEC or ivermectin.

Serous Cavity Filariasis:

Two members of the *Mansonella* species are considered to reside within deeper tissues, including the pleural and peritoneal cavities of humans. Most infections are asymptomatic. *Mansonella ozzardi* can be found in northern parts of South America and Central America. Symptoms can include pruritus, headache, malaise, fever, arthralgia, and pulmonary manifestations. *Treatment*: Ivermectin. *Mansonella perstans* can be found in sub-Saharan Africa and parts of Central and South America. Symptoms can include pruritus, headache, malaise, fever, and arthralgia. Treatment can be challenging, given resistance, and includes doxycycline and albendazole.

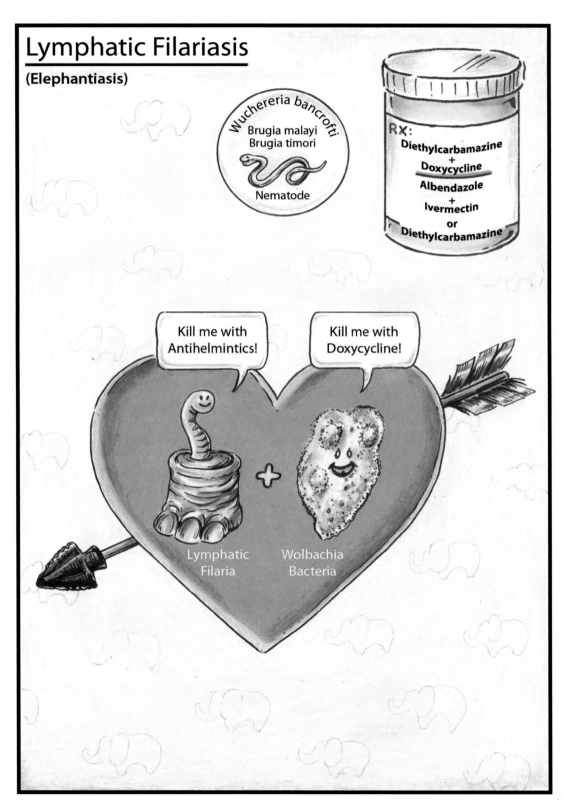

Lymphatic Filariasis
(Elephantiasis)

Subcutaneous Filariasis

Disease	Round Worm	Vector
Loiasis	Loa loa (African Eye Worm)	Horse or Deer fly
Streptocerciasis	Mansonella streptocerca	Midge
River Blindness	Onchocerca volvulus	Black fly

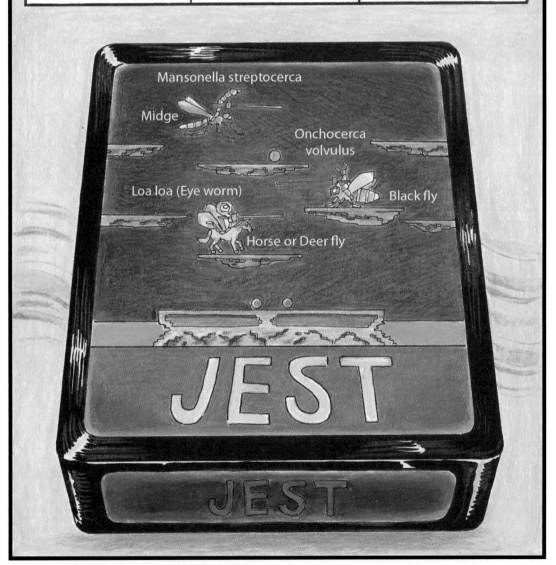

Serous Cavity Filariasis

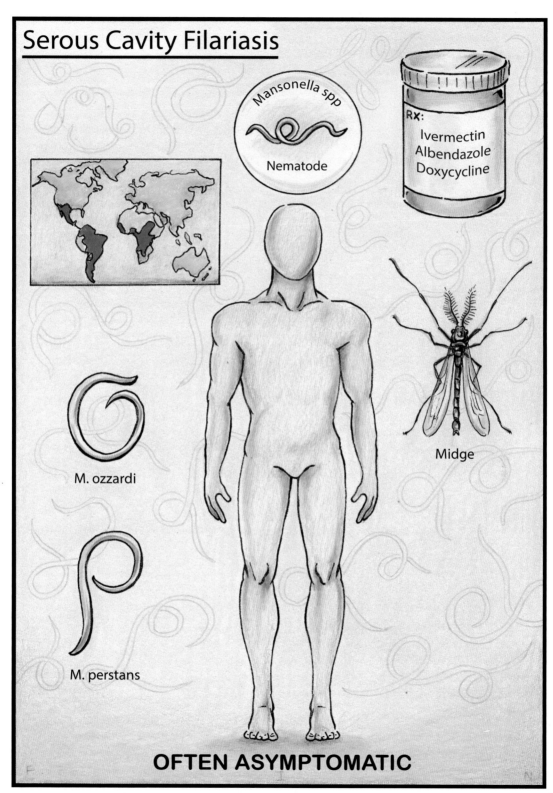

Mansonella spp

Nematode

RX:
Ivermectin
Albendazole
Doxycycline

M. ozzardi

M. perstans

Midge

OFTEN ASYMPTOMATIC

Disease Name: **Onchocerciasis**

Synonym:	River Blindness
Causative Agent:	*Onchocerca volvulus*
Lifecycle:	The disease is spread from infected humans to other humans via the bite of the female black fly. Black flies feed during daytime hours, when microfilaria migrate to the skin. During a blood meal, infectious microfilaria are ingested and migrate to the gut and thoracic muscles of the black fly. The larvae mature over the next week and migrate to the proboscis of the fly. During the next feeding, larvae are passed on to the next host where they migrate to the subcutaneous tissue and mature over the next 6–12 months. Once mature, male and female worms mate and produce approximately 1000 microfilaria per day. These microfilaria then migrate to the skin during the day, awaiting the bite of the black fly to continue their lifecycle.
Geographic Regions Affected:	West Africa, East Africa, Arabian Peninsula, South America
Description:	Onchocerciasis is a nematode infection of humans caused by subcutaneous filarial worms transmitted via the bite of the daytime feeding *Simulium* spp. black fly.
Signs and Symptoms:	Skin changes of varying degrees are common. Acute and chronic papular dermatitis (onchodermatitis), skin atrophy (lizard skin), depigmentation (leopard skin), and lichenification (elephant skin) are characteristic. Pruritus is common. Corneal (eye) involvement includes punctate keratitis that leads to scarring and blindness.
Diagnostic Testing:	Clinical signs and symptoms in individuals from endemic areas lead one to suspect the diagnosis. Slit lamp examination reveals microfilaria in the eye. Skin biopsies plated in saline solution will cause microfilaria to emerge, confirming the diagnosis.
Treatments:	Onchocerciasis mono-infection: ivermection plus doxycycline. If dual infection with either Lymphatic filariasis or Loa loa, treat Onchocerciasis first with ivermectin, followed by diethylcarbamazine (DEC).
Prevention:	Mass treatments with ivermectin and insect control programs have been used with good success in some areas.
Pearls:	Second most common cause of blindness due to infection. Ivermectin is effective at killing the worms within the host, while doxycycline kills off a symbiotic bacteria (*Wolbachia*) within the worms themselves.

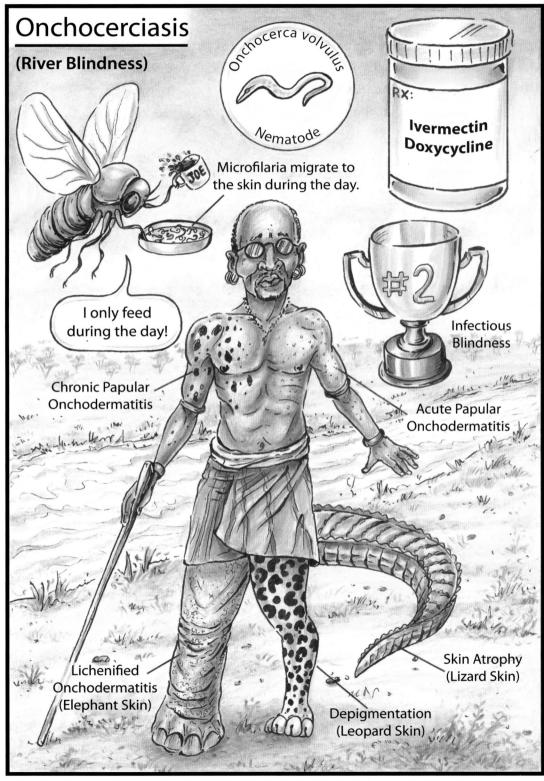

Onchocerciasis
(River Blindness)

Onchocerca volvulus

Nematode

RX:
Ivermectin Doxycycline

Microfilaria migrate to the skin during the day.

JOE

I only feed during the day!

#2

Infectious Blindness

Chronic Papular Onchodermatitis

Acute Papular Onchodermatitis

Lichenified Onchodermatitis (Elephant Skin)

Depigmentation (Leopard Skin)

Skin Atrophy (Lizard Skin)

ROUNDWORMS

Disease Name: **Pinworms**

Synonym: Enterobiasis

Causative Agent: *Enterobius vermicularis*

Lifecycle: Eggs are deposited in the perianal area by female worms, mostly at night. Perianal itching can cause autoinfection and/or eggs can be passed on to others via contaminated fingernails, close contact, aerosolization, or bed linens. Once ingested, eggs will hatch in the duodenum and begin to mature in the bowel. Adult male and female worms mate in the terminal ileum, cecum, and appendix area. The male worm typically dies in the cecum and is passed out with stooling. The female worm migrates to the perianal area to lay eggs and die. The circle of life is completed! Each female produces an average of 10,000 eggs.

Geographic Regions Affected: Worldwide. Pinworms are the most common helminth infection in the United States and Western Europe.

Description: Pinworms is a human nematode infection caused by the ingestion of eggs from the perianal area of infected individuals. Anal itching (pruritus ani) and scratching aids transmission. The disease is most common in children between ages of 5 and 10 years of age.

Signs and Symptoms: Most infections are asymptomatic. Pruritus ani is the most common symptom and is worse at night.

Diagnostic Testing: "Scotch tape test" or paddle test revealing the presence of eggs is diagnostic. In this test, an adhesive tape or paddle is placed on several spots around the perianal area, removing eggs that are identified on microscopy. Samples should be taken over several days, preferably first thing in the morning. Eggs are translucent, bean shaped, and measure 50–60×20–30 μm.

Treatments: Albendazole, mebendazole, or pyrantel pamoate are effective treatment options. At least two rounds of treatment, 2 weeks apart, are required, as the medication only kills the adult worm, not the eggs.

Prevention: Sanitation, handwashing, trimming fingernails, and proper hygiene.

Pearls: Humans are the only animals that get infected, but household pets may carry the eggs on their fur. The female carries the eggs to the perianal area to expose them to a more oxygen-enriched environment. Eggs can live for up to 3 weeks.

Pinworms
(Enterobiasis)

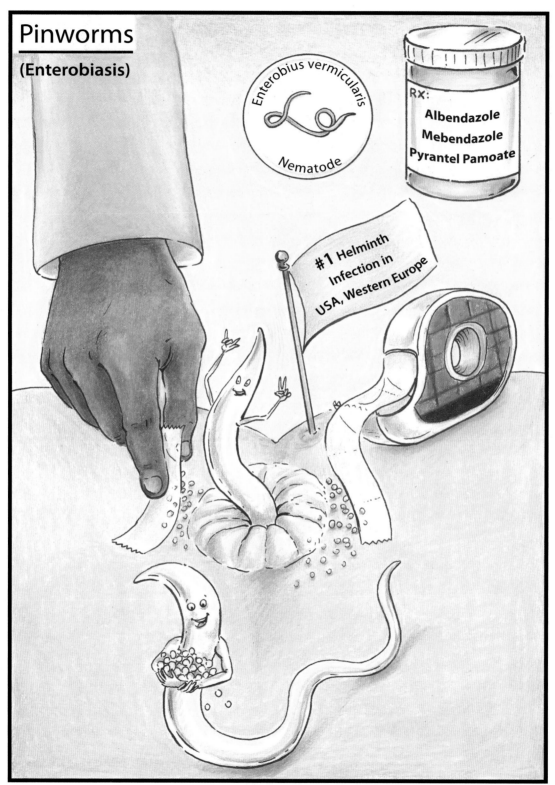

Enterobius vermicularis

Nematode

RX:
Albendazole
Mebendazole
Pyrantel Pamoate

#1 Helminth Infection in USA, Western Europe

ROUNDWORMS

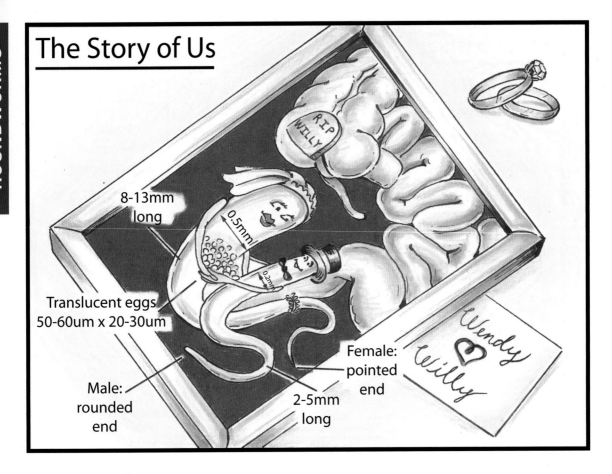

The Story of Us

8-13mm long

0.5mm

Translucent eggs
50-60um x 20-30um

Male:
rounded
end

Female:
pointed
end

2-5mm
long

The Circle of Life

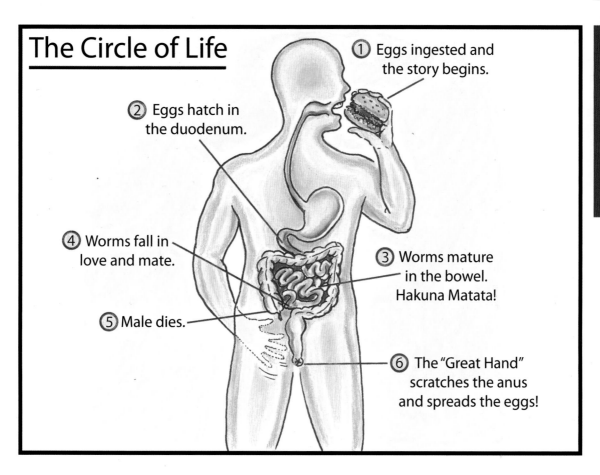

① Eggs ingested and the story begins.

② Eggs hatch in the duodenum.

③ Worms mature in the bowel. Hakuna Matata!

④ Worms fall in love and mate.

⑤ Male dies.

⑥ The "Great Hand" scratches the anus and spreads the eggs!

ROUNDWORMS

Disease Name: # Hookworm

Causative Agents: *Necator americanus, Ancylostoma duodenale*

Lifecycle: The disease is contracted from exposure to fecal contaminated soil. Filariform larvae mature and enter through exposed skin, usually the feet. From here they migrate hematogenously to the lungs where they are coughed up and swallowed. The larvae penetrate the mucosa of the small intestine where they mature and reproduce. Adult *N. americanus* worms can live up to 5 years, while *A. duodenale* lives for about 6 months. Eggs (rhabditiform larvae) are produced and they are excreted with feces. Immature larvae are excreted and mature to filariform larvae to infect others. While both filariform larvae can infect humans by penetrating the skin, *A. duodenale* can cause infection if ingested.

Geographic Regions Affected: Worldwide, now uncommon in United States. *N. americanus*: North and South America, sub-Saharan Africa, Southeast Asia, China. *A. duodenale*: Middle East, North Africa, India. Annual rainfall of 50–60 inches is required for regions to support hookworm.

Description: Hookworm is a nematode infection of the human gastrointestinal (GI) tract that causes intestinal inflammation leading to iron-deficient anemia and protein deficiency.

Signs and Symptoms: Mild infections are often asymptomatic. Acute infections may present with "ground itch" and GI symptoms including nausea, vomiting, and diarrhea. Chronic infection causes iron and protein deficiency secondary to blood loss from the feeding worms.

Diagnostic Testing: Lab tests may reveal eosinophila and microcytic anemia. Serial stool samples are diagnostic. It should be noted that the eggs from the two species are indistinguishable.

Treatments: Effective treatment options include albendazole, mebendazole, or pyrantel pamoate. Iron supplements should be prescribed to treat anemia.

Prevention: Sanitation and proper hygiene, avoid walking barefoot in soil.

Pearls: Eosinophilia is common. Chronic infection can have a profound impact on pregnant women and causes growth retardation in young children. Hookworm is endemic in Haiti, affecting at least 25% of the rural population, if not more. If interested in volunteering in Haiti, please visit Health Corps Haiti at www.medicalstudentmissions.org.

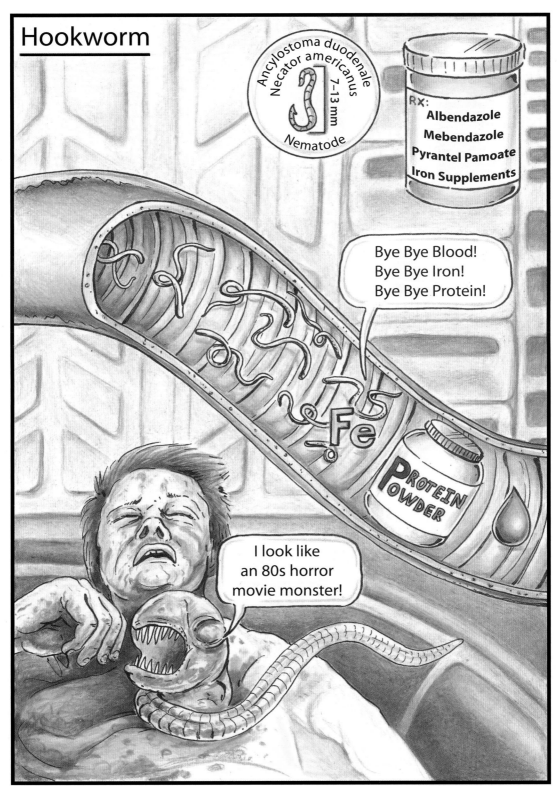

ROUNDWORMS

Disease Name: **Whipworm**

Synonym:	Trichuriasis
Causative Agent:	*Trichuris trichiura*
Lifecycle:	Immature eggs are passed in the feces to soil where they embryonate for 2–4 weeks before becoming infectious. Infectious eggs can be consumed by poor handwashing and sanitation or through ingestion on unwashed vegetables, particularly where human waste is used as fertilizer. Once ingested eggs hatch in the small intestine, the larvae mature and migrate to the cecum and ascending colon where they attached after 2–3 months; 7000–20,000 eggs are released per day, per female worm, and are not infectious until a 2- to 4-week embryonation process is completed in warm, moist soil.
Geographic Regions Affected:	Tropical climates
Description:	Trichuriasis is a human nematode infection caused by the ingestion of embryonated eggs from fecal contaminated soil, water, or vegetables.
Signs and Symptoms:	Most infections are asymptomatic unless there is significant worm burden. Moderate infections cause loose stool and nocturnal stooling. Severe infections can have worms extending to the rectum and can cause rectal prolapse or colitis.
Diagnostic Testing:	Eosinophilia may be present on labs. Stool samples ×3 to identify eggs.
Treatments:	Mebendazole, albendazole, and ivermectin are effective treatment options.
Prevention:	Sanitation and proper hygiene.
Pearls:	Coinfection with ascariasis is not uncommon, since both worms have similar geographic distribution and patterns of infection.

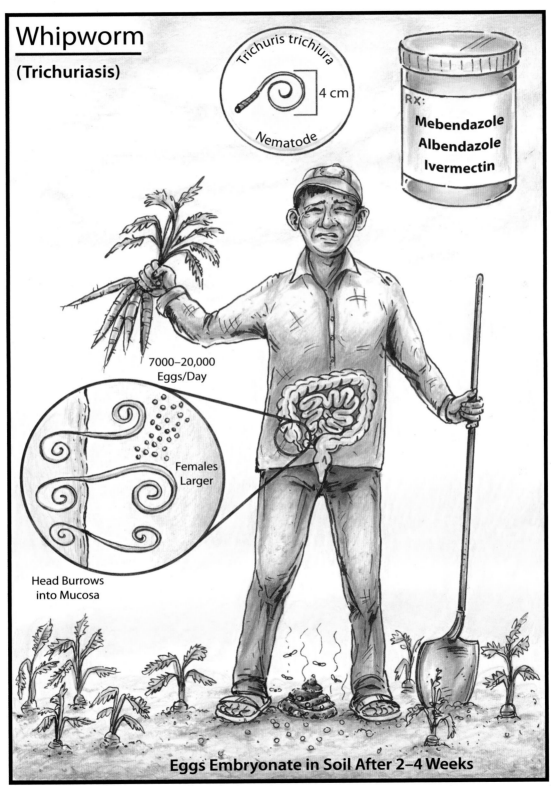

Whipworm
(Trichuriasis)

Trichuris trichiura

4 cm

Nematode

RX:
Mebendazole
Albendazole
Ivermectin

7000–20,000
Eggs/Day

Females
Larger

Head Burrows
into Mucosa

Eggs Embryonate in Soil After 2–4 Weeks

ROUNDWORMS

Disease Name: Trichinosis

Synonym:	Trichinellosis
Causative Agent:	*Trichinella spiralis*

Lifecycle: In humans, the disease is typically acquired from the ingestion of undercooked pork or bear meat containing *Trichinella* cysts. When exposed to gastric acid, these cysts release larvae that burrow into the mucosa of the small intestines. Here the larvae mature and reproduce. After a week, the adult females release newborn larvae that travel through the blood stream, infect striated muscle tissue and form new cysts. Adult worms typically survive for 4 to 6 weeks in the host gastrointestinal (GI) tract before dying off and passing with stool. Meanwhile, encysted larvae can survive in muscle tissue for many years, and the lifecycle repeats itself when infected meat is consumed. Humans, barring cannibalism, are dead-end hosts. Other animals, including rats, foxes, wild boars, and cats, can also become infected. In domesticated pigs the cycle is perpetuated when they are fed infected meat scraps, perform cannibalism, or consume infected rodents.

Geographic Regions Affected: Worldwide. It is uncommon in the U.S. but endemic in Japan and China.

Description: Trichinosis is a nematode infection of the human GI tract in which the parasites' larvae ultimately form cysts in muscle tissue. Symptoms are based on the number of cysts ingested.

Signs and Symptoms: Mild infections are often asymptomatic or mild. Significant infections, seen after an ingestion of meat containing numerous cysts, present with two distinct stages. *Intestinal Stage*: Symptoms begin as early as 2-7 days after exposure and are related to the larvae burrowing into the GI mucosa. Symptoms can include abdominal pain, nausea, vomiting, and diarrhea. *Muscle Stage*: These symptoms typically occur 10 days after infection and are more profound. Symptoms represent the newly formed larvae infecting muscle tissue and include fever, severe muscle pain, swelling, weakness, fever, periorbital edema, and splinter hemorrhages. Myocarditis occurs rarely but is the most-frequent cause of death. The formation of cysts in the diaphragm muscles can potentially compromise breathing and respiration.

Diagnostic Testing: Labs will reveal leukocytosis, eosinophilia, and increased creatine phosphokinase (CPK). ELISA testing can be used to detect IgG antibodies to trichinella, and confirmatory diagnosis is made via muscle biopsy. Eosinophilia doesn't correspond to disease severity.

Treatments: Albendazole or mebendazole combined with oral prednisone is effective for treatment.

Prevention: The U.S. Department of Agriculture recommends cooking pork to an internal temperature of 160° F or 77° C to ensure destruction of any potential trichinae cysts.

Trichinosis
(Trichinellosis)

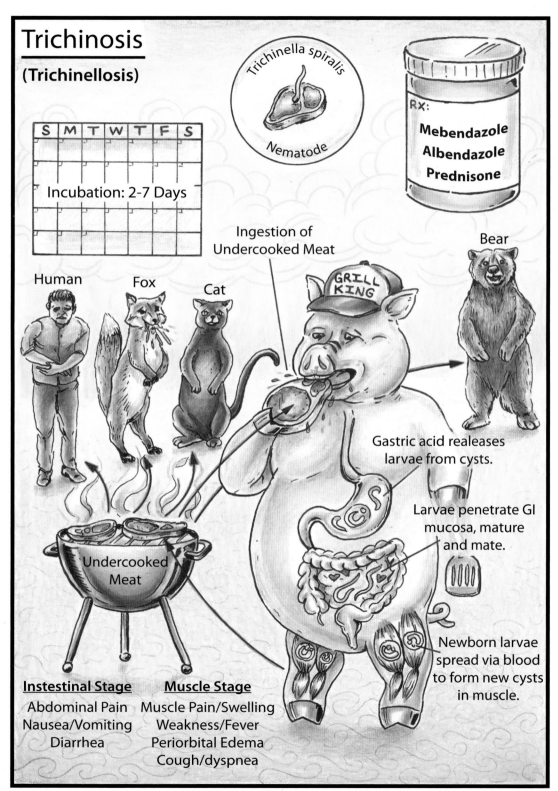

Trichinella spiralis
Nematode

RX:
Mebendazole
Albendazole
Prednisone

Incubation: 2-7 Days

Ingestion of
Undercooked Meat

Bear

Human   Fox   Cat

GRILL KING

Gastric acid realeases
larvae from cysts.

Larvae penetrate GI
mucosa, mature
and mate.

Undercooked
Meat

Newborn larvae
spread via blood
to form new cysts
in muscle.

Instestinal Stage
Abdominal Pain
Nausea/Vomiting
Diarrhea

Muscle Stage
Muscle Pain/Swelling
Weakness/Fever
Periorbital Edema
Cough/dyspnea

ROUNDWORMS

Disease Name: # Dracunculiasis

Synonym: Guinea worm disease

Causative Agent: *Dracunculus medinensis*

Lifecycle: The disease is contracted from the ingestion of unfiltered water that contains copepods or "water fleas" hosting mature, infectious larvae. The ingested copepods die, releasing larvae that then penetrate through the bowels and take up residence in the abdominal cavity and retroperitoneal space. The worms mature over a period of 3 months, mate, and then the male dies. The female worms begin their migration through subcutaneous tissue to the lower extremities about 1 year after mating. Once toward the distal lower extremities, the worms migrate more superficially, creating a papule that ultimately ulcerates, allowing the worms to extend out of the wound and release eggs. The ulceration is quite painful and infected individuals are inclined to dip the affected extremity into water as a means of pain control. Once exposed to water, the worm pokes out, releasing larvae. Small copepods then ingest the larvae, which undergo further development inside the copepod. When infected copepods are ingested by humans, the cycle repeats itself.

Geographic Regions Affected: Africa. However, due largely in part to efforts by the Carter Foundation, global eradication of the Guinea worm is almost complete.

Description: Dracunculiasis is a nematode infection of humans and dogs characterized by a painful ulcer(s) in the lower extremities from where the worm emerges to release larvae when exposed to water.

Signs and Symptoms: Initial infection is asymptomatic. About 1 year later, pregnant females will cause pain in the lower extremities as they migrate distally (fiery serpent). Prior to penetrating out through the skin, a severely painful papule forms that eventually ulcerates. The formation of the papule may be associated with nausea, vomiting, diarrhea, and fever.

Diagnostic Testing: The diagnosis is made clinically and no specific diagnostic tests are required. Once the small painful ulcer develops and the lower extremity is submerged into cool water, the worm will reveal itself.

Treatments: Once the worm reveals itself, its distal end is wrapped around a small twig or piece of gauze. Over the next several days, weeks, or months, the skin is massaged and the twig is slowly rotated drawing more of the worm out being careful to not break the worm. Topical antibiotics may be used to prevent superimposed infections.

Prevention: Proper water filtration using fine cloths or bio-sand filters to remove copepods. Water can also be boiled. Insecticides like temefos can be added to water supplies to kill off water fleas and copepods.

Pearls: When the male worms die they are absorbed by the hosts. Female worms can be quite long, measuring 2 mm wide by 60–100 cm long. Care must be taken to avoid breaking the worm during removal, as the remaining piece can putrefy and cause skin necrosis along the tract. These worms have almost been eradicated from existence and have plagued humans for centuries. Worms have been found in Egyptian mummies, and some speculate that the Staff of Asclepius may represent a Guinea worm wrapped around a small stick.

Dracunculiasis
(Guinea Worm Disease, GWD)

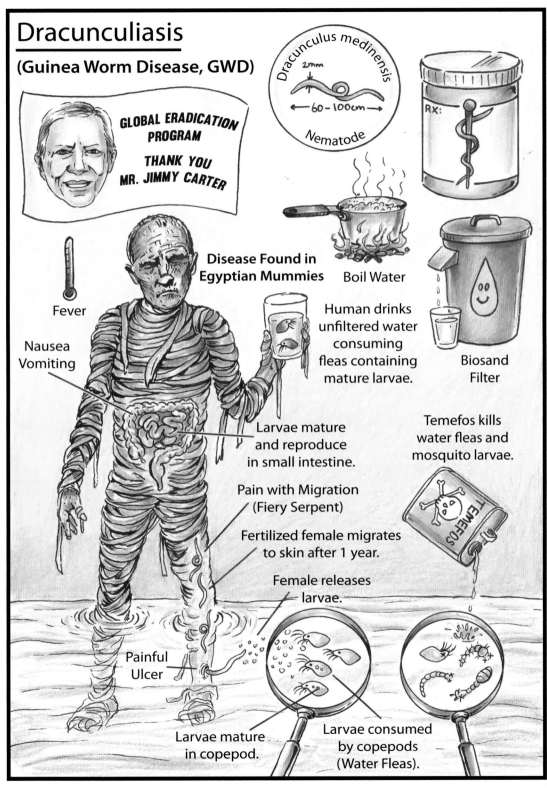

GLOBAL ERADICATION PROGRAM

THANK YOU MR. JIMMY CARTER

Dracunculus medinensis

2mm

←60-100cm→

Nematode

RX:

Fever

Nausea Vomiting

Disease Found in Egyptian Mummies

Boil Water

Human drinks unfiltered water consuming fleas containing mature larvae.

Biosand Filter

Larvae mature and reproduce in small intestine.

Temefos kills water fleas and mosquito larvae.

Pain with Migration (Fiery Serpent)

Fertilized female migrates to skin after 1 year.

TEMEFOS

Female releases larvae.

Painful Ulcer

Larvae mature in copepod.

Larvae consumed by copepods (Water Fleas).

ROUNDWORMS

Disease Name:	# Cutaneous Larva Migrans

Synonyms: CLM, creeping eruption, sandworms, plumber's itch, ground itch

Causative Agent: *Ancylostoma braziliense*

Lifecycle: The disease is contracted from cutaneous penetration of the filariform larvae of hookworms that typically infect dogs and cats. Hookworm eggs are shed from infected dogs or cats into sandy soil and after a 2-week period, develop into infectious filarial larvae. If a dog or cat is exposed, the filarial larvae can penetrate its skin and migrate into deeper tissues. In humans, these specific larvae lack the necessary enzymes to penetrate through the basement membrane to enter into the deeper dermal layers and cannot complete their lifecycle.

Geographic Regions Affected: Worldwide, more frequent in tropical and subtropical nations of Southeast Asia, Africa, South America, Southeastern United States, and the Caribbean.

Description: Cutaneous larva migrans is an incidental, superficial nematode infection of humans caused by larvae from the Ancylostomatidae family of hookworms.

Signs and Symptoms: Patients will develop red and intensely pruritic serpiginous tracks on their lower extremities. Itching may cause secondary bacterial infections. The condition is self-limiting and oral anti-helminthic agents will quickly abate symptoms.

Diagnostic Testing: Eosinophilia may be seen on labs. The diagnosis is typically made with clinical history and classic presentation.

Treatments: Ivermectin and albendazole are effective treatment options.

Prevention: Wear sandals, deworming of dogs and cats, proper disposal of pet feces.

Pearls: "Ground itch" can also be seen with human hookworm and threadworm infections. The cutaneous manifestations of threadworm *(Strongyloides stercoralis)* is referred to as larva currens and is differentiated by its rapid migration, perianal involvement, and wide band of urticaria.

Cutaneous Larva Migrans

(CLM/Creeping Eruption)
(Sandworms)
(Plumber's Itch)
(Ground Itch)

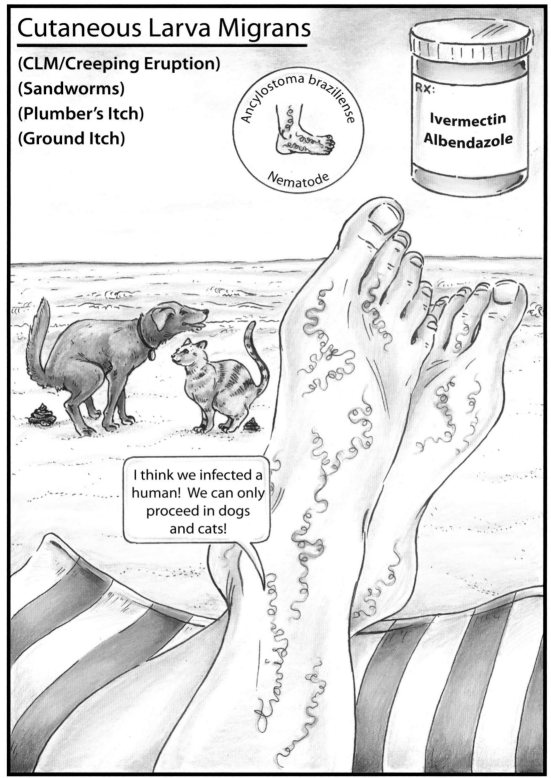

ROUNDWORMS

Disease Name: **Threadworm**

Synonym:	Strongyloidiasis
Causative Agent:	*Strongyloides stercoralis*
Lifecycle:	The disease is contracted from exposure to fecal-contaminated soil. Filariform larvae mature and enter through exposed skin, usually the feet. From there they migrate hematogenously to the lungs, where they are coughed up and swallowed. The larvae penetrate the mucosa of the duodenum and jejunum, where they mature and reproduce. Adult worms can live up to 5 years. Eggs (rhabditiform larvae) are produced and they are excreted with feces. Autoinfection can occur when larvae mature in the gastrointestinal (GI) tract and penetrate the colonic or anal mucosa. Immature larvae are excreted and mature to filariform larvae to infect others.
Geographic Regions Affected:	Tropical and subtropical areas of the world with poor sanitation; Vietnam, Cambodia, Laos, some parts of Africa, Brazil, and Central America.
Description:	Threadworm is a nematode infection of the human GI tract.
Signs and Symptoms:	Most immunocompetent adults are asymptomatic. Cutaneous symptoms can include pruritus, burning, edema, and inflammation at the site of infection. Pulmonary symptoms may include cough, dyspnea, hemoptysis, and a Loffler-like syndrome. GI symptoms include epigastric pain, nausea, vomiting, and diarrhea. *Hyperinfection syndrome*: Immunocompromised patients may suffer from autoinfection and develop significant worm burden. Fever, severe nausea, vomiting, abdominal pain, and pulmonary symptoms would manifest, potentially leading to multisystem organ failure, sepsis, shock, and death.
Diagnostic Testing:	Identification of rhabditiform larvae in stool samples. Up to three stool samples are usually required and specialized techniques, such as the agar plate method, increase sensitivity. Using the agar plate method, plates are inoculated with stool and incubated for 2 days. Larvae will migrate from the stool, creating bacterial trails along the way. If negative, a string test can be performed. Here the patient swallows a capsule attached to a long string and when removed, the string is tested for larvae. IgM/IgG serology can also be obtained.
Treatments:	Ivermectin is the preferred treatment. Albendazole can be used as an alternative, but it is less effective. For hyperinfections, treatment needs to be repeated after 15 days.
Prevention:	Proper sanitation and hygiene, handwashing.
Pearls:	Eosinophilia is common.

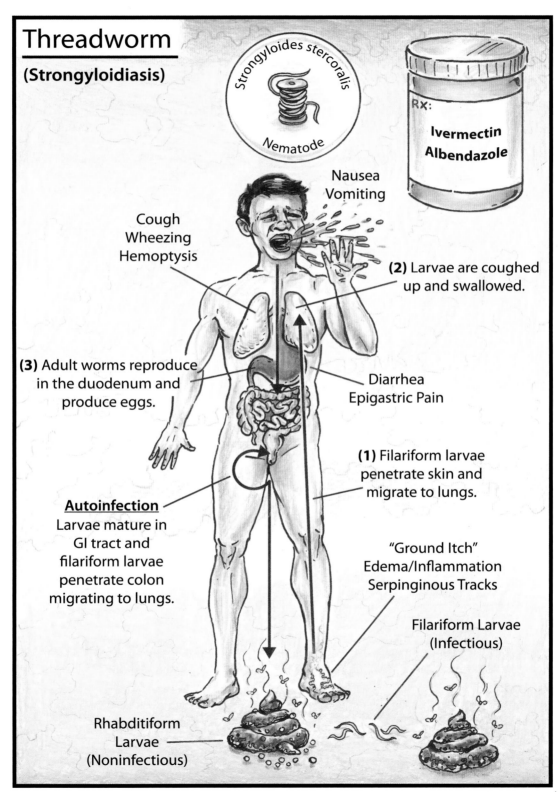

Threadworm
(Strongyloidiasis)

Strongyloides stercoralis

Nematode

RX:

Ivermectin
Albendazole

Nausea
Vomiting

Cough
Wheezing
Hemoptysis

(2) Larvae are coughed
up and swallowed.

(3) Adult worms reproduce
in the duodenum and
produce eggs.

Diarrhea
Epigastric Pain

(1) Filariform larvae
penetrate skin and
migrate to lungs.

Autoinfection
Larvae mature in
GI tract and
filariform larvae
penetrate colon
migrating to lungs.

"Ground Itch"
Edema/Inflammation
Serpinginous Tracks

Filariform Larvae
(Infectious)

Rhabditiform
Larvae
(Noninfectious)

Section **2**

TAPEWORMS

TAPEWORMS

Causative Agent: *Taenia solium*

Lifecycle: Pork tapeworm disease is contracted from ingestion of infected "measly" pork containing cysticerci. Once inside the human intestine, the cysts hatch, releasing protoscolices that attach to the intestinal wall, becoming the heads (scolex) of adult tapeworms. Hermaphroditic proglottids form off the scolex, mature, become pregnant, produce eggs, and eventually break off the tapeworm. Degraded proglottids release eggs into the passed stools. Contaminated human feces are consumed by pigs, the eggs hatch in their gastrointestinal (GI) tract, and then the larvae seek out striated muscle, forming cysticerci. Humans can serve as intermediate hosts if they consume *Taenia solium* eggs through fecal contamination or autoinoculation. This could cause the more-severe condition *cysticercosis*, the development of cysticerci in human muscle or brain tissue *(neurocysticercosis)*.

Geographic Regions Affected: Worldwide. Common in places where humans live in close contact with pigs and could eat undercooked pork: Central and South America, India, and Asia.

Description: *Pork tapeworm* is a cestode infection of the human GI tract, which is often asymptomatic. *Cysticercosis* is the more severe infection characterized by cyst formation in the brain, eyes, and/or striated muscles.

Signs and Symptoms: *Pork tapeworm* is often asymptomatic. Significant worm burden may cause nausea, abdominal discomfort, and malaise. *Cysticercosis* may remain asymptomatic for years until the cysts degrade and activate the host's immune system. *Neurocysticercosis* can present as altered mental status, seizures, or symptoms associated with hydrocephalus such as headache, nausea, and blurred vision.

Diagnostic Testing: Serial stool samples looking for eggs is diagnostic for tapeworm, and serologic testing can be a useful adjunct. CT or MRI neuroimaging is necessary for the evaluation and diagnosis of neurocysticercosis.

Treatments: *Tapeworm:* Praziquantel or niclosamide are effective treatment options. *Cysticercosis:* Albendazole combined with praziquantel and steroids or albendazole alone or combined with steroids is necessary for treatment.

Prevention: Sanitation and proper hygiene, proper cooking of pork, and/or freezing pork to −15°C for at least 20 days. Pickling pork does not kill the cysticerci.

Pearls: Humans are the only definitive host for *Taenia solium* and pigs or humans serve as intermediate hosts. Worms measure 2–8 m in length on average, have hooks on their scolex, live for several years, and produce eggs that can survive for about 2 months in the environment.

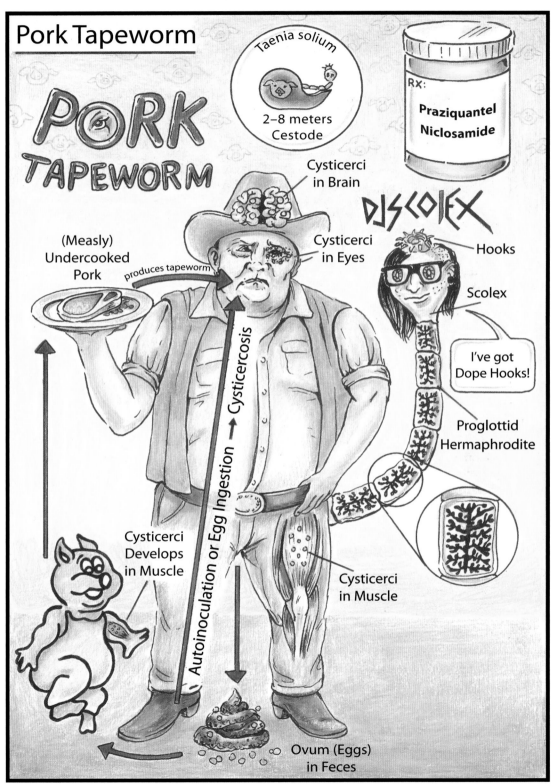

TAPEWORMS

TAPEWORMS

Disease Name: **Broad Fish Tapeworm**

Causative Agent: *Diphyllobothrium latum*

Lifecycle: Broad fish tapeworm disease is contracted from the ingestion of infected undercooked fish. Once ingested, plerocercoids develop into adult worms and attach themselves to the lining of the small intestine. Reproduction is asexual, as the worm is a hermaphrodite. When mature, pregnant proglottids release eggs into the stool. Immature eggs develop into embryos in fresh water and become coracidium. These coracidium are consumed by small crustaceans/copepods (first intermediate host) and develop into proceroid larvae. Copepods are then consumed by small fish like minnows (second intermediate host) and the proceroids infect the fish and develop into pleroceroid larvae. Many of these small fish are consumed by larger predator fish. Humans (definitive host) are infected by the ingestion of the undercooked small fish or larger predator fish (most common). Once in the human, the pleroceroid develops into adult worms and the cycle is repeated.

Geographic Regions Affected: Worldwide. Common in Europe, Russia, Japan.

Description: Broad fish tapeworm is a cestode infection of the human gastrointestinal tract, which is often asymptomatic. The disease is contracted via the ingestion of raw or undercooked fish. Common dishes include sushi, sashimi, and ceviche.

Signs and Symptoms: Often asymptomatic. Significant worm burden may cause nausea, vomiting, abdominal discomfort, diarrhea, and malaise. After years of infection, human hosts may develop B12 megaloblastic anemia. This is because the worm consumes most of the host's ingested B12—the worm essentially steals it!

Diagnostic Testing: Serial stool samples looking for eggs and proglottids are diagnostic. Long-term infections can cause B12 deficiency anemia, sometimes quite significant, presenting with neurologic findings.

Treatments: Praziquantel and niclosamide are effective treatment options. Vitamin B12 supplementation may be necessary to treat anemia.

Prevention: Avoid ingestion of undercooked fish.

Pearls: Worms measure 10–25 m in length on average and are the largest tapeworms to infect humans. Their bodies have a unique scolex with two ventral grooves used to attach to the intestinal wall, a neck, and proglottids that are wider than they are long. Canines, felines, and bears can also serve as definitive hosts.

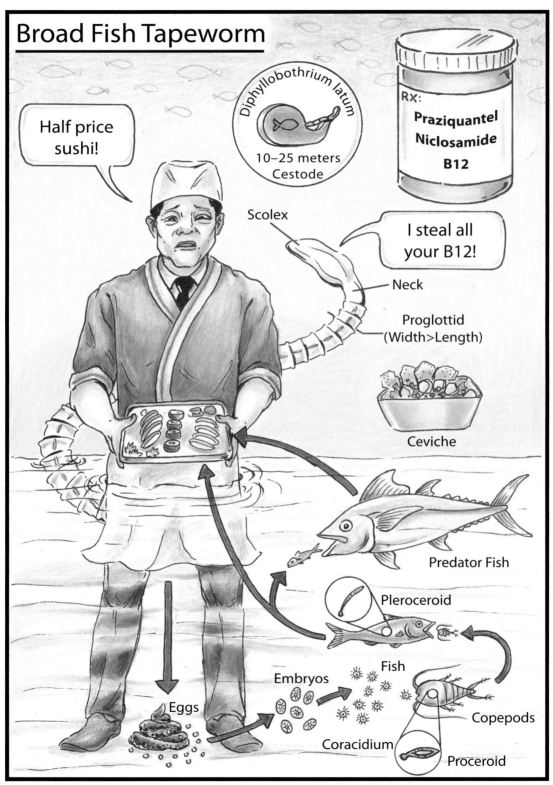

TAPEWORMS

Disease Name: **Beef Tapeworm**

Causative Agent: *Taenia saginata*

Lifecycle: Beef tapeworm disease is contracted from ingestion of infected "measly" beef containing cysticerci. Once inside the human intestine, the cysts hatch, releasing protoscolices that attach to the intestinal wall, becoming the heads (scolex) of adult tapeworms. Hermaphroditic proglottids form off the scolex, mature, become pregnant, produce eggs, and eventually break off the tapeworm. Degraded proglottids release eggs into the passed stools. Contaminated human feces are consumed by cattle, the eggs hatch in their gastrointestinal (GI) tract, and then the larvae seek out striated muscle, liver, and/or lung tissue to form cysticerci. Unlike the pork tapeworm, humans cannot serve as intermediate hosts for beef tapeworm.

Geographic Regions Affected: Worldwide. Common in Central and South America, Europe, Africa, and Asia.

Description: Beef tapeworm is a cestode infection of the human GI tract, which is often asymptomatic.

Signs and Symptoms: Often asymptomatic. Significant worm burden may cause nausea, abdominal discomfort, and malaise.

Diagnostic Testing: Serial stool samples looking for eggs are diagnostic for tapeworms. *Taenia* (beef and pork tapeworm) eggs cannot be distinguished morphologically, but their proglottids have different appearances under microscopy. India ink staining highlights the ovaries and testicles of the proglottids.

Treatments: Praziquantel and niclosamide are effective treatment options.

Prevention: Sanitation and proper hygiene, proper cooking of beef, and/or deep-freezing beef long enough to kill cysticerci.

Pearls: Humans are the only definitive host for *T. saginata,* and cattle serve as intermediate hosts. Worms measure 4–12 m in length on average, but they can be larger. Beef tapeworms are larger than pork tapeworms, and their scolex has four suckers and lacks hooks. Worms can live for several years and produce eggs that survive for about 2 months in the environment.

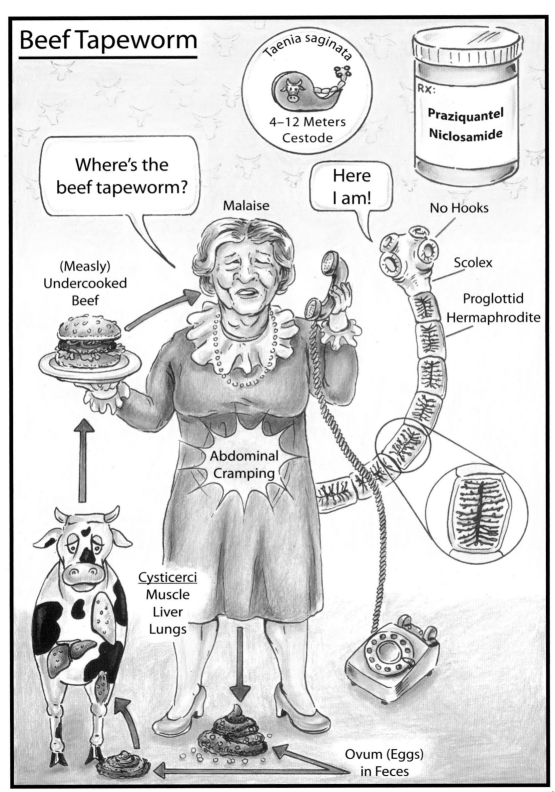

Disease Name: Echinococcosis

Synonyms: Dog tapeworm, cystic echinococcosis (CE), alveolar echinococcosis (AE)

Causative Agents: *Echinococcus granulosus* (CE), *E. multilocularis* (AE)

Lifecycle: *E. granulosus* causes cystic echinococcosis (AKA: hydatid disease); mature worms in definitive hosts (dogs) release infectious eggs, which are consumed by incidental (human) or intermediate hosts (sheep, cattle, goats, horses, camels, swine). *E. multilocularis* causes alveolar echinococcosis; mature worms in definitive hosts (foxes, coyotes) release infectious eggs, which are consumed by incidental (human) or intermediate hosts (rodents).

Geographic Regions Affected: *E. granulosus* (CE): South and Central America, Middle East. *E. multilocularis* (AE): North America, Western China, Russia.

Description: Echinococcosis is an incidental human cestode infection caused by ingestion of infectious eggs released in the stool of definitive hosts.

Signs and Symptoms: *Cystic echinococcosis (CE)*: Initial infection is asymptomatic and might not cause symptoms for decades. Cysts are often singular and affect one organ, most commonly the liver (50%–70%) or lung (20%–30%). CNS, renal, and bone cysts can also occur. Cysts will enlarge over time, causing pain and symptoms in their respective organ systems. Many patients remain asymptomatic for their lifetime, with disease discovered incidentally at autopsy. Ruptured cysts may cause anaphylaxis. *Alveolar echinococcosis (AE)*: The vast majority of cysts (>99%) are hepatic and symptomatic. Symptoms are vague and include fatigue, malaise, and right upper quadrant pain from liver capsule enlargement. If untreated, the mortality rate is high.

Diagnostic Testing: Diagnostic imaging including CT scan, MRI, and ultrasound can be used to locate and visualize cysts. After cyst detection, serology can confirm the diagnosis. ELISA serology for antibody detection is more sensitive than serology for antigen detection.

Treatments: Treatment options include observation, chemotherapy, surgery, or puncture-aspiration-injection-reaspiration (PAIR). PAIR combined with albendazole is the recommended treatment for single liver cysts caused by *E. granulosus*. Surgery is currently the only effective treatment for *E. multilocularis*.

Prevention: Sanitation and proper hygiene.

Pearls: To associate respective intermediate and definitive host relationships, remember that dogs herd cattle and sheep, while foxes and coyotes eat rodents.

TAPEWORMS

Echinococcosis

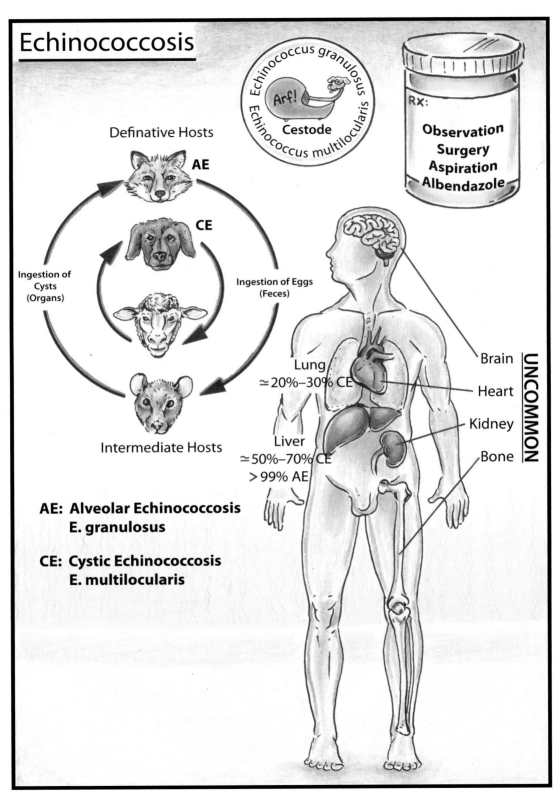

Definative Hosts

AE

CE

Echinococcus granulosus
Echinococcus multilocularis

Arf!

Cestode

RX:

**Observation
Surgery
Aspiration
Albendazole**

Ingestion of
Cysts
(Organs)

Ingestion of Eggs
(Feces)

Intermediate Hosts

Lung
≃ 20%–30% CE

Liver
≃ 50%–70% CE
> 99% AE

Brain

Heart

Kidney

Bone

UNCOMMON

TAPEWORMS

**AE: Alveolar Echinococcosis
E. granulosus**

**CE: Cystic Echinococcosis
E. multilocularis**

TAPEWORMS

Disease Name: Dwarf Tapeworm

Causative Agent: *Hymenolepis nana*

Lifecycle: The disease is contracted from the ingestion of infected insects (beetles and mealworms) serving as intermediate hosts or by the direct ingestion of eggs in contaminated soil, food, or water. The ingested eggs release oncospheres that penetrate the intestine villus and form cystircercoid larvae. These larvae then develop into adult tapeworms and attach to the lining of the ileum. Eggs are produced and released into passing stool. Since eggs are infectious without further development, autoinoculation can occur. The dwarf tapeworm is unique because it can complete its entire lifecycle in the human or with the assistance of small arthropods serving as the intermediate hosts.

Geographic Regions Affected: Worldwide. Common in Egypt, Sudan, Thailand, India, and South America.

Description: Dwarf tapeworm is an infection of the human gastrointestinal tract, which is often asymptomatic.

Signs and Symptoms: Often asymptomatic. Significant infections are more common in children and may present with nausea, diarrhea, abdominal pain, and pruritus ani.

Diagnostic Testing: Serial stool samples looking for eggs are diagnostic.

Treatments: Praziquantel and niclosamide are effective treatment options.

Prevention: Sanitation and proper hygiene.

Pearls: Eosinophilia is common. Chronic infection can have a profound impact on pregnant women and causes growth retardation in young children. Rodents that consume infected beetles or meal worms (intermediate hosts) can also serve as definitive hosts for this parasite.

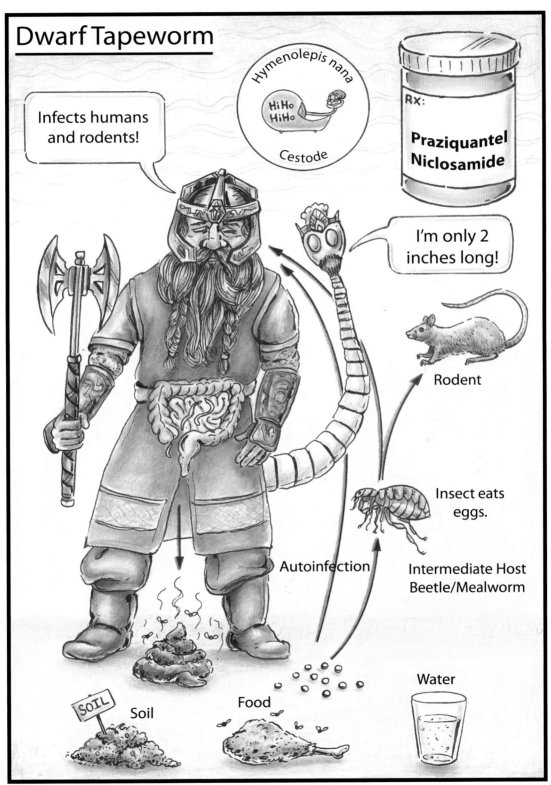

Dwarf Tapeworm

Hymenolepis nana

Cestode

Infects humans and rodents!

RX:

Praziquantel Niclosamide

I'm only 2 inches long!

Rodent

Insect eats eggs.

Autoinfection

Intermediate Host Beetle/Mealworm

Soil

Food

Water

FLATWORMS

Disease Name: Schistosomiasis

Synonym:	Snail fever
Causative Agents:	Blood flukes: *Schistosoma haematobium, S. japonicum, S. mansoni*
Lifecycle:	The disease is contracted via the penetration of schistosoma cercariae through exposed skin when wading or bathing in fresh, slow flowing, snail-infested water. Eggs are passed through infected human feces *(S. japonicum, S. mansoni)* or urine *(S. haematobium)*. Once in fresh water, eggs hatch and release miracidia that penetrate specific snails (intermediate host). Once in the snail, miracidia reproduce asexually over the next 4–6 weeks and mature into cercariae. When cercariae are released from the snail, they seek out a definitive host. Once penetrating the human skin, miracidia transform to schistosomula and migrate to the lungs, where they mature over the next 5–6 weeks before descending into their respective venous environments. The worms reproduce sexually and release eggs into human feces or urine, depending on species. Adult worms live an average of 3–5 years.
Geographic Regions Affected:	Africa and Middle East *(S. haematobium)*; China, Thailand, Indonesia *(S. japonicum)*; South America, Africa, Caribbean *(S. mansoni)*
Description:	Schistosomiasis is a trematode infection of humans caused by a blood fluke with preference for the portal and mesenteric venous system *(S. japonicum, S. mansoni)* or urinary bladder venous plexus *(S. haematobium)*.
Signs and Symptoms:	Most infections are asymptomatic, with severity of illness based on worm burden. "Swimmers itch" or schistosome dermatitis occurs when the cercariae penetrate the skin and cause urticaria, pruritus, and a macular rash. Previously sensitized individuals may have more pronounced symptoms. Acute schistosomiasis may cause *Katayama fever*, specifically from *S. japonicum* and *S. mansoni*. Several weeks after exposure, patients may develop fever, chills, malaise, abdominal pain, diarrhea, hematochezia, chest pain, cough, and hepatosplenomegaly. Chronic infections can cause granulomatous changes in the liver *(S. japonicum, S. mansoni)* and hematuria *(S. haematobium)*. *S. haematobium* can cause bladder calcification and ureteral reflux, leading to kidney damage.
Diagnostic Testing:	Labs will reveal eosinophilia. Serial stool and urine samples are required to identify the excreted eggs. Urine antigen testing is available in some countries.
Treatments:	Praziquantel is the preferred treatment for all forms of schistosomiasis.
Prevention:	Avoid standing water in endemic countries.
Pearls:	Respective species can increase incidence of hepatocellular *(S. japonicum, S. mansoni)* and bladder cancer *(S. haematobium)*.

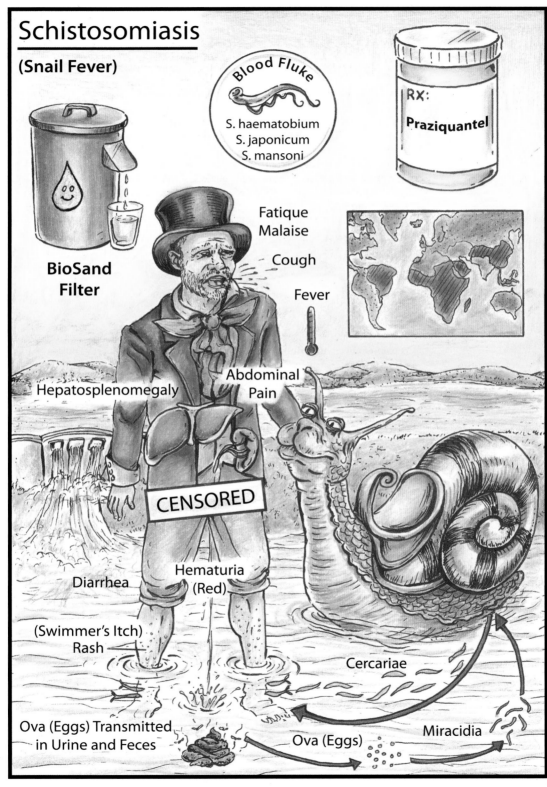

Schistosomiasis
(Snail Fever)

Blood Fluke

S. haematobium
S. japonicum
S. mansoni

RX:
Praziquantel

BioSand Filter

Fatique
Malaise

Cough

Fever

Hepatosplenomegaly

Abdominal Pain

CENSORED

Diarrhea

Hematuria (Red)

(Swimmer's Itch) Rash

Cercariae

Ova (Eggs) Transmitted in Urine and Feces

Ova (Eggs)

Miracidia

Disease Name: **Liver Fluke**

Synonym:	Chinese liver fluke
Causative Agents:	*Clonochis sinensis, Opisthorchis viverrini, Opisthorchis felineus*
Lifecycle:	The disease is contracted from ingestion of undercooked fish. From infected humans, embryonated eggs are passed into the environment through feces. The eggs are consumed by specific snails (first intermediate host), wherein they hatch to form miracidia. The miracidia reproduce inside the snail and produce large numbers of cercariae. The cercariae are eventually released into the water and penetrate fish (second intermediate host), wherein they form metacercarial cysts. Once humans ingest the undercooked fish, metacercarial cysts hatch, migrate through the upper GI tract, and take up residence in the gallbladder and bile ducts. There they feed on bile, reproduce, and can live for up to 30 years.
Geographic Regions Affected:	East and Southeast Asia (*C. sinensis*), Southeast Asia (*O. viverrini*), Russia (*O. felineus*)
Description:	The Chinese liver fluke is a trematode infection of humans with preference for the bile ducts and gallbladder.
Signs and Symptoms:	Patients may initially be asymptomatic or develop fever, nausea, vomiting, diarrhea, and abdominal pain within 4 weeks of initial infection. Chronic symptoms are associated with worm burden and feeding within the bile ducts and include right upper quadrant pain, jaundice, elevated liver enzymes, malaise, and weight loss. Long-standing infections can cause periductal fibrosis and increased incidence of biliary ductal carcinoma.
Diagnostic Testing:	Labs will reveal eosinophilia, elevated liver enzymes, and increased bilirubin levels. Eggs can be identified in serial stool samples, duodenal aspirates, or bile specimens. Diagnostic imaging including US, CT, and MRI will reveal biliary ductal dilation and wall thickening. Worms may be visualized swimming in the gallbladder on US.
Treatments:	Praziquantel and albendazole are effective treatment options.
Prevention:	Avoid undercooked fish in endemic areas.
Pearls:	Chronic infection increases the likelihood of developing biliary duct and gallbladder carcinoma.

FLATWORMS

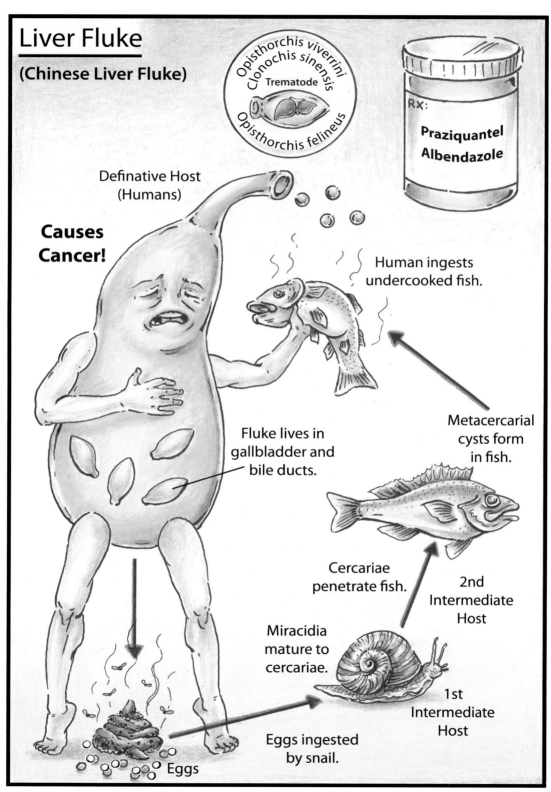

Liver Fluke

(Chinese Liver Fluke)

Opisthorchis viverrini
Clonochis sinensis
Trematode
Opisthorchis felineus

RX:

**Praziquantel
Albendazole**

Definative Host
(Humans)

**Causes
Cancer!**

Human ingests
undercooked fish.

Metacercarial
cysts form
in fish.

Fluke lives in
gallbladder and
bile ducts.

Cercariae
penetrate fish.

2nd
Intermediate
Host

Miracidia
mature to
cercariae.

1st
Intermediate
Host

Eggs ingested
by snail.

Eggs

FLATWORMS

145

Disease Name: **Lung Fluke**

Synonyms:	Paragonimiasis, Japanese lung fluke, oriental lung fluke
Causative Agent:	*Paragonimus westermani*
Lifecycle:	The disease is contracted from the ingestion of undercooked crabs (crayfish in the United States). Starting in the definitive host (humans), unembryonated eggs are coughed up from the lungs and excreted in the sputum or swallowed and pass with stool. Once in the external environment, the eggs become embryonated and hatch into miracidia. Next the miracidia find and penetrate small snails (first intermediate host). In the snails, further development occurs over the next 3–5 months until the snail releases cercariae. The cercariae penetrate small crabs and crayfish (second intermediate host), wherein they form metacercarial cysts. Once humans ingest the undercooked crustacean, metacercarial cysts hatch, penetrate through the duodenum, and ultimately migrate to the lungs through the diaphragm, where they encapsulate and begin egg production. Worms can live in humans for up to 20 years.
Geographic Regions Affected:	East Asia *(P. westermani)*, South America *(P. mexicanus)*, and North America *(P. kellicotti)*
Description:	Paragonimiasis is a trematode infection of humans with preference for the lungs.
Signs and Symptoms:	Symptoms of acute infection occur within 2 weeks and include abdominal pain and diarrhea, followed by fever, chills, cough, and urticaria. Chronic symptoms are associated with the shedding of eggs into the bronchial tree and include cough, pleuritic chest pain, and hemoptysis.
Diagnostic Testing:	Labs will reveal eosinophilia. Serial stool and sputum samples are required to identify the excreted eggs. Serology and enzyme immunoassay testing are available.
Treatments:	Praziquantel or triclabendazole are effective treatment options.
Prevention:	Avoid undercooked crabs and crayfish.
Pearls:	Can be confused with pulmonary TB and/or lung cancer.

FLATWORMS

Lung Fluke

(Paragonimiasis)
(Japanese Lung Fluke)
(Oriental Lung Fluke)

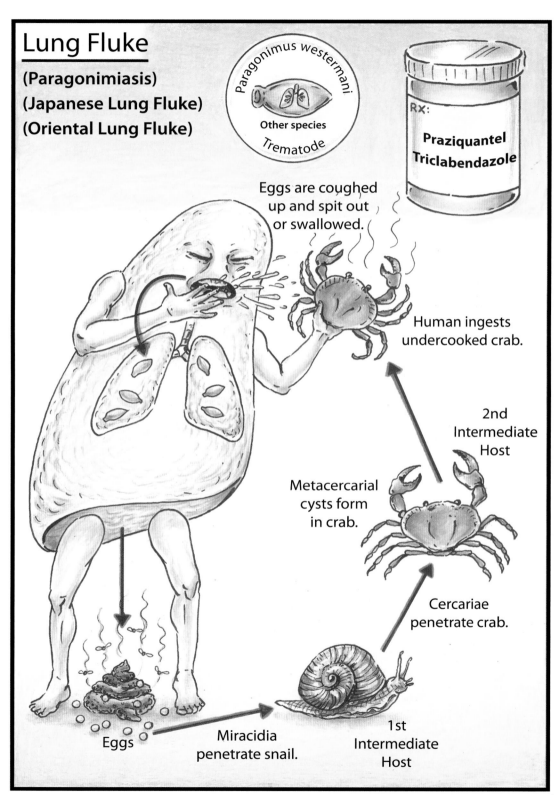

Paragonimus westermani

Other species

Trematode

RX:

Praziquantel
Triclabendazole

Eggs are coughed up and spit out or swallowed.

Human ingests undercooked crab.

2nd Intermediate Host

Metacercarial cysts form in crab.

Cercariae penetrate crab.

Eggs

Miracidia penetrate snail.

1st Intermediate Host

PART 6

FUNGAL

Disease Name: Sporotrichosis

Synonym: Rose gardener's disease

Causative Agent: *Sporothrix schenkii*

Incubation: 1–12 weeks; Average: 3 weeks

Geographic Regions Affected: Worldwide, more common in tropical and subtropical locales.

Description: Sporotrichosis is a cutaneous, lymphocutaneous, pulmonary, or disseminated fungal disease caused by the dimorphic fungi *Sporothrix schenkii*. Dimorphic fungi are human pathogens that grow as a mold at 25°C and as a yeast at 37°C. The fungi are commonly found in or on soil, hay, peat moss, plants, and on rose thorns. Cats can carry and spread the disease via their claws. The disease is not contagious.

Signs and Symptoms: Cutaneous sporotrichosis is the most-common disease manifestation and typically presents as a small, painless, nodular lesion on the finger, hand, or arm, which eventually ulcerates. Lymphocutaneous sporotrichosis occurs as the infection spreads up the lymph channels and secondary lesions occur and eventually ulcerate as well. Lesions may wax and wane over months to years if left untreated. Primary pulmonary sporotrichosis is a rare disease caused by the inhalation of spores. Patients present with cough, mediastinal lymphadenopathy, pulmonary fibrosis, lung nodules and cavitations. Disseminated disease can occur via hematogenous spreading of the disease to the joints (osteoarticular sporotrichosis—most common), lung (secondary pulmonary sporotrichosis), or central nervous system (CNS) (sporotrichosis meningitis). Multifocal disseminated disease can occur in the immunocompromised.

Diagnostic Testing: The diagnosis should be considered based on occupational exposure and disease pattern or presentation. Fungal culture is the gold standard for diagnosis, and samples should be obtained from several sites. Pathologic examination of biopsied lesions will reveal a pyogranulomatous response and the classic "cigar body"–shaped yeast.

Treatments: Itraconazole is the treatment of choice in most cases, except for pregnancy and severe infections. Severe pulmonary, disseminated, or CNS infections should be treated with amphotericin B followed by itraconazole. Alternative treatments include saturated solution of potassium iodide or terbinafine.

Pearls: When seen under microscopy, the mold has a "daisy wheel" appearance and the yeast has a "cigar body" shape. Dimorphic fungi grow as a "Mold in the Cold and a Yeast in the Beast (Heat)."

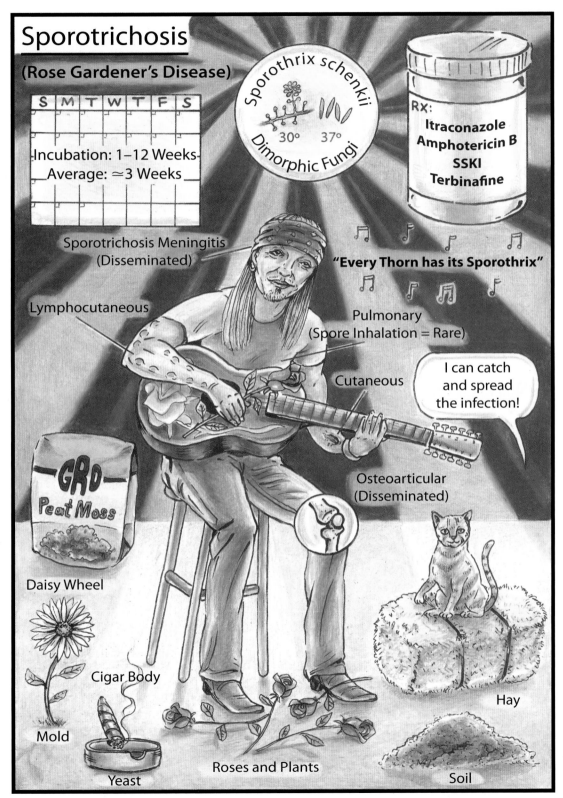

Sporotrichosis
(Rose Gardener's Disease)

Incubation: 1–12 Weeks
Average: ≃3 Weeks

Sporothrix schenkii
30° 37°
Dimorphic Fungi

RX:
Itraconazole
Amphotericin B
SSKI
Terbinafine

Sporotrichosis Meningitis
(Disseminated)

"Every Thorn has its Sporothrix"

Lymphocutaneous

Pulmonary
(Spore Inhalation = Rare)

Cutaneous

I can catch and spread the infection!

Osteoarticular
(Disseminated)

GRO Peat Moss

Daisy Wheel

Cigar Body

Mold

Yeast

Roses and Plants

Hay

Soil

Disease Name: **Paracoccidioidomycosis**

Synonym: South American blastomycosis

Causative Agents: *Paracoccidioides brasiliensis, Paracoccidioides lutzii*

Incubation: 1 month to 9 years

Geographic Regions Affected: Central and South America. Most cases have been reported in Brazil.

Description: Paracoccidioidomycosis is a systemic fungal infection caused by the dimorphic fungi *Paracoccidioides spp.* Dimorphic fungi are human pathogens that grow as a mold at 25°C and as a yeast at 37°C. The disease is spread via the inhalation of conidia, small single-cell molds, swept up into the air of disturbed soil. The initial exposure is often asymptomatic. The disease presents in either the acute/subacute "juvenile" (≈5%–10% of cases) or chronic "adult" form (≈90% of cases). The disease is not contagious (it is not spread from person to person).

Signs and Symptoms: The acute or subacute disease manifestations are more common in younger patients and the immunocompromised. The acute form presents as a significant illness with fever, chills, malaise, weight loss, lymphadenopathy, hepatosplenomegaly, cough, dyspnea, and multiple skin and mucocutaneous lesions. Chronic disease causes cough and pulmonary fibrosis or emphysematous changes, chronic ulcers of the mucous membranes, mouth, nasopharynx, or larynx, cervical lymphadenopathy, and cutaneous skin lesions. Adrenal insufficiency is also common in the chronic setting.

Diagnostic Testing: Direct microscopy of sputum, skin lesions, lymph node aspirates or tissues using KOH prep or calcofluor stains will often reveal yeast with a "pilot's wheel" of "Mickey Mouse head" appearance. Fungal cultures can be prepared from sputum or lymph node aspirates. Serologic tests can aid in diagnosis and titers can be followed to assess treatment response. Chest radiographs often show fibrosis and emphysematous changes in chronic disease.

Treatments: Itraconazole is recommended for mild to moderate disease; duration of therapy is based on disease severity. Amphotericin B followed by itraconazole is recommended for severe disease. Alternative regiments include ketoconazole or sulfonamides (TMP/SMX). TMP/SMX may require several years of treatment for maximum effectiveness and/or to prevent relapse.

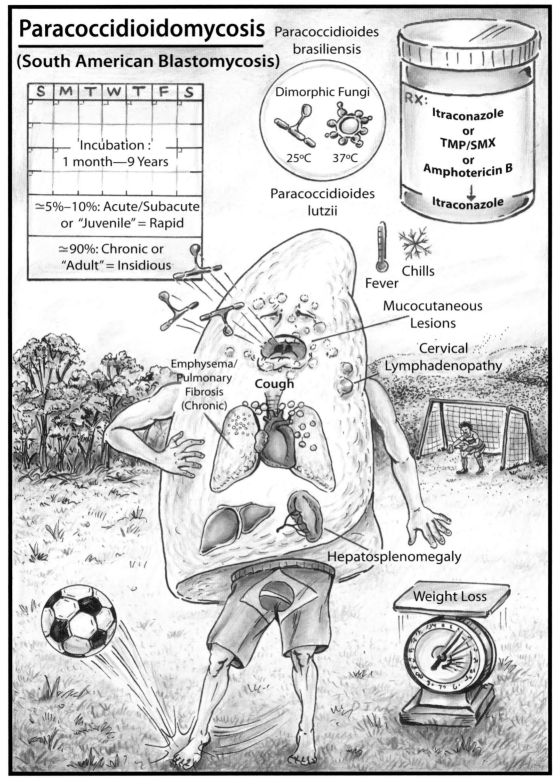

Paracoccidioidomycosis
(South American Blastomycosis)

Paracoccidioides brasiliensis

S	M	T	W	T	F	S
		Incubation :				
		1 month—9 Years				

≃5%–10%: Acute/Subacute or "Juvenile" = Rapid

≃90%: Chronic or "Adult" = Insidious

Dimorphic Fungi

25°C 37°C

Paracoccidioides lutzii

RX: **Itraconazole** or **TMP/SMX** or **Amphotericin B** ↓ **Itraconazole**

Fever

Chills

Mucocutaneous Lesions

Cervical Lymphadenopathy

Emphysema/ Pulmonary Fibrosis (Chronic)

Cough

Hepatosplenomegaly

Weight Loss

Disease Name: Coccidioidomycosis

Synonym: San Joaquin Valley fever

Causative Agents: *Coccidioides immitis, Coccidioides posadasii*

Incubation: 7–21 days

Geographic Regions Affected: Desert regions in the western hemisphere, most commonly in the United States and parts of Mexico. The two U.S. states with the most cases are Arizona and California. Other states include Nevada, New Mexico, Utah, and Texas.

Description: Coccidioidomycosis is primarily a pulmonary fungal infection caused by the dimorphic fungi *Coccidioides spp*. Dimorphic fungi are human pathogens that grow as a mold at 25°C and as a yeast at 37°C. The disease is spread via the inhalation of arthroconidia, small single-cell molds, swept up into the air of disturbed soil, often after heavy rainstorms, vigorous hiking, or construction. Once inhaled, the mold transforms into yeast and begins reproduction in the host, triggering an immune response and the signs and symptoms of infection. The disease is not contagious (it is not spread from person to person).

Signs and Symptoms: More than half of all infections are asymptomatic or mild. In those that are symptomatic, acute infection often mimics community-acquired pneumonia and symptoms can include fever, chills, malaise, headache, chest pain, cough, shortness of breath, migratory arthralgia, myalgia, rash, and erythema nodosum. The disease is often self-limiting after several weeks, but fatigue can persist for months. More severe disease is often seen in the immunocompromised and/or those with a large arthroconidial inoculum. About 5% of infections become chronic, exemplified by severe pulmonary manifestations and/or disseminated disease with meningeal, bone, or joint space involvement. Desert rheumatism is the triad of arthralgia, fever, and erythema nodosum.

Diagnostic Testing: IgM/IgG serology can be obtained. Sputum samples can be sent for fungal culture and direct examination microscopy using KOH or calcofluor staining. For patients with early infection, isolating the organism in culture may be the only way to diagnose since antibodies take weeks to months to develop. Titers determined by complement-fixing antibody tests can be obtained to confirm diagnosis and anticipate likelihood of extrapulmonary dissemination (titers ≥1:16 indicate a high likelihood of dissemination). Chest x-ray findings in chronic disease can include mediastinal lymphadenopathy, nodules, granulomas, and cavitary lesions. Spontaneous pneumothorax may occur if cavitary lesions or blebs rupture. These findings may mimic tuberculosis (TB) or cancer.

Treatments: Mild infections are often self-limiting and resolve spontaneously. Indications for treatment proposed by the Infectious Disease Society of America include >10% weight loss, night sweats >3 weeks, significant pulmonary infiltrates, prominent hilar lymphadenopathy, titers ≥1:16, inability to work, and/or symptoms longer than 2 months. Itraconazole and fluconazole are effective treatments for mild to moderate disease. Amphotericin B is recommended for severe infections or disseminated disease.

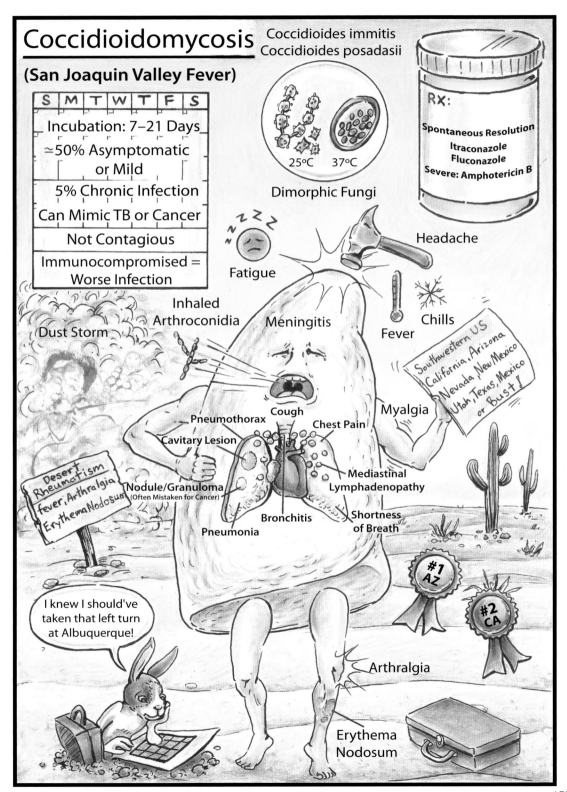

Disease Name: **Blastomycosis**

Synonyms:	Gilchrist's disease, North American blastomycosis
Causative Agent:	*Blastomyces dermatitidis*
Incubation:	1–3 months
Geographic Regions Affected:	Predominantly found in the Ohio, Mississippi, and St. Lawrence River Valleys, as well as the Great Lakes Region of the United States.
Description:	Blastomycosis is primarily a pulmonary fungal infection caused by the dimorphic fungi *Blastomyces dermatitidis*. Dimorphic fungi are a human pathogen that grow as a mold at 25°C and as a yeast at 37°C. The disease is spread via the inhalation of conidia, small single-cell molds, swept up into the air of disturbed soil. In addition to pulmonary manifestations, blastomycosis can also present as skin, bone, genitourinary, or laryngeal lesions. The disease also infects dogs and is not contagious (it is not spread from person to person).
Signs and Symptoms:	Up to 50% of cases are asymptomatic. When symptomatic, blastomycosis can present in a variety of ways in the acute and chronic settings. From a pulmonary perspective, it can present as mild flu-like illness, pneumonia, or acute respiratory distress syndrome (ARDS). Chronic pulmonary manifestations on chest x-ray can include nodules, granulomas, mediastinal lymphadenopathy, or cavitary lesions, all potentially mimicking tuberculosis (TB) or cancer. Since blastomycosis is an insidious and often slowly progressive disease, dissemination is not uncommon, specifically in the immunocompromised. Disseminated disease can present cutaneously as verrucous or ulcerative skin lesions, as osteomyelitis in the bones, as disseminated lesions in the genitourinary system, or as meningitis-causing lesions in the central nervous system (CNS).
Diagnostic Testing:	Fungal culture is the gold standard for the diagnosis of blastomycosis. Direct microscopy can detect yeast in biopsied tissues and respiratory secretions. Enzyme immunoassay (EIA) antigen detection studies can be performed on urine, serum, and bronchoalveolar washings. Serologic testing is not useful for the diagnosis of blastomycosis.
Treatments:	The authors recommend consultation with the Infectious Disease Society of America guidelines. Overall, the guidelines encourage the treatment of all infected individuals to prevent disseminated disease and recommend treatment for all patients with moderate to severe pneumonia, disseminated disease, and compromised immune systems. Mild to moderate pulmonary and disseminated disease can be treated with oral itraconazole. Severe disease should be treated more aggressively with amphotericin B followed by oral itraconazole. CNS infections are treated with amphotericin B followed by oral fluconazole, itraconazole, or voriconazole, often for a 12-month duration.
Pearls:	Under microscopy, the hyphae branch at 90 degrees and the conidia resemble lollipops. Untreated blastomycosis has a high mortality in the immunocompromised and in patients who develop ARDS as a result of infection.

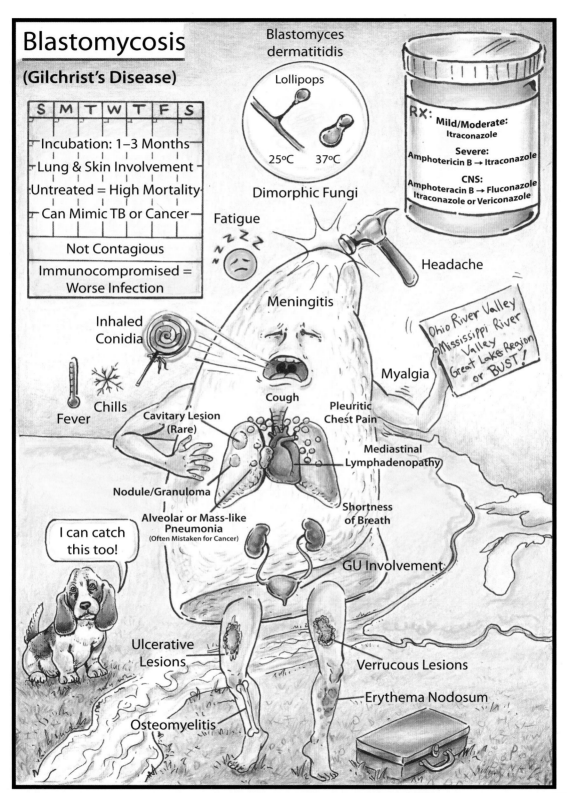

Blastomycosis
(Gilchrist's Disease)

Blastomyces dermatitidis

Lollipops

25°C   37°C

Dimorphic Fungi

RX:
Mild/Moderate:
Itraconazole

Severe:
Amphotericin B → Itraconazole

CNS:
Amphoteracin B → Fluconazole
Itraconazole or Vericonazole

S	M	T	W	T	F	S

Incubation: 1–3 Months
Lung & Skin Involvement
Untreated = High Mortality
Can Mimic TB or Cancer
Not Contagious
Immunocompromised = Worse Infection

Fatigue

Headache

Meningitis

Inhaled Conidia

Ohio River Valley Mississippi River Valley Great Lakes Region or BUST!

Myalgia

Fever   Chills

Cough

Pleuritic Chest Pain

Cavitary Lesion (Rare)

Mediastinal Lymphadenopathy

Nodule/Granuloma

Shortness of Breath

Alveolar or Mass-like Pneumonia
(Often Mistaken for Cancer)

I can catch this too!

GU Involvement

Ulcerative Lesions

Verrucous Lesions

Erythema Nodosum

Osteomyelitis

157

Disease Name: Histoplasmosis

Synonyms:	Spelunker's lung, cave disease
Causative Agent:	*Histoplasma capsulatum*
Incubation:	3–17 days
Geographic Regions Affected:	Worldwide, predominantly found in river valleys. In the United States, most cases are found in the Midwest and Southeastern states (Ohio and Mississippi River Valleys). There is a positive association with this disease and cave exploration in the United States and Central and South America.
Description:	Histoplasmosis is primarily a pulmonary fungal infection caused by the dimorphic fungi *Histoplasma capsulatum*. Dimorphic fungi are a human pathogen that grows as a mold at 25°C and as a yeast at 37°C. The disease is spread via the inhalation of conidia, small single-cell molds, swept up into the air of disturbed soil, often contaminated with bat guano or feces from starlings or black birds. Once inhaled, the mold transforms into yeast and begins reproduction in the host, triggering an immune response and the signs and symptoms of infection. The disease is not contagious (it is not spread from person to person).
Signs and Symptoms:	The vast majority of patients (≈90%) are asymptomatic or have mild disease and don't seek medical attention. Symptomatic patients may develop fever, chills, headache, substernal chest pain, and nonproductive cough. Malaise, fatigue, myalgia, arthralgia, and erythema nodosum may also occur. Patients can also develop pericarditis, mediastinitis, and/or hepatosplenomegaly. Mediastinal lymphadenopathy can occur, but it is uncommon (5% to 10% of patients). The disease is often self-limiting, but moderate to severe pulmonary, disseminated, and central nervous system (CNS) infections require antifungal treatment. More-severe disease is often seen in the immunocompromised and/or those patients with a large conidial inoculum. About 5% of infections become chronic, exemplified by the development of pulmonary cavitary disease with low-grade fever, cough, and dyspnea mimicking tuberculosis (TB). Chronic cavitary disease is more common in those with preexisting emphysema.
Diagnostic Testing:	Enzyme immunoassay (EIA) antigen detection studies can be performed on urine, serum, and bronchoalveolar washings. Titers determined by complement-fixing antibody tests can be obtained to confirm diagnosis. Fungal cultures can be performed on respiratory secretions. Acute chest x-ray findings may reveal patchy pneumonitis and mediastinal lymphadenopathy. Chest x-ray findings in chronic disease can include mediastinal lymphadenopathy, nodules, granulomas, and cavitary lesions. These findings may mimic TB or cancer.
Treatments:	Mild infections are often self-limiting and resolve spontaneously. Indications and recommendations for treatment are based on the severity of illness and the authors recommend consultation with the Infectious Disease Society of America guidelines. Itraconazole is effective for mild to moderate disease with symptoms lasting longer than 1 month. Amphoteracin B is indicated for severe infections.

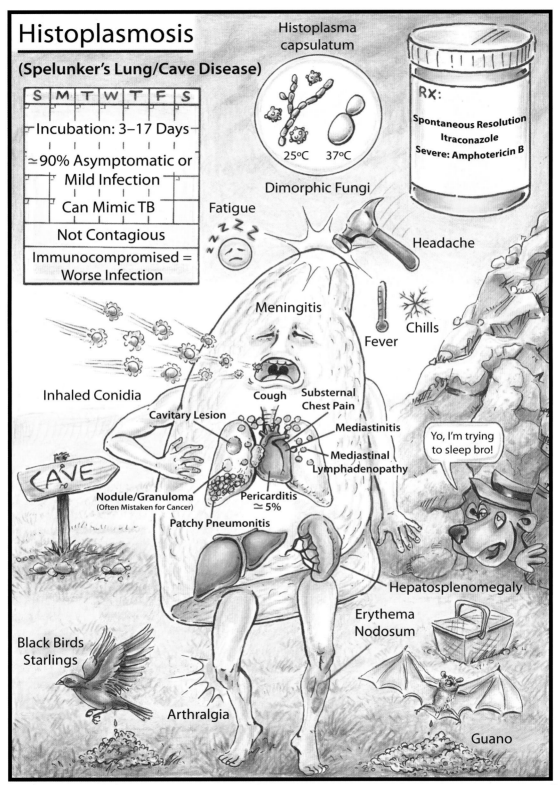

Histoplasmosis
(Spelunker's Lung/Cave Disease)

S	M	T	W	T	F	S

Incubation: 3–17 Days

≈90% Asymptomatic or Mild Infection

Can Mimic TB

Not Contagious

Immunocompromised = Worse Infection

Histoplasma capsulatum

25°C   37°C

Dimorphic Fungi

RX:
Spontaneous Resolution
Itraconazole
Severe: Amphotericin B

Fatigue

Headache

Meningitis

Chills

Fever

Inhaled Conidia

Cough

Substernal Chest Pain

Cavitary Lesion

Mediastinitis

Mediastinal Lymphadenopathy

Yo, I'm trying to sleep bro!

Nodule/Granuloma
(Often Mistaken for Cancer)

Pericarditis ≈5%

Patchy Pneumonitis

CAVE

Hepatosplenomegaly

Erythema Nodosum

Black Birds Starlings

Arthralgia

Guano

Disease Name: Tinea Infections of the Skin

Tinea Pedis (Athlete's Foot): This is the most common dermatophytosis, and it affects the foot, often in the interdigital web spaces. It is more common in adolescents and young adults and is associated with sweating. It is commonly transmitted in areas of shared bathing and showering (gyms, college dorms, military barracks, prisons, etc.). Wearing shower shoes or flip flops and good foot hygiene can limit infections and transmission. For treatment, topical creams or ointments are usually sufficient. Terbinafine, fluconazole, griseofulvin, or ketoconazole can be prescribed and taken orally for severe infections.

Tinea Corporis (Ringworm): Fungal infection of the trunk or extremities, commonly appear as a raised, red ring with a central clearing. The infection can be spread from person to person or acquired as a zoonosis from dogs, cats, cattle, and other animals. The disease is more common in hot and humid climates. Treatment is similar to that for tinea pedis.

Tinea Cruris (Jock Itch): Fungal infection of the groin and inguinal region, more common in athletic males. Tinea cruris is often bilateral and spares the penis and scrotum. It can be distinguished from *Candida* largely by the absence of satellite lesions. Treatment is similar to that for tinea pedis.

Tinea Manuum: Fungal infection of the hand(s). Treatment is similar to that for tinea pedis.

Tinea Faciei/Tinea Barbae: Fungal infection of the face, neck, or beard area. Folliculitis, sycosis barbae, and pseudofolliculitis barbae should be considered in the differential. Given the involvement of numerous hair follicles, oral therapy is the preferred treatment.

Tinea Capitis: Fungal infection of the scalp characterized by pruritic, annular patches of alopecia. The condition is most common in young children and can occur with or without inflammation. The hair shafts in tinea capitis are infected in one of two ways. In ectothrix infections, spores are formed on the exterior of the hair shafts and hairs break off several millimeters above the scalp. In endothrix infections, spores are formed within the individual hair shafts and this causes the hairs to break at the level of the scalp, often appearing as clusters of black dots. If inflammation is significant, a raised, boggy, soft tissue mass known as a kerion may form. Kerions are occasionally mistaken for bacterial abscesses. Oral antifungals are required for treatment and include griseofulvin, terbinafine, itraconazole, and fluconazole.

Tinea Unguium/Onychomycosis: Fungal infection of fingernails and/or toenails. Treatment is mostly for cosmetic purposes, and oral medications are the most effective, including itraconazole, fluconazole, and terbinafine. Some medications may require pulsed dosing, and toenails typically require a longer duration of treatment than fingernails. There are some lacquers (ciclopirox or amorolfine) available for treatment, but they have limited effectiveness.

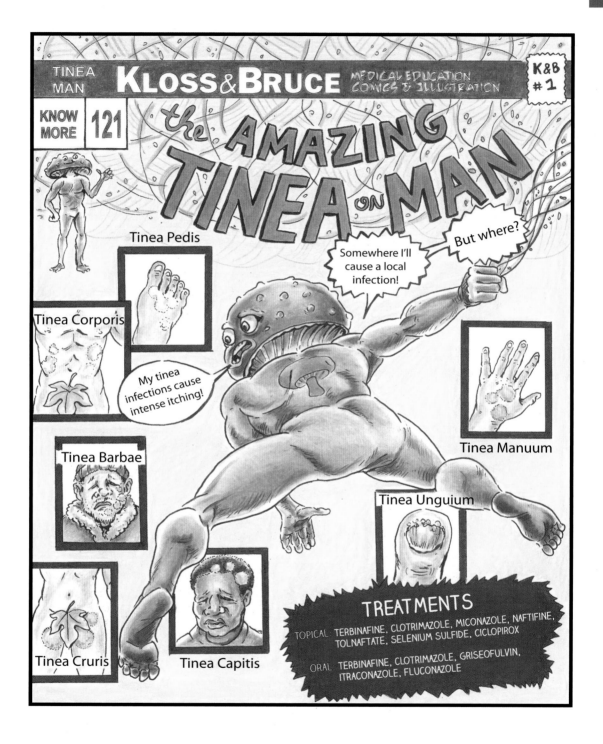

Disease Name: **Tinea Versicolor**

Synonym:	Pityriasis versicolor
Causative Agents:	*Malassezia globosa, Malassezia furfur*
Incubation:	Unknown/Varied
Geographic Regions Affected:	Worldwide. More common in tropical and subtropical regions.
Description:	Tinea versicolor is a cutaneous overgrowth of a common topical yeast, often more pronounced in warm, humid environments and during the summer months.
Signs and Symptoms:	Lesions have sharp boarders, are nonpruritic, and tend to affect the trunk and proximal extremities. In lighter-skinned people, lesions may be hyperpigmented, whereas hypopigmentation occurs more commonly in darker-skinned people. Tanning tends to enhance the appearance of these lesions.
Diagnosis:	This is typically a visual diagnosis. Microscopy with KOH preparation will reveal the characteristic "spaghetti and meatballs" appearance of round yeasts with short hyphae filaments. Lesions will fluoresce yellow-green under a Wood's lamp.
Treatments:	Topical azole antifungal or terbinafine creams are effective and inexpensive. Less effective treatments include topical selenium sulfide lotion. Severe cases can be treated with oral itraconazole, ketoconazole, or fluconazole.
Pearls:	Telling an attractive young female that she has a noncontagious skin infection does not make for a good introduction or icebreaker. This has been confirmed by independent research on at least two separate occasions.

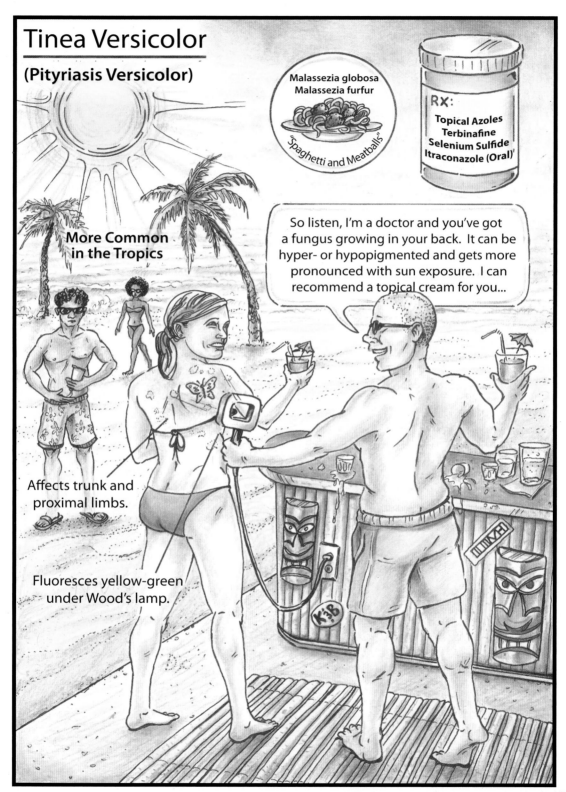

Disease Name: Aspergillosis

Causative Agents:	*Aspergillus fumigatus, Aspergillus flavus*
Incubation:	Unknown/Varied
Geographic Regions Affected:	Worldwide

Description: Aspergillosis incorporates a wide variety of mycotic infections caused by molds of the *Aspergillus* genus. Infections can be localized or disseminated and mostly occur in patients with preexisting tuberculosis (TB), chronic obstructive pulmonary disease (COPD), or compromised immune systems (AIDS, stem cell or whole organ transplant recipients).

Aspergilloma or "Fungus Ball": A localized collection or "ball" of noninvasive *Aspergillus* can occur in the sinuses (maxillary is most common) or in a preexisting pulmonary cavity (typically in the apex of the lung) in patients with bullous emphysema, TB, or sarcoidosis. Treatment is surgical.

Otomycosis: Noninvasive chronic otitis externa infection caused by *Aspergillus* spp. *A. niger* will have a blackish coloration and/or drainage, whereas *A. fumigatus* will have a greenish hue.

Allergic Bronchopulmonary Aspergillosis (ABPA): ABPA is a noninvasive, exaggerated immune response to *Aspergillus* in patients with preexisting asthma or cystic fibrosis. *Aspergillus fumigatus* is the most common causative agent. Over time, patients develop bronchiectasis, mucous plugging, and pulmonary infiltrates that do not respond to antibiotic treatment. Patients will have peripheral eosinophilia, elevated IgE levels, positive skin test reactivity to *Aspergillus*, and IgG antibodies against *Aspergillus*. Treatment includes antifungals and corticosteroids.

Invasive Pulmonary Aspergillosis (IPA): IPA is an invasive, florid *Aspergillus* infection of the lungs in immunocompromised patients, typically those with significant neutropenia. Signs and symptoms include fever, cough, dyspnea, and chest pain. Chest x-ray will reveal diffuse infiltrates and CT scan of the chest may reveal the "halo" (ground glass appearance surrounding a nodule) or "air crescent" signs.

Cerebral Aspergillosis: Cerebral spread of *Aspergillus* has an extremely high mortality and presents as headaches, focal neurologic deficits, and altered mental status. CT scans may reveal ring-enhancing lesions and localized edema.

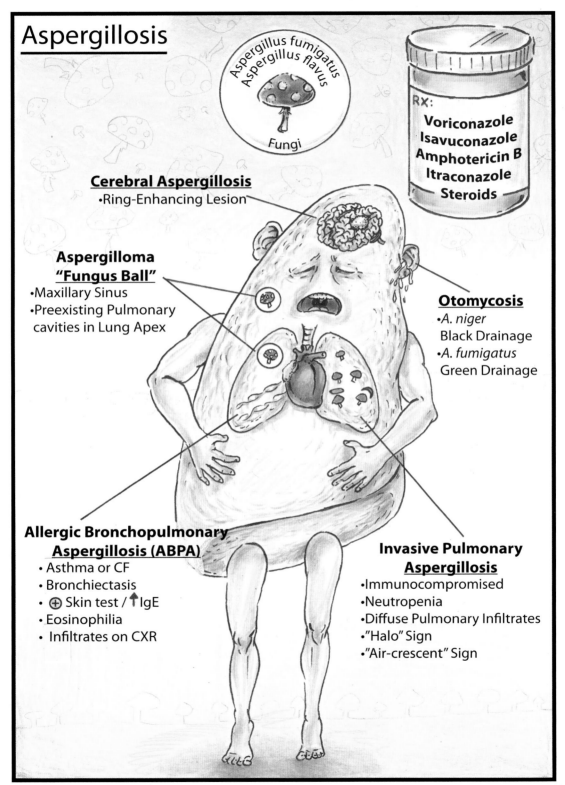

Aspergillosis

Aspergillus fumigatus
Aspergillus flavus

Fungi

RX:
Voriconazole
Isavuconazole
Amphotericin B
Itraconazole
Steroids

Cerebral Aspergillosis
•Ring-Enhancing Lesion

Aspergilloma "Fungus Ball"
•Maxillary Sinus
•Preexisting Pulmonary cavities in Lung Apex

Otomycosis
•*A. niger* Black Drainage
•*A. fumigatus* Green Drainage

Allergic Bronchopulmonary Aspergillosis (ABPA)
• Asthma or CF
• Bronchiectasis
• ⊕ Skin test / ↑IgE
• Eosinophilia
• Infiltrates on CXR

Invasive Pulmonary Aspergillosis
•Immunocompromised
•Neutropenia
•Diffuse Pulmonary Infiltrates
•"Halo" Sign
•"Air-crescent" Sign

Disease Name: **Mucormycosis**

Synonym:	Zygomycosis
Causative Agents:	*Mucor* spp., *Rhizopus* spp., *Lichtheimia* spp., *Cunninghamella* spp.
Incubation:	Unknown/Varied
Geographic Regions Affected:	Worldwide

Description: Mucormycosis is a rare, severe angioinvasive fungal infection that predominantly infects the sinuses or lungs of people with uncontrolled diabetes or a compromised immune system. Rhinocerebral mucormycosis begins in the sinuses, can spread to the orbits and brain, and is more common in diabetics. Pulmonary mucormycosis affects the lungs and is more common in cancer patients or stem cell or whole-organ transplant recipients. Infants who ingest spores may develop gastrointestinal (GI) mucormycosis, and a cutaneous form can infect wounds and burns.

Signs and Symptoms: *Rhinocerebral*: Symptoms are progressive and initially consistent with sinusitis. Fever, headache, unilateral facial swelling/pain/numbness, sinus congestion, unilateral ocular abnormalities (blindness), and eventually, hard palate ulcerations and eschar formation secondary to ischemic necrosis. *Pulmonary*: Fever, chills, cough, dyspnea, chest pain, hemoptysis, and pulmonary infiltrates are hallmarks. Presentation may be indistinguishable from invasive pulmonary aspergillosis. However, in pulmonary mucormycosis, patients will often have concurrent rhinocerebral symptoms. *Cutaneous*: Infection begins as an area of erythema that progresses to a black eschar. Given the angioinvasive properties of the fungi, necrotizing fasciitis can occur. *GI*: Abdominal pain, nausea, vomiting, GI bleeding. Necrotizing enterocolitis can occur and is often fatal. *Disseminated infections*: Signs and symptoms of dissemination are organ specific. Central nervous system (CNS) manifestations include altered mental status and coma.

Diagnosis: Patient history, risk factors, clinical presentation, and signs and symptoms suggest the diagnosis. Fluid washings from the sinuses and/or lungs can be sent for microscopy or fungal culture. Tissue biopsies can also be obtained and examined by pathology.

Treatments: Early identification of the disease process followed by surgical debridement of infected tissues and cavities and treatment with antifungal medications improves outcomes. Mucormycosis is resistant to fluconazole and voriconazole. Effective medications include amphotericin B, posaconazole, and isavuconazole.

Pearls: Risk factors for mucormycosis include uncontrolled diabetes, diabetic ketoacidosis (DKA), compromised immune systems, hematologic malignancies, stem cell and whole organ transplant recipients, and treatment with deferoxamine for chelation of iron overloaded states.

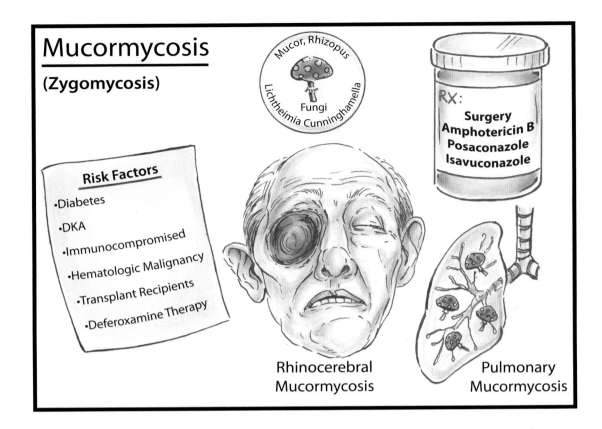

Mucormycosis

(Zygomycosis)

Mucor, Rhizopus

Lichtheimia Cunninghamella

Fungi

RX:
**Surgery
Amphotericin B
Posaconazole
Isavuconazole**

Risk Factors

- Diabetes
- DKA
- Immunocompromised
- Hematologic Malignancy
- Transplant Recipients
- Deferoxamine Therapy

Rhinocerebral
Mucormycosis

Pulmonary
Mucormycosis

PART 7

SEXUALLY TRANSMITTED DISEASES

Disease Name: **Gonorrhea**

Synonym: The Clap

Causative Agent: *Neisseria gonorrhoeae*

Incubation: 1–14 days; Average: 2–5 days

Geographic Regions Affected: Worldwide

Description: Gonorrhea is a common cause of urethritis in men and cervicitis in women. It is the second-most–common reportable sexually transmitted disease in the United States.

Signs and Symptoms: Men typically develop urethritis and present with a purulent urethral discharge and dysuria. Unilateral testicular pain and swelling are indicative of epididymitis and/or epididymo-orchiditis.

In women, the infection often affects the cervix and can progress into the upper genital tract causing salpingitis and pelvic inflammatory disease (PID). In cervicitis, symptomatic women may complain of discharge, intermenstrual bleeding, dyspareunia, urethritis, dysuria, and pelvic pain. On exam, cervical discharge and friability are likely to be present. In PID women will have more frank abdominal pain with systemic symptoms such as fever, chills, nausea, and vomiting. Physical exam in PID will reveal signs of cervicitis, cervical motion tenderness, adnexal tenderness, and peritonitis. Tubo-ovarian abscess can occur as a late complication of untreated PID. PID can also lead to infertility or increased risk of ectopic pregnancy and can cause perihepatic adhesions (Fitz-Hugh-Curtis syndrome).

Extragenital infection can occur in the rectum, pharynx, and conjunctiva. Lastly, disseminated gonococcal infection (DGI) can occur and classically presents as either (1) a triad of polyarthritis, tenosynovitis, and dermatitis, or (2) septic arthritis. In septic arthritis, the knee is most commonly affected. Disseminated gonococcal meningitis and endocarditis can also occur, but are rare.

Diagnostic Testing: Culture and nucleic acid amplification testing (NAAT) are available for the diagnosis of gonorrhea. Since NAAT is not FDA approved for the diagnosis of rectal, oropharyngeal, or conjunctival gonorrhea, culture is indicated. Gram stain (male urethral discharge only) will reveal polymorphonuclear leukocytes with intracellular gram-negative diplococci.

Treatments: The Centers for Disease Control and Prevention (CDC) recommends treatment of uncomplicated gonococcal infections with ceftriaxone 250 mg IM and 1 g of oral azithromycin. Azithromycin empirically covers for chlamydia and is thought to reduce the likelihood of emerging gonococcal resistance to cephalosporins. Epididymo-orchitis, prostatitis, and proctitis are treated with IM ceftriaxone and 10 days of oral doxycycline. Conjunctivitis should be treated with 1 g of ceftriaxone IM and 1 g of oral azithromycin. Disseminated gonorrhea requires more-frequent and higher doses of ceftriaxone. PID is treated with ceftriaxone and doxycycline +/− metronidazole. IV administration and hospital admission may be required.

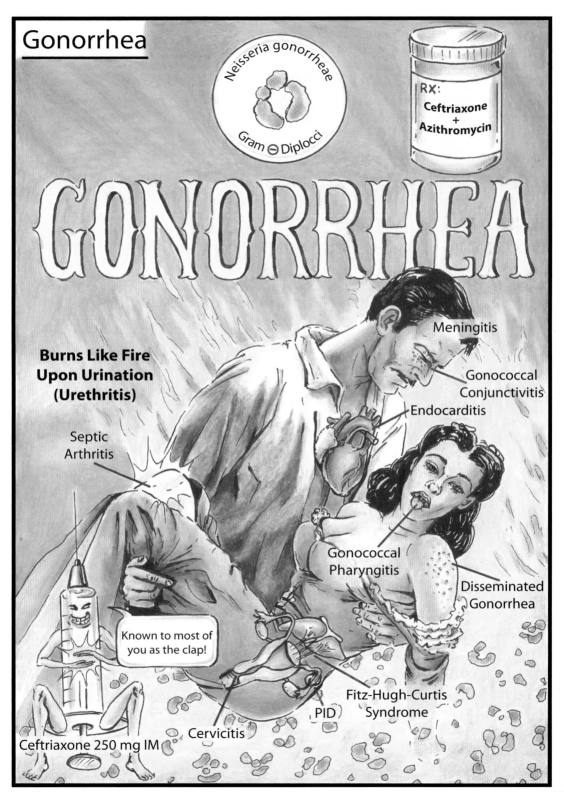

Disease Name: Condylomata Acuminata

Synonyms: Genital warts, anogenital warts

Causative Agent: Human papillomavirus (HPV)

Incubation: 2 weeks to 8 months

Geographic Regions Affected: Worldwide

Description: Human papillomavirus is a dsDNA virus and is considered the most common sexually transmitted infection worldwide. There are more than 200 types of HPV, each with an inherent risk of causing cancer. HPV 6 and HPV 11 are highly associated with anogenital warts, causing about 90% of cases. HPV 16 and HPV 18 are closely linked to cervical cancer, with HPV 16 also highly associated with oropharyngeal, anal, vulvovaginal, and penile cancers.

Signs and Symptoms: Many HPV infections are subclinical or asymptomatic. When anogenital warts occur, they can appear externally on the foreskin, glans penis, penile shaft, scrotum, perineum, anus, and vulva. Internal warts may appear within the pharynx, intravaginally, on the cervix, or within the rectum. Warts tend to be painless but can become inflamed or pruritic. Warts may be single or multiple, flat, raised, pedunculated, and/or cauliflower-like in appearance. Color can vary from hypopigmented, skin toned, erythematous, to hyperpigmented.

Diagnostic Testing: This is typically a visual diagnosis. Biopsy can be obtained to confirm the diagnosis and to rule out cancer. Women should be screened with Pap testing (cytology) to look for abnormal cells in accordance with the American College of Obstetricians and Gynecologists (ACOG) guidelines. Abnormal Pap testing is typically followed by colposcopy and tissue biopsy. In 2014 the FDA approved a DNA test that screens cells obtained from the cervix for high-risk HPV strains (hrHPV). Co-testing with Pap and hrHPV is recommended every 5 years for women age 30 and older.

Treatments: For external warts, provider-administered treatments include trichloroacetic acid (TCA), bichloroacetic acid (BCA), cryotherapy with liquid nitrogen, surgical removal, curettage, or electrocautery. Patient-administered treatments include podophyllotoxin 0.5% solution or gel or imiquimod 3.75% or 5% cream. Intraurethral, intravaginal, cervical, and intra-anal warts must be removed by providers. There are several HPV vaccines on the market, with the human papillomavirus 9-valent vaccine providing the broadest coverage.

Condylomata Acuminata

(Anogenital Warts)

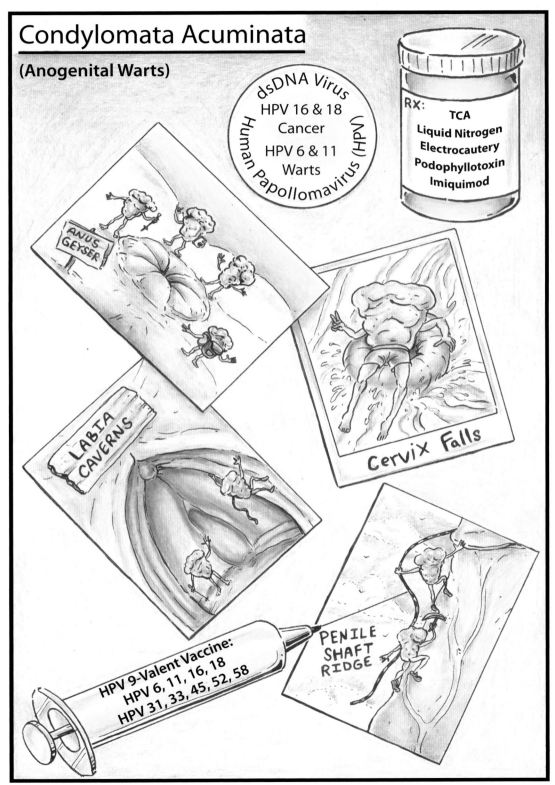

dsDNA Virus
HPV 16 & 18
Cancer
HPV 6 & 11
Warts
Human Papollomavirus (HPV)

RX:
TCA
Liquid Nitrogen
Electrocautery
Podophyllotoxin
Imiquimod

ANUS GEYSER

LABIA CAVERNS

Cervix Falls

PENILE SHAFT RIDGE

HPV 9-Valent Vaccine:
HPV 6, 11, 16, 18
HPV 31, 33, 45, 52, 58

Disease Name: **Pubic Lice**

Synonyms:	Crabs, phthiriasis pubis, pediculosis pubis, pediculosis ciliaris
Causative Agent:	*Phthris pubis*—pubic louse
Lifecycle	The adult pubic louse is infectious and passed from human to human by close contact. Adult females will lay and attach eggs (nits) to hair shafts. These eggs hatch and release nymphs that go through three molts before becoming adults. Adults need a blood meal to survive and can only live off of humans for 2 days.
Incubation:	About 12 hours to 7 days
Geographic Regions Affected:	Worldwide
Description:	Pubic lice (*Phthris pubis*) are topical ectoparasites that commonly attach to pubic hair and are sexually transmitted. They are 1–3 mm long, broad bodied, and resemble crabs when magnified (hence the name). In addition to pubic hair, they can also affect the eyelashes (pediculosis ciliaris), beards, mustache, and hair in the axilla or lower abdomen. Shared bedding, towels, or clothing may also be modes of transmission. However, despite what your friend tells you, pubic lice cannot be transmitted via a toilet seat.
Signs and Symptoms:	The saliva of the louse causes intense itching. Small spots of blood may be noticed in an infected individual's undergarments.
Diagnostic Testing:	Diagnosis is made via the visualization of nits (eggs) or pubic lice attached to hair shafts on a person's body. A magnifying glass is often helpful in making the diagnosis.
Treatments:	Permethrin 1% lotion can be applied to the affected area and washed off after 10 minutes. The affected area should be retreated 10 days after the first treatment. Alternative regimens recommended by the Centers for Disease Control and Prevention (CDC) include malathion 0.5% lotion applied and left on for 8–12 hours prior to being washed off or ivermectin 250 mcg/kg orally once and repeated 2 weeks later. For pediculosis ciliaris, apply petroleum jelly to affected eyelids 4 times a day for 10 days. Sexual partners within the previous 30 days should be offered treatment.

Pubic Lice

(Crabs)

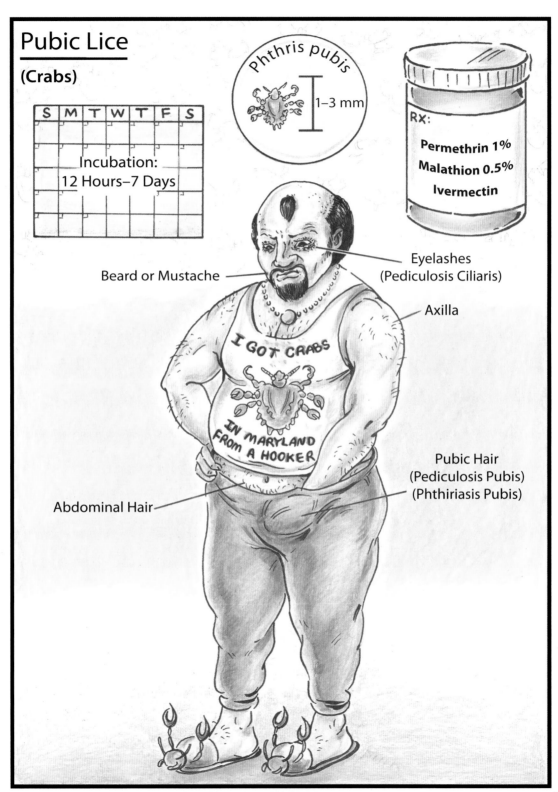

Incubation:
12 Hours–7 Days

Phthris pubis

1–3 mm

RX:

Permethrin 1%

Malathion 0.5%

Ivermectin

Beard or Mustache

Eyelashes
(Pediculosis Ciliaris)

Axilla

I GOT CRABS

IN MARYLAND
FROM A HOOKER

Pubic Hair
(Pediculosis Pubis)
(Phthiriasis Pubis)

Abdominal Hair

Disease Name:	**Syphilis**

Synonym: The Great Imitator

Causative Agents: *Treponema pallidum* subsp. *pallidum*

Incubation: 10–90 days, Average: 3 weeks

Geographic Regions Affected: Worldwide

Description: Syphilis is a sexually transmitted disease caused by the gram-negative spirochete *Treponema pallidum* subsp. *pallidum*. Infections can be chronic and progress through four stages: primary, secondary, latent, and tertiary. In the United States, men who have sex with men (MSM) are at greatest risk of acquiring the infection. Syphilis can also be acquired congenitally.

Signs and Symptoms: Primary infection is characterized by the presence of one or more firm, painless, nonpruritic chancre(s). Without treatment, secondary syphilis will occur 4–10 weeks later and often presents as a symmetric, nonpruritic, reddish-pink rash on the trunk, palms, and soles. Lesions known as condyloma latum may also appear on the mucous membranes. Without treatment, these symptoms resolve over 3–6 weeks, and the disease enters a latent (dormant) phase. Without treatment, about one third of patients will develop tertiary syphilis sometime over the next 3–15 years. Tertiary disease presents as either gummatous syphilis, neurosyphilis, or cardiovascular syphilis. Gummas are soft, noncancerous growths that often occur in the skin, liver, or bone. Some signs of neurosyphilis include poor balance, tabes dorsalis, and Argyll Robertson pupils. Syphilitic aortitis, resulting in an aortic aneurysm, is the most common form of cardiac syphilis. Congenital syphilis is discussed elsewhere, but some signs of disease include saddle nose, snuffles, saber shins, Clutton joints, and notched Hutchinson teeth.

Diagnostic Testing: Darkfield microscopy or direct fluorescent antibody testing can be performed on fluid or smears from lesions. Serological tests are either nontreponemal (screening) or treponemal specific (confirmatory). RPR, VDRL, and TRUST tests are used for screening purposes. Positive results should be followed up with confirmatory, treponemal-specific testing, such as *T. pallidum* enzyme immunoassay (TP-EIA) or fluorescent treponemal antibody absorption (FTA-ABS). Rapid finger-stick diagnostic tests are also available. Patients who have previously had and been treated for syphilis will continue to test positive for the disease using these various antibody tests.

Treatments: The treatment of choice is benzathine penicillin G 2.4 million units IM × 1 for primary, secondary, or latent infections less than 1 year's duration. Latent infections of more than 1 year's duration or of an indeterminate age and tertiary infections other than neurosyphilis should receive benzathine penicillin G 2.4 million units IM weekly × 3. Neurosyphilis is very difficult to treat and requires 18–24 million units continuous IV infusion for 10–14 days. Penicillin-allergic patients should be desensitized and treated with penicillin. Azithromycin as a 2-g single oral dose is an alternative option for early infection; however, resistance is possible. Doxycycline and ceftriaxone can be used as alternative treatments; however, benzathine penicillin G remains the preferred treatment.

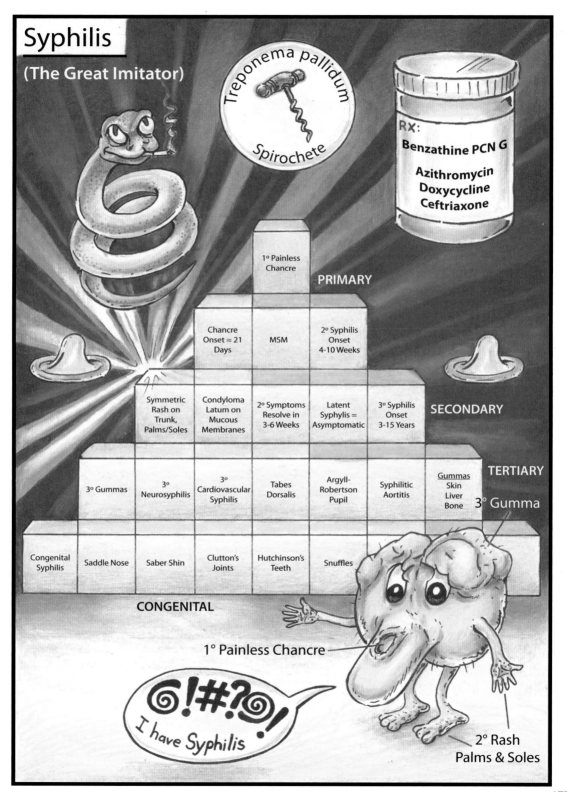

Disease Name: Chlamydia

Causative Agent: *Chlamydia trachomatis*

Incubation: Variable; Average: 1–3 weeks

Geographic Regions: Worldwide

Description: Chlamydia is a common cause of urethritis in men and cervicitis in women. It is the most common reportable sexually transmitted disease in the United States and is frequently asymptomatic in both men and women. Given its "silent" and asymptomatic nature, all sexually active women <25 years old and women ≥25 years old at higher risk of infection should be screened for chlamydia annually.

Signs and Symptoms: Symptomatic men typically develop urethritis and present with dysuria and a clear, scant urethral discharge. Epididymitis and/or epididymo-orchiditis can also occur, causing unilateral testicular pain and swelling. Chlamydia may cause prostatitis in some men.

In women, the infection often affects the cervix and can progress into the upper genital tract, causing salpingitis and pelvic inflammatory disease (PID). In cervicitis, symptomatic women may complain of discharge, intermenstrual bleeding, dyspareunia, and pelvic pain. Dysuria can occur with urethritis. On examination, cervical discharge and friability may be present. Pelvic inflammatory disease can be asymptomatic and insidious or acute. Acutely, women with PID will have frank pelvic or abdominal pain with systemic symptoms like fever, chills, nausea, and vomiting. Physical exam findings consistent with PID include signs of cervicitis, cervical motion tenderness, adnexal tenderness, and peritonitis. Tubo-ovarian abscess can occur as a late complication of untreated PID. PID can also lead to infertility or increased risk of ectopic pregnancy and can cause perihepatic adhesions (Fitz-Hugh-Curtis syndrome).

Chlamydia can cause proctitis as a result of recipient anal intercourse and conjunctivitis if the eyes are exposed to infectious secretions. Chlamydial infections can lead to reactive arthritis in some patients, mostly Caucasian males who are HLA-B27 positive.

Diagnostic Testing: Nucleic acid amplification testing (NAAT) is now considered the gold standard for diagnosing chlamydia, and a rapid version is available that can provide results in 90 minutes.

Treatments: For uncomplicated chlamydial urethritis or cervicitis, the Centers for Disease Control and Prevention (CDC) recommends treatment with a single 1-g oral dose of azithromycin or doxycycline 100 mg orally, twice a day for 7 days. Alternate antibiotic choices include erythromycin, levofloxacin, and ofloxacin. To cover for gonorrhea, 250 mg of IM ceftriaxone is often given empirically. Epididymo-orchitis, prostatitis, and proctitis should be treated with IM ceftriaxone and 10 days of oral doxycycline. PID is treated with ceftriaxone and doxycycline +/− metronidazole. IV administration and hospital admission may be required.

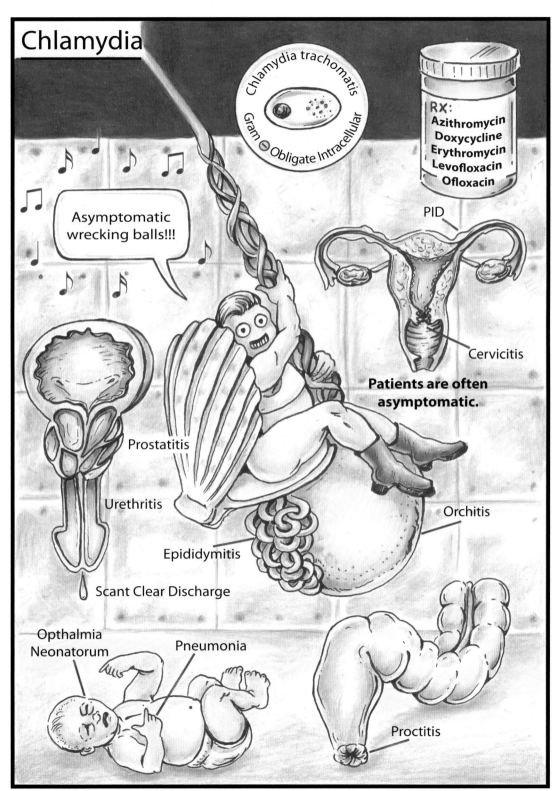

Disease Name: Trachoma

Causative Agent: *Chlamydia trachomatis* serotypes A, B, and C

Incubation: 5–10 days

Geographic Regions Affected: Poor and resource-limited areas of Africa, Asia, the Middle East, Australia, Pacific Islands, Central and South America. The highest incidence is in Africa.

Description: Trachoma is a chlamydial infection of the eye characterized by repeated infections, scarring of the conjunctiva, inversion of the eyelids, opacification of the cornea, and blindness. The disease is easily spread in close quarters via hand-to-eye contact or via transmission by eye-seeking flies. Trachoma is the number one cause of infectious blindness worldwide.

Signs and Symptoms: Trachoma and its manifestations are categorized as either acute (active and inflammatory) or chronic (cicatricial and characterized by scarring). Active trachoma is most common in young children and is often asymptomatic or manifests as conjunctivitis with ocular discharge. Inflammation leads to the formation of characteristic follicles on the upper tarsal conjunctiva (undersurface of the upper eyelid). Over time, the tarsal conjunctiva forms scar tissue, distortion of the eyelid, and trichiasis (inversion of the eyelashes). This is the cicatricial or chronic stage of the disease. In chronic trachoma the inverted eyelashes cause continued irritation of the eye, corneal opacification, and blindness.

Diagnostic Testing: The disease is often diagnosed clinically through screening programs in endemic areas of the world. The World Health Organization (WHO) has developed The Simplified WHO Trachoma Grading System to categorize the severity of disease based on ocular findings on clinical exam.

Treatments: The WHO recommends one of two antibiotic treatments for trachoma. Oral azithromycin given as a single 20 mg/kg dose in children or 1 g dose for adults is the preferred treatment. It is safe, easily tolerated, clears the nasopharynx of infectious organisms, and as a single dose has excellent compliance rates. The alternative is 1% topical tetracycline ophthalmic ointment applied twice daily for 6 weeks. The topical is less expensive but has a lower rate of compliance given the duration of therapy and the discomfort associated with application. Surgery is indicted when trichiasis is present.

Pearls: The WHO is working diligently to eliminate blindness caused by trachoma by 2020 and has developed the **SAFE** initiative. This is a combination of efforts that includes **S**urgery, **A**ntibiotics, **F**acial cleanliness, and **E**nvironmental improvement. For more information, please visit the International Trachoma Initiative website at www.trachoma.org.

Trachoma

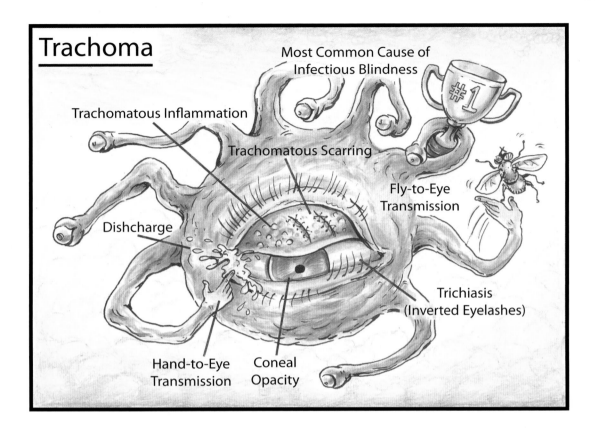

Most Common Cause of Infectious Blindness

Trachomatous Inflammation

Trachomatous Scarring

Fly-to-Eye Transmission

Dishcharge

Trichiasis (Inverted Eyelashes)

Hand-to-Eye Transmission

Coneal Opacity

Disease Name: **Reactive Arthritis**

Synonym:	Reiter syndrome
Causative Agents:	*Chlamydia trachomatis, Chlamydia pneumoniae, Campylobacter spp., Salmonella spp., Escherichia coli, Yersinia spp., Shigella spp., Clostridium difficile*
Incubation:	1–4 weeks after initial infection
Geographic Regions Affected:	Worldwide

Description: Reactive arthritis is a rheumatoid factor (RF) seronegative, HLA-B27–linked, inflammatory arthritic syndrome following a genitourinary or gastrointestinal illness. The condition is more common in Caucasian males between the ages of 20 and 50, most of whom are HLA-B27 positive.

Signs and Symptoms: The classic triad of nongonococcal urethritis, conjunctivitis, and asymmetric oligoarthritis gave rise to the mnemonic: "Can't see, can't pee, can't climb a tree." Mucocutaneous lesions (aphthous stomatitis), enthesitis (heel pain, plantar fasciitis, Achilles tendonitis), and cardiac manifestations may also occur. The condition may resolve spontaneously after several weeks to months or can become chronic.

Diagnostic Testing: The workup is similar to that of rheumatoid arthritis. Labs would include a complete blood cell count, complete metabolic panel, CRP, SED rate, HLA-B27 marker, rheumatoid factor, and anti-cyclic citrullinated peptide (anti-CCP) test. A urine test for chlamydia and stool sample for infectious enteropathies can also be obtained as part of the workup. Arthrocentesis performed on a joint with effusion would be gram stain and culture negative for bacteria.

Treatments: Antibiotics may be prescribed to treat any underlying residual infection. Nonsteroidal antiinflammatory drugs (NSAIDs) are the mainstay of therapy. Additional rheumatologic treatments may be indicated for severe disease including oral corticosteroids, sulfasalazine, methotrexate, and/or tumor necrosis factor (TNF) inhibitors.

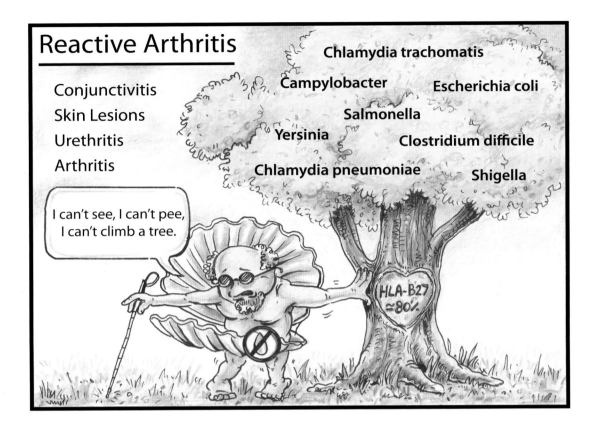

Disease Name: # Herpes Simplex

Causative Agents: Herpes simplex virus 1 & 2 (HSV-1 & HSV-2)

Incubation: 2–12 days; Average: 4 days

Geographic Regions Affected: Worldwide

Description: Herpes simplex is a life-long viral infection caused by either the HSV-1 or HSV-2 virus. Infections are classified as either primary or recurrent. Primary infections occur when a patient is initially infected with either HSV-1 or HSV-2 for the first time; recurrent infections or "outbreaks" occur when the HSV infection is reactivated. Recurrent infections can occur under stress, tend to be milder than initial infections, heal more quickly, and depending on frequency, may benefit from suppressive therapy. Since HSV viral shedding can occur without obvious lesions, people might not realize they are infectious.

Signs and Symptoms: Herpetic lesions appear the same in both primary and recurrent infections. They begin as papules, then progress to vesicles, ulcerations, and then crust over and heal without scaring. In addition to localized herpetic lesions, primary infections often include systemic symptoms such as fever, malaise, headache, and regional lymphadenopathy. Recurrent infections or "outbreaks" often have a prodromal burning or tingling sensation that precedes the appearance of a herpetic lesion. HSV-1 transmission via skin-to-skin or skin-to-mat contact in wresting is known as herpes gladiatorum. Herpes gingivostomatitis is a herpes simplex infection of the mouth and gums, herpes simplex of the finger is known as whitlow, and herpes simplex keratitis is an infection of the cornea.

Diagnostic Testing: Viral culture, PCR testing, direct fluorescent antibody (DFA) testing, and/or IgM/IgG serology can be obtained. A Tzanck smear, a microscopy slide prepared with scrapings from an unroofed blister, can be obtained to look for multinucleated giant cells. Tzanck smears are an outdated mode of testing but are included for historical purposes.

Treatments: Acyclovir, valacyclovir, or famciclovir can be taken orally to decrease the duration of symptoms, hasten healing, and decrease viral shedding. The dosages and duration of treatment required for episodic recurrences are less than those required for initial episodes. Medications can be prescribed for chronic daily suppression for those with frequent outbreaks. Acyclovir is available for oral, topical, and IV administration. Foscarnet can be used in cases of acyclovir resistance. IV acyclovir is used in cases of herpes meningitis.

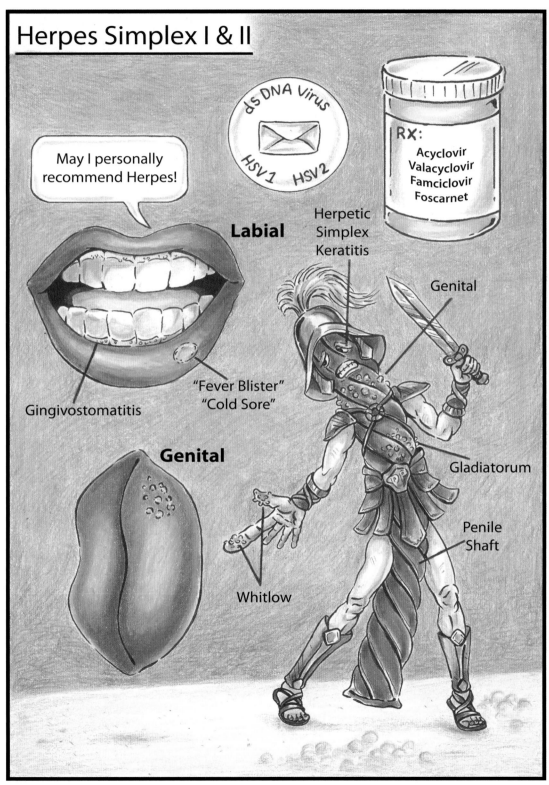

Herpes Simplex I & II

dS DNA Virus

HSV 1 HSV 2

May I personally recommend Herpes!

RX:
Acyclovir
Valacyclovir
Famciclovir
Foscarnet

Labial

Herpetic Simplex Keratitis

Genital

Gingivostomatitis

"Fever Blister"
"Cold Sore"

Gladiatorum

Genital

Penile Shaft

Whitlow

Disease Name: Trichomoniasis

Synonyms:	Trich, Trichomonas Vaginalis, TV
Causative Agent:	*Trichomonas vaginalis*
Incubation:	4–28 days
Geographic Regions Affected:	Worldwide
Description:	Trichomoniasis is a common sexually transmitted disease caused by the flagellated protozoan *T. vaginalis*.
Signs and Symptoms:	Trichomoniasis tends to cause more symptoms in women than in men: about 50% of infected women are symptomatic compared to 25% of infected men. In addition, infected women often develop symptoms over time, whereas men can often clear the infection spontaneously. Symptomatic women may complain of pelvic pain, dysuria, dyspareunia, vaginal burning, itching, and a scant, frothy green, malodourous discharge. On speculum exam, the cervix may have punctate hemorrhages referred to as "strawberry cervix." Men, when symptomatic, can present with dysuria and a urethral discharge.
Diagnostic Testing:	On saline wet mount, motile trichomonads may be seen swimming among a sea of increased white blood cells. Vaginal pH tends to be >4.5. Additional tests include nucleic acid amplification tests (NAATs), rapid antigen detection tests, and culture. Culture has essentially been replaced by the newer molecular detection tests.
Treatments:	As per recommendations from the Centers for Disease Control, metronidazole or tinidazole as a single 2 g oral dose is the recommended regimen. The alternative regimen calls for metronidazole 500 mg orally, twice daily, for 7 days. Current sex partners should be referred for treatment.

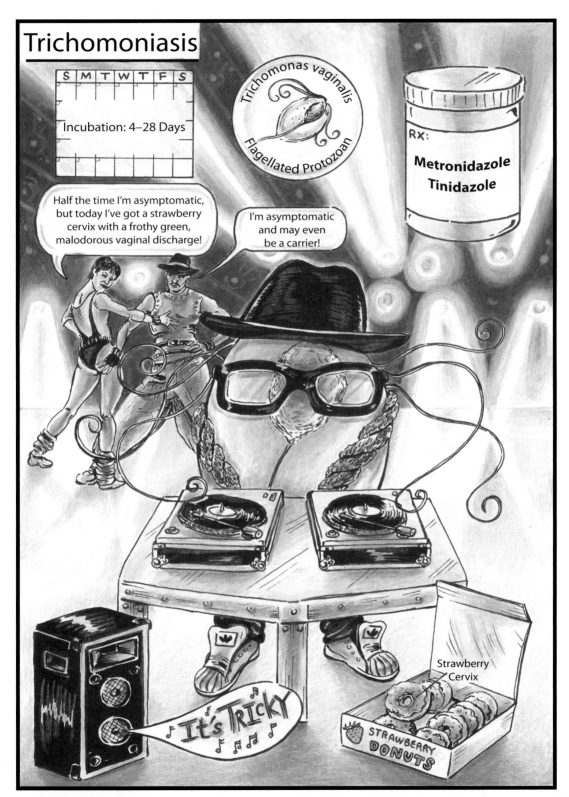

Disease Name: Scabies

Synonym:	7-year itch
Causative Agent:	*Sarcoptes scabiei* var. *hominis*—human itch mite
Incubation:	Initial infection: 2–6 weeks; repeat exposure: Rapid onset
Geographic Regions Affected:	Worldwide

Description: Scabies (*Sarcoptes scabiei*) is a topical ectoparasite spread by close personal contact. The disease is characterized by intense pruritus (itching) caused by sensitization to the mite's feces. Initial infections have a longer incubation and delayed onset of pruritus, whereas repeat infections (the patient is already sensitized) have a more rapid onset of symptoms. Severe infections with extremely high mite burdens are referred to as Norwegian or crusted scabies and are more common in the infirm, elderly, immunocompromised, and homeless.

Signs and Symptoms: The hallmark symptom is intense pruritus, often worse at night. Patients may also develop a small papular rash at infected areas and fine burrows may be visualized in the interdigital web spaces. Common sites of infection include the wrists, elbows, axilla, groin, waist, small of back, popliteal regions, and between the shoulder blades. The face and scalp are typically spared, except in severe cases with high mite burden. Infants and the elderly may have facial involvement.

Diagnostic Testing: Diagnosis is often made via history and characteristic skin findings. Skin scrapings can be obtained for definitive diagnosis.

Treatments: Topical application of permethrin 5% cream applied to all areas of the body, sparing the face, and left on for 8–14 hours followed by a shower and repeated in 1–2 weeks. Oral ivermectin 200 μg/kg as a single dose and repeated 2 weeks later is an alternative first-line regiment. Lindane 1% can be applied and left to sit on the body for 8 hours before washing off as well. Lindane should never be used in infants and children, as it can cause seizures and is considered a second- or third-line agent in adults given its neurotoxicity. Norwegian scabies requires treatment with daily topical permethrin and frequent doses of oral ivermectin. Antihistamines can decrease pruritus. Since the pruritus is caused by a reaction to the feces and not the mite itself, itching can continue for weeks after initial treatment.

Pearls: Scabies can spread rapidly in crowded conditions such as nursing homes, prisons, homeless shelters, and refugee camps. Crusted or Norwegian scabies is highly contagious. Scabies mites cannot survive off of the human body for more than 3 days.

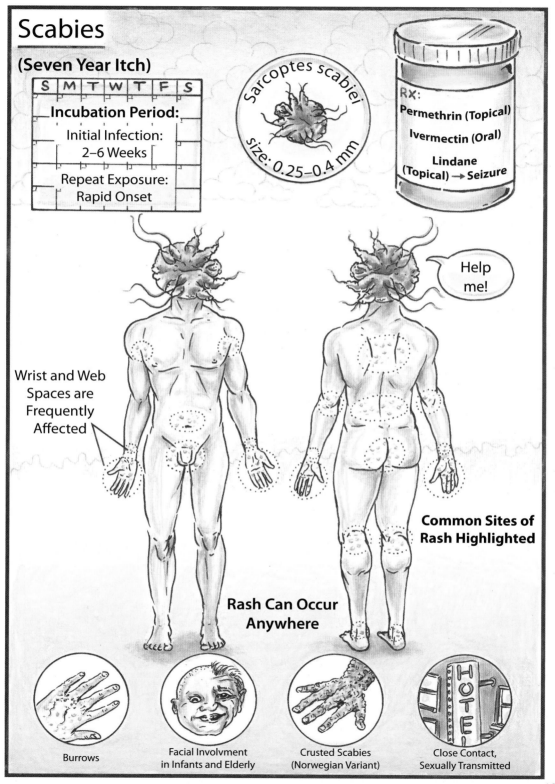

Scabies
(Seven Year Itch)

Incubation Period:

Initial Infection:
2–6 Weeks

Repeat Exposure:
Rapid Onset

Sarcoptes scabiei
size: 0.25–0.4 mm

RX:
Permethrin (Topical)

Ivermectin (Oral)

Lindane
(Topical) → Seizure

Help me!

Wrist and Web Spaces are Frequently Affected

Common Sites of Rash Highlighted

Rash Can Occur Anywhere

Burrows

Facial Involvment in Infants and Elderly

Crusted Scabies (Norwegian Variant)

Close Contact, Sexually Transmitted

Disease Name: **Chancroid**

Synonym:	Soft chancre
Causative Agent:	*Haemophilus ducreyi*
Incubation:	4–10 days
Geographic Regions Affected:	Some subtropical and tropical regions of the world including the Caribbean and Africa. The disease is sporadic and rare in the United States.
Description:	Chancroid is a sexually transmitted disease that causes painful, well-circumscribed, nonindurated (soft), genital ulcers with ragged edges and inguinal lymphadenopathy. In contrast, syphilis causes painless, indurated (hard), genital ulcers. Chancroid is more common in men, associated with prostitution, sex workers, and drug use and increases the likelihood of HIV transmission.
Signs and Symptoms:	Chancroid begins as a papule or nodule at the site of inoculation that evolves into a painful, well-circumscribed, nonindurated, genital ulcer with ragged edges. Autoinoculation can occur. About 50% of men will have a single ulcer, whereas for women, multiple ulcers is the norm (kissing ulcers). Tender inguinal lymphadenopathy is common and suppurative lymphadenopathy and significant tissue destruction can occur with untreated disease progression.
Diagnostic Testing:	On Gram stain, organisms often appear in long, parallel trails with a "school of fish" appearance. If culture is pursued, chocolate agar works best. Since *H. ducreyi* is extremely difficult to culture, most cases are diagnosed based on clinical findings and ruling out other, more common, causes of genital ulcers. In chancroid, one or more painful genital ulcers are suggestive of the disease, painful genital ulcers with tender lymphadenopathy are highly suggestive of the disease, and painful ulcers with suppurative lymphadenopathy is pathognomonic. A presumptive diagnosis of chancroid can be made in patients with any of the above presentations, a negative darkfield or serology for syphilis *(Treponema pallidum)*, and a negative herpes simplex (HSV) PCR or viral culture.
Treatments:	As per the Centers for Disease Control and Prevention (CDC) STD Treatment Guidelines, a variety of antibiotics are effective at treating this condition. The recommended regimen is azithromycin 1 g orally as a single dose, ceftriaxone 250 mg IM as a single dose, ciprofloxacin 500 mg twice daily for 3 days, or erythromycin 500 mg orally three times a day for 7 days. Azithromycin or ceftriaxone have the convenience of single-dose therapy.

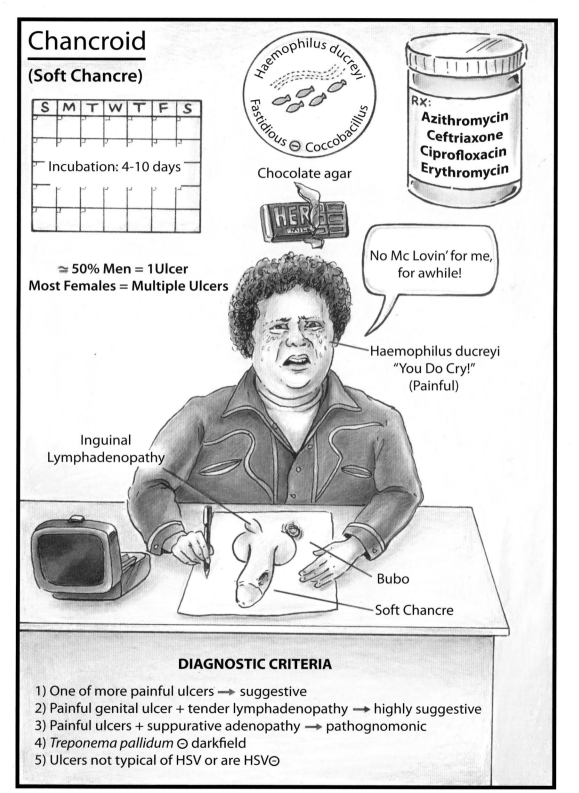

Chancroid
(Soft Chancre)

Incubation: 4-10 days

Haemophilus ducreyi
Fastidious ⊖ Coccobacillus

Chocolate agar

RX:
Azithromycin
Ceftriaxone
Ciprofloxacin
Erythromycin

≃ 50% Men = 1 Ulcer
Most Females = Multiple Ulcers

No Mc Lovin' for me, for awhile!

Haemophilus ducreyi
"You Do Cry!"
(Painful)

Inguinal Lymphadenopathy

Bubo

Soft Chancre

DIAGNOSTIC CRITERIA

1) One of more painful ulcers → suggestive
2) Painful genital ulcer + tender lymphadenopathy → highly suggestive
3) Painful ulcers + suppurative adenopathy → pathognomonic
4) *Treponema pallidum* ⊖ darkfield
5) Ulcers not typical of HSV or are HSV⊖

Disease Name: **Donovanosis**

Synonym:	Granuloma inguinale
Causative Agent:	*Klebsiella granulomatis*
Incubation:	1–12 weeks
Geographic Regions Affected:	Some tropical regions of the world including Papua New Guinea, the Caribbean, central Australia, India, Brazil, and southern Africa. The disease is rare in the United States.
Description:	Donovanosis is a sexually transmitted disease that causes painless, slowly progressive, chronic, beefy-red ulcerations on the genital and perineal areas without significant lymphadenopathy.
Signs and Symptoms:	Donovanosis begins as a small, painless papule or nodule that evolves into a beefy-red, friable ulcer. The ulcer is also painless, has a granulomatous base, expands slowly, and can spread via autoinoculation. Satellite lesions can occur and lymphadenopathy is notably absent or minimal. As the ulcer heals, scar tissue can develop, causing lymphedema and disfigurement of the genital.
Diagnostic Testing:	The organism is extremely difficult to culture and most cases are diagnosed based on clinical appearance. A smear or crush preparation can be obtained from the margin of an active ulcer and prepared for microscopy using Giemsa, Wright, or Leishman stain. Microscopy often reveals the pathognomonic Donovan bodies: large, intracytoplasmic, encapsulated bodies, found within macrophages swabbed from the site of ulceration.
Treatments:	As per the Centers for Disease Control and Prevention (CDC) STD Treatment Guidelines, a variety of antibiotics are effective at treating this condition. The recommended regimen is azithromycin 1 g orally per week or 500 mg orally per day for at least 3 weeks and until all lesions have completely healed. Doxycycline, ciprofloxacin, erythromycin, or TMP/SMX can all be used as alternative single-agent daily regimens for at least 3 weeks and continued until all lesions have completely healed. Long-term antibiotic treatment may be necessary for the ulcers to completely heal, and partial treatment can lead to disease reoccurrence.

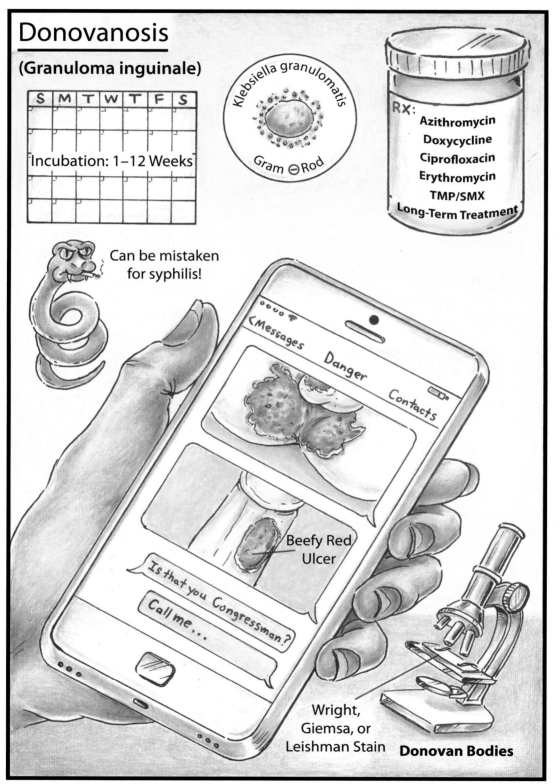

Donovanosis
(Granuloma inguinale)

Incubation: 1–12 Weeks

Klebsiella granulomatis

Gram ⊖ Rod

RX:
Azithromycin
Doxycycline
Ciprofloxacin
Erythromycin
TMP/SMX
Long-Term Treatment

Can be mistaken for syphilis!

‹Messages   Danger   Contacts

Beefy Red Ulcer

Is that you Congressman?

Call me...

Wright, Giemsa, or Leishman Stain   **Donovan Bodies**

Disease Name: **Vaginitis**

Vaginitis: Vaginitis is a generic term for inflammation of the vagina caused by infection, atrophy, and/or changes in the normal flora. Signs and symptoms of vaginitis can include pain, pruritus, dyspareunia, dysuria, and discharge. The chart and below text summarize the three most common infectious agents that cause vaginitis.

Candida Vulvovaginitis: Candidiasis is an overgrowth of *Candida albicans* or *C. glabrata* yeast within the lower genital tract. It is often associated with antibiotic use. Women often complain of intense pruritus and a thick, white, curd-like, vaginal discharge. Vaginal pH is <4.5 and KOH test is positive for pseudohyphae and candida buds. Wet mount is negative for trichomonads and Gram stain will reveal increased white blood cells. Treatment includes topical azole antifungals or oral fluconazole.

Trichomoniasis: A common sexually transmitted disease caused by the flagellated protozoan *Trichomonas vaginalis*. Discharge is typically thin, frothy, greenish in color, and malodorous. Vaginal pH is >4.5, KOH test is negative for pseudohyphae or candida buds, wet mount may reveal trichomonads, and Gram stain will reveal increased white cells. Preferred treatment is metronidazole or tinidazole as a single 2 g oral dose. The alternative regimen calls for metronidazole 500 mg orally, twice daily for 7 days.

Bacterial Vaginosis: BV occurs when there is a shift in the normal vaginal flora from Lactobacillus to other, mostly anaerobic, species including *Gardnerella vaginalis*, Ureaplasma, Mobiluncus, Mycoplasma, and Prevotella. BV has a higher prevalence in minority populations and females with multiple sex partners. Infected women often complain of a fishy vaginal odor, usually more noticeable after sexual intercourse. Discharge is typically thin, copious, grayish-white to yellow, and has a fishy odor. Vaginal pH is increased >4.5, KOH test is negative for pseudohyphae or candida buds, but does have a "fishy" or amine smell (+whiff test). Wet mount is negative for trichomonads and Gram stain will reveals clue cells (vaginal epithelial cells covered with coccobacilli bacteria). Preferred treatment is metronidazole 500 mg by mouth twice daily for 7 days, intravaginal metronidazole gel 0.75% daily for 5 days, or intravaginal clindamycin cream 2% daily for 7 days.

Vaginitis

Name	Vulvovaginitis	Trichomoniasis	Bacterial Vaginosis
Disharge	Curdy, White	Frothy, Green	Thin, Fishy, Yellow
Symptoms	Burning Itching	Burning Itching	Fishy Odor No Itching
pH	<4.5	>4.5	>4.5
KOH	Pseudohyphae	⊖	⊕ Whiff Test
Wet Mount Gram Stain	⊕ WBC	Trichomonads ⊕ WBC	Clue Cells ⊖ WBC
Rx	Topical Azole Fluconazole	Metronidazole Tinidazole	Metronidazole Clindamycin

Disease Name: Molluscum Contagiosum

Synonyms: MC, water warts

Causative Agents: Molluscum contagiosum virus (MCV), genotypes 1–4, with genotype 1 responsible for the vast majority of infections.

Incubation: 2–7 weeks

Geographic Regions Affected: Worldwide

Description: Molluscum contagiosum is a viral infection of the skin that gives rise to small, raised, waxy, flesh-colored lesions with a central dimple. The virus is spread via skin-to-skin contact and lesions can arise anywhere on the skin except palms and soles. Lesions are often found on the face, trunk, axilla, and popliteal regions. When occurring on the genitals, the lesions may be the result of sexual transmission. The disease is common in children, the immunocompromised, and those who participate in contact sports.

Signs and Symptoms: Molluscum contagiosum is diagnosed by the presence of characteristic appearing dome-shaped, umbilicated, waxy appearing papules measuring 2–5 mm in size. The lesions may be pruritic and become inflamed over time. Lesions often resolve spontaneously without treatment over several months and tend not to scar.

Diagnostic Testing: Molluscum contagiosum is often a visual diagnosis.

Treatments: Conservative treatment and reassurance can be provided. If patients wish to pursue more aggressive treatments, options include cryotherapy, curettage, cantharidin, and podophyllotoxin.

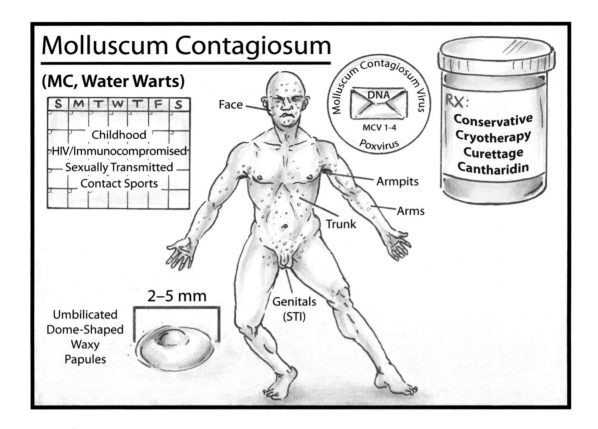

Molluscum Contagiosum

(MC, Water Warts)

S	M	T	W	T	F	S
	Childhood					
HIV/Immunocompromised						
Sexually Transmitted						
Contact Sports						

Molluscum Contagiosum Virus

DNA

MCV 1-4

Poxvirus

RX:
**Conservative
Cryotherapy
Curettage
Cantharidin**

Face

Armpits

Arms

Trunk

Genitals
(STI)

2–5 mm

Umbilicated
Dome-Shaped
Waxy
Papules

Disease Name: **Lymphogranuloma Venereum**

Causative Agent: *Chlamydia trachomatis* serotypes L1, L2, L3

Incubation: Primary LGV: 3–30 days; Secondary LGV: 2–6 weeks.

Geographic Regions Affected: Subtropical and tropical regions of the world. There is an increasing incidence among men who have sex with men (MSM) in the United States, the European Union, and Australia.

Description: Lymphogranuloma venereum (LGV) is classically a subtropical and tropical sexually transmitted disease caused by *C. trachomatis* serotypes L1, L2, L3. LGV is a disease of the lymph tissue and can progress through primary, secondary, and tertiary stages if left untreated.

Signs and Symptoms: *Primary LGV* presents as a painless papule or shallow ulcer at the site of inoculation 3–30 days after initial exposure. The ulcer can be present on the penis, vaginal wall, or rectal mucosa and often heals over a 10-day period. Treatment is often delayed, given the painless nature of the lesion and/or lack of awareness of its presence. *Secondary LGV* can present either classically as swollen unilateral inguinal lymphadenopathy (buboes) or as proctocolitis with pain, tenesmus, and rectal bleeding. The latter presentation is more common in MSM and is the result of having contracted the disease via receptive anal intercourse. *Tertiary or late-stage LGV* is the result of chronic, untreated disease and presents as perirectal abscesses, fistulas, anal strictures, and/or lymphedema of the genitals.

Diagnostic Testing: Clinical presentation and sexual and travel history should heighten suspicion for the disease. Urine, rectal swabs, and/or lymph node aspirates can be tested for *C. trachomatis* by culture, direct immunofluorescence, or nucleic acid detection (NAAT).

Treatments: The Centers for Disease Control and Prevention (CDC) STD Treatment Guidelines recommend doxycycline twice daily for 21 days as the preferred regimen or erythromycin four times daily for 21 days as the alternative. Azithromycin 1 g orally once a week for 3 weeks may also have some efficacy.

Lymphogranuloma Venereum

(LGV)

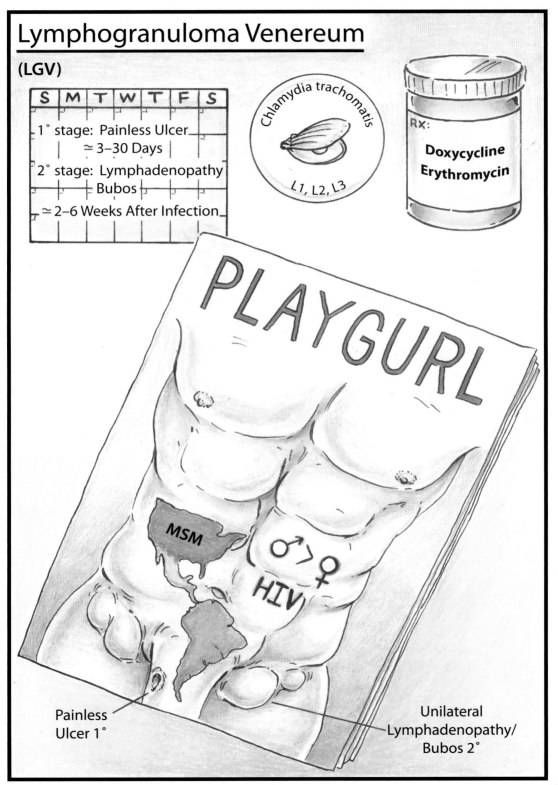

S	M	T	W	T	F	S

1° stage: Painless Ulcer
≃ 3–30 Days

2° stage: Lymphadenopathy Bubos
≃ 2–6 Weeks After Infection

Chlamydia trachomatis

L1, L2, L3

RX:
Doxycycline
Erythromycin

PLAYGURL

MSM

♂ > ♀

HIV

Painless Ulcer 1°

Unilateral Lymphadenopathy/ Bubos 2°

PART 8

PULMONARY

Disease Name: Middle Eastern Respiratory Syndrome

Synonym:	MERS
Causative Agent:	MERS Coronavirus, MERS-CoV
Reservoir:	Possibly the Egyptian Tomb Bat
Incubation:	2–14 days; Average: 5–6 days
Geographic Regions Affected:	All cases of MERS have been linked to exposure to the Arabian Peninsula.
Description:	MERS is a severe respiratory tract infection caused by a novel coronavirus. The first reported case occurred in Saudi Arabia in 2012 and the largest outbreak outside the Middle East occurred in South Korea in 2015. The disease is thought to be transmitted from camels to humans, but it can also be transmitted from person to person.
Signs and Symptoms:	Infections from MERS-CoV are not fully understood and may cause a wide spectrum of illness, with less-severe cases avoiding clinical detection. Those patients with severe illness often present with fever, chills, malaise, myalgia, headache, shortness of breath (SOB), and nonproductive cough. Nausea, vomiting, abdominal pain, and diarrhea may also occur. Some patients may present atypically with gastroenteritis preceding severe pneumonia. MERS can cause severe pneumonia, adult respiratory distress syndrome (ARDS), renal failure, and death. The Centers for Disease Control and Prevention (CDC) reports a high mortality rate, somewhere between 30% and 40%.
Diagnostic Testing:	The CDC recommends obtaining several specimens of bodily fluid for testing with polymerase chain reaction (PCR) in patients under investigation (PUI) for MERS. Specimens should be obtained via nasopharyngeal swab, sputum sample or broncheoalveolar lavage (BAL), and serum. Those with symptoms for more than 14 days prior to presentation and/or testing can also have blood sent for serology. More information on diagnostic testing is available on the CDC website.
Treatment:	Supportive. Intubation and mechanical ventilation may be indicated in severe disease.
Pearls:	To reduce the likelihood of contracting MERS, the World Health Organization encourages people with comorbidities and/or compromised immune systems to avoid contact with camels while visiting the Arabian Peninsula. Good handwashing and hygiene are encouraged for all people with contact with camels and, in general, people are discouraged from drinking camel milk or urine.

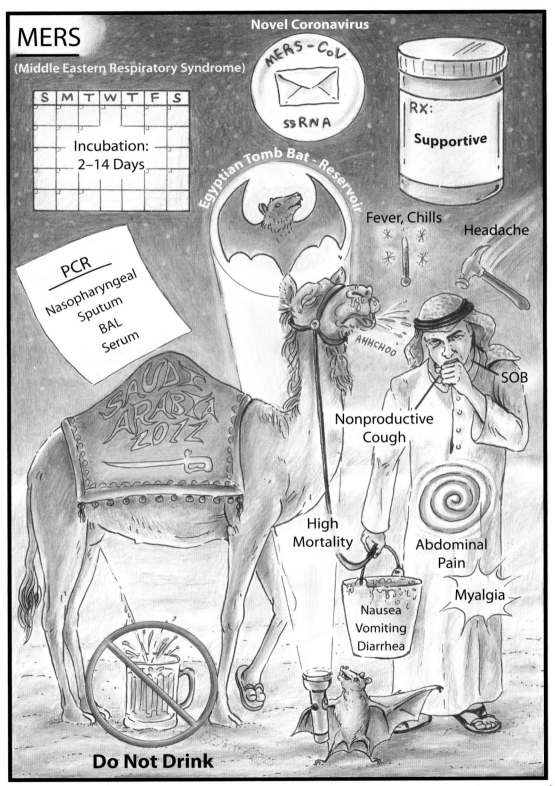

Disease Name: Tuberculosis

Synonyms:	Consumption, TB
Causative Agent:	*Mycobacterium tuberculosis*
Reservoir:	Humans
Incubation:	2–12 weeks from exposure to positive purified protein derivative (PPD) test
Geographic Regions Affected:	Worldwide, more common in developing nations

Description:

Tuberculosis (TB) is primarily a bacterial disease of the lung caused by the aerobic, nonmotile, acid-fast, bacillus *M. tuberculosis*. TB is spread via airborne droplets and is notoriously difficult to treat, given the bacteria's slow reproductive rate. Initial or primary TB infections either are suppressed by the immune system or cause active disease. A primary infection that results in active disease is referred to as primary progressive TB. Suppression of TB occurs in 90% of primary infections and results in latent TB. Latent TB can remain dormant for many years and, if not treated, will become active (reactivation TB or progressive secondary TB) in about 10% of those infected. Latent TB is not contagious, whereas active TB is. Risk factors for TB include homelessness, incarceration, and HIV.

Signs and Symptoms:

Active pulmonary TB causes fever, malaise, fatigue, night sweats, weight loss, cough, dyspnea, pleuritic chest pain, and hemoptysis. Symptom onset is often more gradual in cases of reactivation TB. Disease that spreads outside the lungs is referred to extrapulmonary TB and is more common in children and the immunocompromised. Common sites of extrapulmonary TB include the pleura, meninges, lymphatic system, genitourinary (GU) system, and the bones.

Diagnostic Testing:

PPD screening tests determine if the patient had ever had a previous exposure to TB. Chest x-rays may show signs of active disease and may reveal miliary lesions, consolidation, cavitary lesions, pleural effusions, nodular infiltrates, granulomas, and mediastinal lymphadenopathy. TB has a preference for the lung apices, predominantly on the right side. When testing for active disease, sputum samples should be obtained for acid-fast bacilli (AFB) staining using the Ziehl-Neelsen (ZN) stain, plated for culture and sensitivity, and tested using polymerase chain reaction (PCR). Culture is the gold standard for diagnosis, but it takes up to 4–8 weeks for results. Rapid diagnostic tests are available for use in developing nations.

Treatments:

Latent TB is often treated with daily isoniazid with or without supplemental pyridoxine for 9 months. Alternative regimens exist, including daily rifampin for 4 months. Treatment of active and/or extrapulmonary TB requires multiple drugs including, but not limited to, isoniazid, rifampin, ethambutol, streptomycin, and pyrazinamide. Each drug has specific and common side effects, included on our illustration.

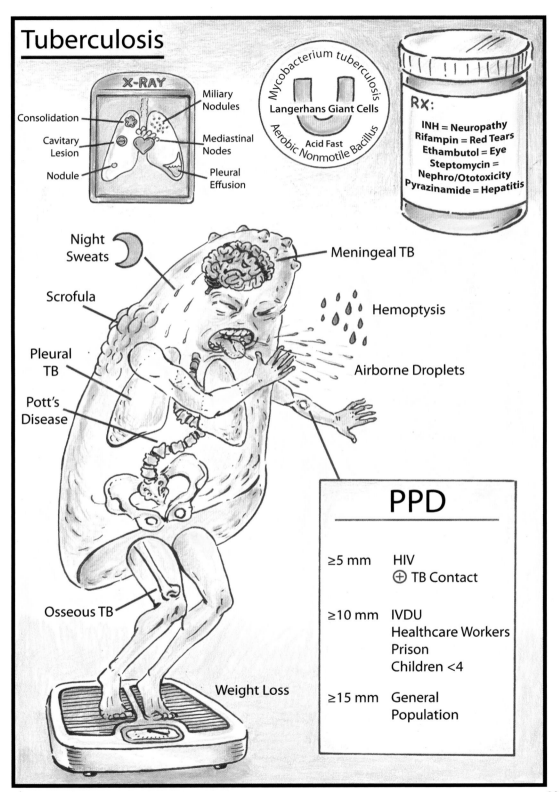

Tuberculosis

X-RAY

Consolidation
Cavitary Lesion
Nodule

Miliary Nodules
Mediastinal Nodes
Pleural Effusion

Mycobacterium tuberculosis
Langerhans Giant Cells
Acid Fast
Aerobic Nonmotile Bacillus

RX:

INH = Neuropathy
Rifampin = Red Tears
Ethambutol = Eye
Steptomycin =
Nephro/Ototoxicity
Pyrazinamide = Hepatitis

Night Sweats

Scrofula

Pleural TB

Pott's Disease

Osseous TB

Meningeal TB

Hemoptysis

Airborne Droplets

Weight Loss

PPD

≥5 mm HIV
⊕ TB Contact

≥10 mm IVDU
Healthcare Workers
Prison
Children <4

≥15 mm General
Population

Disease Name: **Legionnaires' Disease**

Synonym:	Legionellosis
Causative Agent:	*Legionella pneumophila* is most common, other *Legionella* spp.
Reservoir:	*Legionella* can reside and replicate in amoebas found in aquatic environments.
Incubation:	2–10 days; Average 4–6 days
Geographic Regions Affected:	Worldwide
Description:	Legionnaires' disease is an acute consolidating pneumonia occurring after the inhalation and/or microaspiration of *Legionella*-contaminated aerosolized water, often from air conditioner cooling towers. It can occur sporadically or in epidemic outbreaks. The elderly, males, cigarette smokers (COPD), and immunocompromised are most at risk. The disease was first recognized when it caused an epidemic at the 1976 Legionnaires' Convention at the Bellevue-Stratford Hotel in Philadelphia, Pennsylvania.
Signs and Symptoms:	Fever, severe headache, malaise, and myalgia are often the first presenting symptoms. Nausea, vomiting, and diarrhea can also occur. Cough is often productive, with occasional blood-tinged sputum and/or hemoptysis. There may be a relative bradycardia and chest x-ray will reveal consolidated pneumonia. Confusion and seizures may also occur.
Diagnostic Testing:	Labs will reveal hyponatremia, hypophosphatemia, elevated liver enzymes, leukopenia/leukocytosis, thrombocytopenia, increased lactic dehydrogenase (LDH), disseminated intravascular coagulation (DIC), and possible acute kidney injury. Confirmatory diagnosis is established by urinary antigen, cultures of endotracheal aspirates or sputum, immunofluorescence microscopy, detection of serum antibodies, and/or molecular amplification by polymerase chain reaction (PCR).
Treatments:	Azithromycin is the preferred antibiotic. Levofloxacin or moxifloxacin can be used as an alternative.
Pearls:	Hyponatremia and relative bradycardia are hallmarks of Legionnaires' disease, but not confirmatory. Pontiac fever is a brief, febrile, upper respiratory illness caused by the inhalation of *Legionella* spp. aerosolized from contaminated water or potting soil. It has a short incubation period of several hours to 3 days and is more common in people in their 30s. Pontiac fever is self-limiting, and treatment is supportive.

Legionnaires' Disease

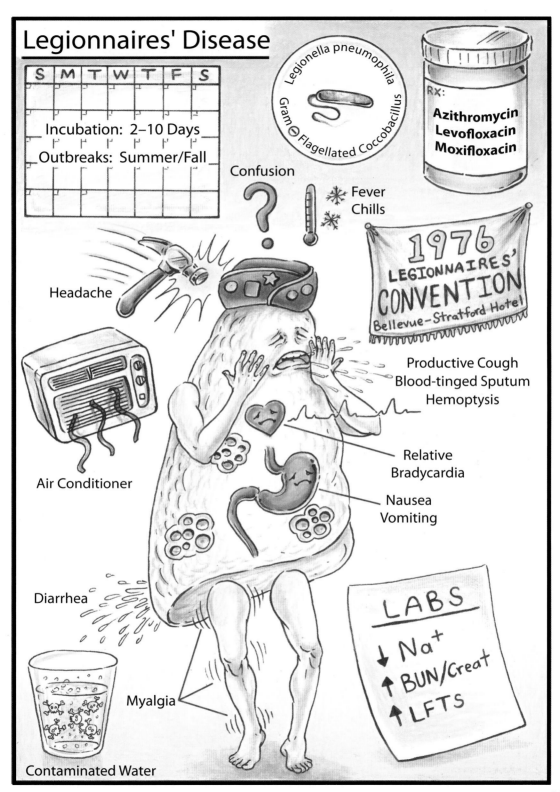

S M T W T F S

Incubation: 2–10 Days

Outbreaks: Summer/Fall

Legionella pneumophila

Gram ⊖ Flagellated Coccobacillus

RX:
Azithromycin
Levofloxacin
Moxifloxacin

Confusion

Fever
Chills

Headache

1976
LEGIONNAIRES'
CONVENTION
Bellevue-Stratford Hotel

Air Conditioner

Productive Cough
Blood-tinged Sputum
Hemoptysis

Relative
Bradycardia

Nausea
Vomiting

Diarrhea

LABS
↓ Na⁺
↑ BUN/Creat
↑ LFTS

Myalgia

Contaminated Water

Disease Name: Psittacosis

Synonyms:	Parrot fever, Ornithosis
Causative Agent:	*Chlamydia psittaci*
Reservoir:	Birds
Incubation:	5–19 days
Geographic Regions Affected:	Worldwide

Description: Psittacosis is a rare acute bacterial zoonosis contracted by exposure to *C. psittaci* bacteria from the aerosolized feces of certain birds, specifically parrots. Pigeons, geese, ducks, and chickens can also carry the bacteria. The disease often presents as an atypical pneumonia with severe headache and is more common in young and middle-aged adults. Those with increased exposure to birds (veterinarians, pet shop owners, zoo keepers, poultry workers, farmers, etc.) are at greatest risk of infection.

Signs and Symptoms: The disease can vary in presentation from asymptomatic or mild to severe respiratory illness and pneumonia. Patients most commonly present with symptoms of atypical pneumonia including acute fever, severe headache with photophobia, and nonproductive cough. Cough characteristically presents later in the course of illness. Given the variations in disease presentation, symptoms are occasionally nonspecific and, in addition to the above, can also include chills, malaise, myalgia, arthralgia, epistaxis, abdominal pain, nausea, vomiting, and diarrhea. Hepatosplenomegaly, hepatitis, and disseminated intravascular coagulation (DIC) may also occur.

Diagnostic Testing: Diagnosis should be considered in those patients with classic symptoms and a history of exposure to birds. Chest x-ray can reveal any number of abnormalities, with lower lobe consolidation the most common finding. Labs will reveal normal to mildly increased WBC with a shift to the left. Liver enzymes are often elevated. Diagnosis is often based on history of bird exposure and a rise of serum antibody titers. When psittacosis is suspected, cultures are discouraged, as the bacteria is highly infectious and can put lab workers at risk.

Treatments: Doxycycline or tetracycline are effective treatments and once initiated, patients tend to improve within 24 hours. Azithromycin or erythromycin are considered second-line agents and can be considered when tetracycline antibiotics are not tolerable.

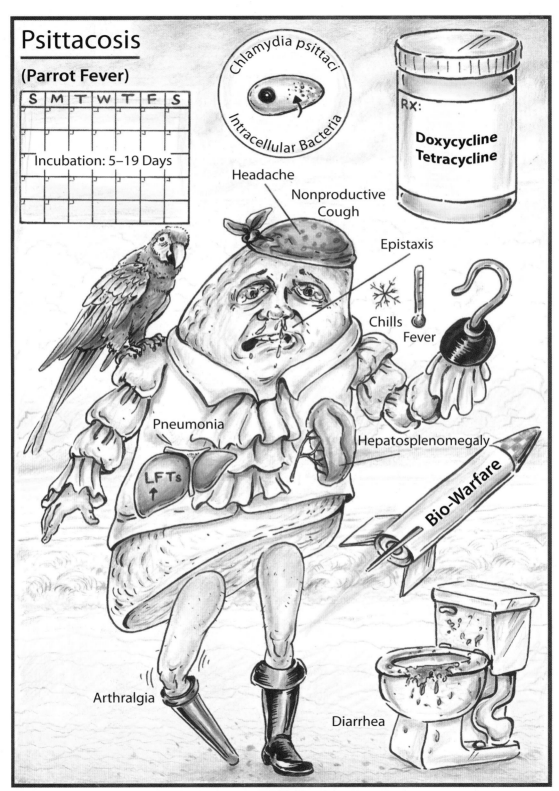

Psittacosis

(Parrot Fever)

Incubation: 5–19 Days

Chlamydia psittaci
Intracellular Bacteria

RX:
Doxycycline
Tetracycline

Headache

Nonproductive Cough

Epistaxis

Chills Fever

Pneumonia

LFTs ↑

Hepatosplenomegaly

Bio-Warfare

Arthralgia

Diarrhea

Disease Name: Avian Influenza

Synonyms: Bird flu, Avian flu, Asian Avian Influenza A

Causative Agents: Avian Influenza A Viruses: Asian H5N1 and Asian H7N9

Reservoir: Wild aquatic birds and waterfowl such as gulls, tern, ducks, geese, and swans are the natural reservoirs. The virus can infect domesticated birds and poultry causing disease, which can then potentially spill over to the human population.

Incubation: A(H5N1): 2–17 days; Average: 2–5 days
A(H7N9): 1–10 days; Average: 5 days

Geographic Regions Affected: Asia, China, Middle East

Description: Avian influenza is a viral infection in birds caused by certain strains of the Influenza A virus. While these specific strains are typically limited to bird-to-bird transmission, bird-to-human transmission can occur and result in disease. Human-to-human transmission has been reported but is extremely rare and, fortunately, not sustained. If sustained human-to-human transmission were to occur, it could cause a global pandemic.

Avian Influenza A viruses are classified as low pathogenic avian influenza (LPAI) or high pathogenic avian influenza (HPAI). Birds infected with LPAI viruses can be asymptomatic or have mild symptoms including changes to egg production. In contrast, those birds infected with HPAI strains often have a more severe illness, which can include respiratory symptoms and death. If introduced into a domestic flock, avian influenza can spread rapidly and requires the eradication of infected flocks and the quarantine of those flocks in close proximity to the outbreak.

Signs and Symptoms: In humans, Avian Influenza A (H5N1) and A (H7N9) are known to cause severe disease. Infected patients will develop fever, chills, malaise, myalgia, headache, and cough. Nausea, vomiting, abdominal pain, and diarrhea may occur in some patients. These viruses have a high likelihood of causing severe pneumonia, shock, adult respiratory distress syndrome (ARDS), multisystem organ failure, and death. Mortality is as high as 60%.

Diagnostic Testing: Nasopharyngeal swabs can be tested for novel influenza viruses using polymerase chain reaction (PCR). More information is available on the Centers for Disease Control and Prevention (CDC) website.

Treatments: The CDC recommends the use or oral oseltamivir in all human cases of suspected infection with novel influenza viruses, including avian influenza, even if more than 48 hours has passed since symptom onset. A 10-day duration of treatment may be advisable in immunocompromised patients and those with severe illness. Outpatient prophylaxis for 5 days with oral oseltamivir is recommended for those who have had contact with infected patients.

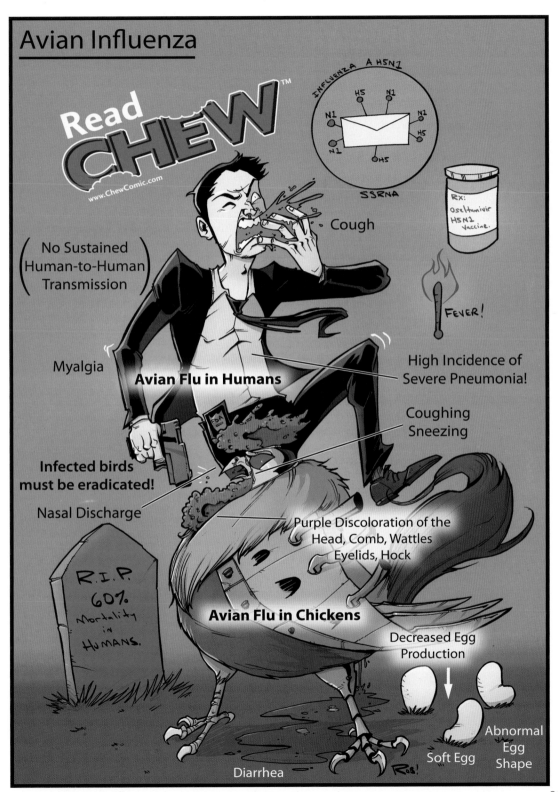

Avian Influenza

Read **CHEW**™
www.ChewComic.com

INFLUENZA A H5N1

SSRNA

RX:
Oseltamivir
H5N1
Vaccine.

Cough

FEVER!

No Sustained
Human-to-Human
Transmission

Avian Flu in Humans

Myalgia

High Incidence of
Severe Pneumonia!

Coughing
Sneezing

**Infected birds
must be eradicated!**

Nasal Discharge

Purple Discoloration of the
Head, Comb, Wattles
Eyelids, Hock

R.I.P.
60%
Mortality
in
Humans.

Avian Flu in Chickens

Decreased Egg
Production

Soft Egg

Abnormal
Egg
Shape

Diarrhea

Disease Name: **Influenza**

Synonyms:	The Flu
Causative Agent:	Influenza A & B viruses
Reservoir:	Humans
Incubation:	1–4 days; Average: 2 days
Geographic Regions Affected:	Worldwide

Description:

Influenza is an acute febrile viral respiratory tract infection most common in temperate climates during the winter. The disease is spread via respiratory droplets, causes periodic epidemics, and has the potential to cause global pandemics. Pandemics occur when a new strain of influenza emerges for which humans have had little to no previous exposure. There are three types of influenza virus (A–C) based on the core protein, with only types A and B causing significant disease in humans. Type A viruses are further classified based on two specific antigens, hemagglutinin (HA or H) and neuraminidase (NA or N), found on the surface of the virus. These antigens are responsible for the HN classifications often seen on annual vaccines. Since influenza viruses are constantly undergoing genetic changes via antigenic drift (frequent and minor) and antigenic shift (infrequent and significant), new and updated vaccinations are required each year.

Signs and Symptoms:

Infected patients will develop acute fever, chills, rigors, malaise, myalgia, headache, rhinorrhea, and nonproductive cough. Nausea, vomiting, and diarrhea may occur in some patients, more so in children. The immunocompromised, extremes of age, pregnant women, residents of long-term care facilities, and those with preexisting medical conditions are more likely to have severe disease and complications. Pneumonia, either from the influenza virus directly or secondarily from bacteria, is one potential complication.

Diagnostic Testing:

Rapid influenza diagnostic tests (RIDT) are immunoassays that detect Influenza A and B viral antigens. Nasopharyngeal swabs can be tested for influenza viruses using polymerase chain reaction (PCR).

Treatments:

There are two classes of drugs used to treat influenza. The adamantanes include amantadine and rimantadine, which target and inhibit function of the M2 protein and are only effective against Influenza A. Given the increased resistance to these drugs over the years and efficacy against both Influenza A and B, neuraminidase inhibitors are preferred for the treatment and prophylaxis of influenza. Neuraminidase inhibitors include oseltamivir, zanamivir, and peramivir. Oseltamivir is taken orally and zanamivir is an inhaled powder. A newer drug, peramivir, is indicated for treatment only (no indication for prophylaxis) and is given as a single intravenous (IV) dose. These medications are thought to decrease the duration and severity of illness and are only effective when initiated within 48 hours of symptom onset.

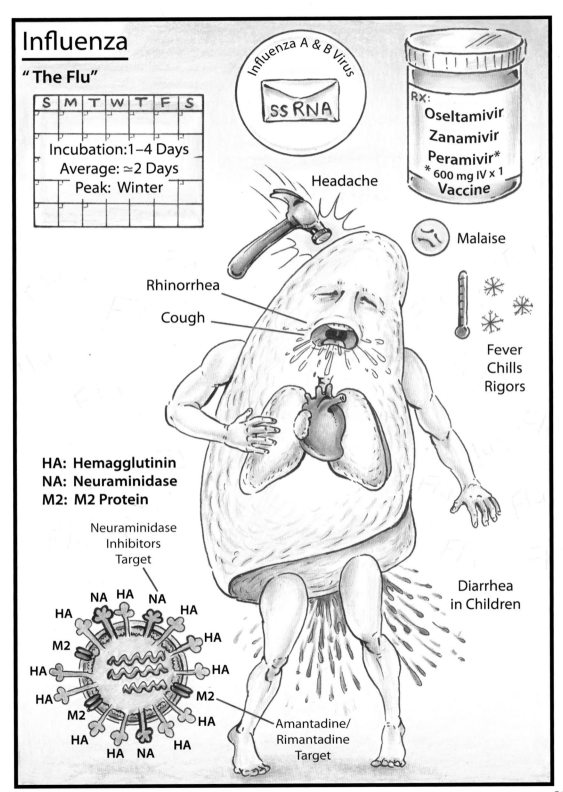

Influenza

" The Flu"

S	M	T	W	T	F	S

Incubation: 1–4 Days
Average: ≃2 Days
Peak: Winter

Influenza A & B Virus

SS RNA

RX:
Oseltamivir
Zanamivir
Peramivir*
* 600 mg IV x 1
Vaccine

Headache

Malaise

Fever
Chills
Rigors

Rhinorrhea

Cough

HA: Hemagglutinin
NA: Neuraminidase
M2: M2 Protein

Neuraminidase
Inhibitors
Target

NA HA NA
HA   HA
M2   HA
HA   HA
HA   M2
M2   HA
HA NA HA

Diarrhea
in Children

Amantadine/
Rimantadine
Target

Disease Name: Severe Acute Respiratory Syndrome

Synonym: SARS

Causative Agent: SARS coronavirus (SARS CoV)

Reservoirs: Possibly the palm civet and horseshoe bat

Incubation: 2–7 days

Geographic Regions Affected: The first cases of SARS have been traced back to the Guangdong Providence of China and Hong Kong in 2002. From there, SARS quickly spread to other countries around the region and world before being contained.

Description: SARS is a severe respiratory tract infection caused by a novel coronavirus. The disease was initially thought to have been transmitted from palm civets to humans. However, since person-to-person transmission is highly effective, the disease can quickly spread.

Signs and Symptoms: Most patients have a several-day prodrome of fever, chills, malaise, headache, and myalgia before developing a nonproductive cough. The cough typically gets worse and can ultimately progress to pneumonia, adult respiratory distress syndrome (ARDS), multisystem organ failure, and/or death.

Diagnostic Testing: Labs often reveal decreased lymphocytes and platelets with increased AST and lactic dehydrogenase (LDH). Chest x-ray, depending on severity of illness, can reveal bilateral infiltrates to signs of severe ARDS. Respiratory secretions, blood/serum/plasma, and stool samples should be collected for polymerase chain reaction (PCR) testing in accordance with Centers for Disease Control and Prevention (CDC) guidelines. Serology is only helpful in the convalescent phase of the disease. More information on diagnostic testing is available on the CDC website.

Treatment: Supportive. Intubation and mechanical ventilation may be indicated in severe disease.

Pearls: In the Western hemisphere, Toronto, Canada, was hit particularly hard by SARS. Kopi luwak, a coffee from Indonesia, is famous as the most expensive in the world and is made from the feces of palm civets fed coffee cherries. Since many of these animals are kept confined to small cages and force fed, the authors encourage you to boycott this product.

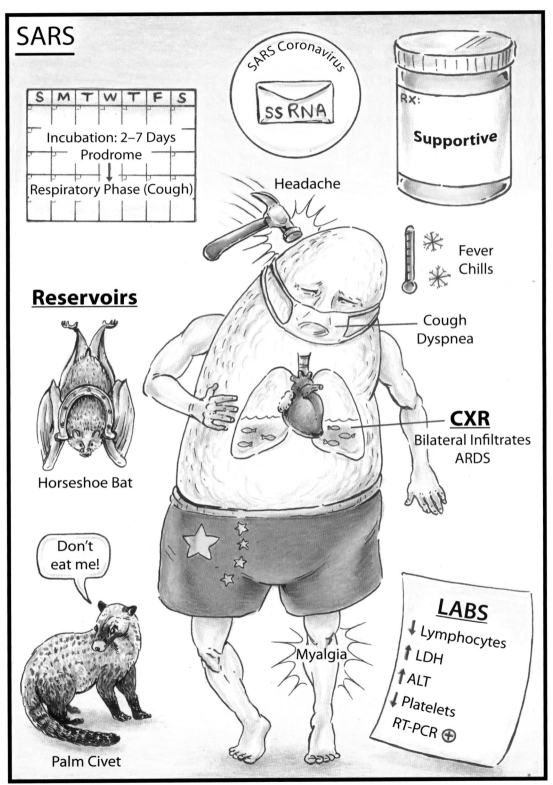

SARS

Reservoirs

Horseshoe Bat

"Don't eat me!"

Palm Civet

SARS Coronavirus
ss RNA

RX: **Supportive**

Incubation: 2–7 Days
Prodrome
↓
Respiratory Phase (Cough)

Headache

Fever
Chills

Cough
Dyspnea

CXR
Bilateral Infiltrates
ARDS

Myalgia

LABS
↓ Lymphocytes
↑ LDH
↑ ALT
↓ Platelets
RT-PCR ⊕

PART 9

MOSQUITO-BORNE ILLNESSES

Disease Name: **Zika Fever**

Synonyms:	Zika, Zika virus disease
Causative Agent:	Zika virus (ZIKV)
Vectors:	*Aedes aegypti, Aedes albopictus*
Reservoir:	Human and nonhuman primates
Incubation:	3–12 days

Geographic Regions Affected: Tropical and subtropical regions are at risk, as well as any regions that may support the *Aedes* spp. mosquito. Most U.S. cases are in returning travelers; however, the Centers for Disease Control and Prevention (CDC) has confirmed several cases of local mosquito-borne Zika in Florida and Texas.

Description: Zika is an acute febrile mosquito-borne illness similar to but milder than dengue. Infection is characterized by fever, arthralgia, myalgia, headache, conjunctivitis, and a pruritic maculopapular rash that begins on the face and spreads to the rest of the body. Most patients (~80%) are asymptomatic or have mild disease. When symptomatic, symptoms last for about 3–7 days. Zika infections during pregnancy have been implicated in microcephaly and other fetal brain defects, with Brazil being hit the hardest. Guillian-Barré syndrome has also been reported following some Zika infections.

Signs and Symptoms: Often asymptomatic, but classic signs of infection include fever, arthralgia, conjunctivitis, and rash. The fever in Zika is low grade, unlike the high fevers of dengue and chikungunya.

Diagnostic Testing: Symptomatic, non-pregnant individuals should receive testing of both urine and serum by Zika virus RNA NAT (nucleic acid testing) and IgM serology tests. NAT and serology tests for dengue and chikungunya should also be considered for individuals at risk of exposure and presenting with compatible illness. Patients presenting within 14 days of symptom onset can undergo NAT testing on both serum and urine. A positive result on either or both confirms the diagnosis. Negative NAT testing should be followed by serology. For patients presenting ≥14 days after symptom onset, NAT testing is not indicated, and only serology should be obtained. Negative IgM serology rules out acute infection, and positive IgM serology should be followed by plaque neutralization reduction testing (PNRT) for disease confirmation. More detailed information and testing algorithms for pregnant females is available on the CDC website.

Treatments: Supportive. NSAIDs should be avoided until dengue has been ruled out.

Prevention: Avoid mosquitos. Zika can be transmitted sexually, via blood transfusion, and passed vertically from mother to child during pregnancy. The CDC has recommended that men and women who traveled to areas where Zika is common should avoid sex or use condoms for at least 8 weeks after return from travel and for 8 weeks (women) and up to 6 months (men) if they had Zika or similar symptoms.

Pearls: Zika can be detected in semen for as long as 3–6 months after initial infection.

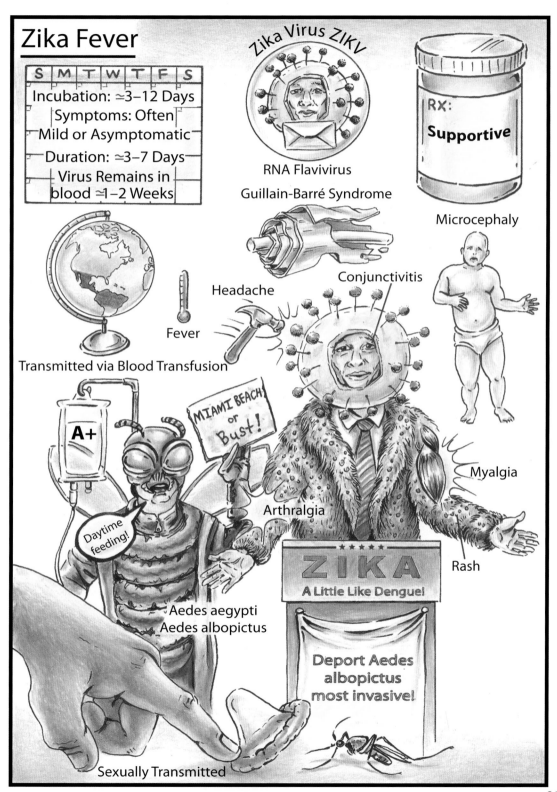

Disease Name:	**Dengue**
Synonyms:	Dengue hemorrhagic fever, breakbone fever
Causative Agent:	Dengue fever virus (DENV)—four major serotypes
Vector:	*Aedes* spp.—*A. aegypti* is the principal vector, but *A. albopictus* and *A. polynesiensis* can also transmit the virus. These are all daytime-feeding mosquitos.
Reservoir:	Human and nonhuman primates. Monkeys in West Africa and Southeast Asia.
Incubation:	3–14 days
Geographic Regions Affected:	Tropical and subtropical regions are at risk, as well as any regions that may support the *Aedes* spp. mosquito.
Description:	Dengue is an acute febrile mosquito-borne viral illness.
Signs and Symptoms:	Dengue fever (DF) is an acute febrile illness characterized by retroorbital headache, malaise, severe myalgia, arthralgia, and rash. The disease is most often asymptomatic or mild but can be severe and progress to hemorrhage (dengue hemorrhagic fever [DHF]) or shock (dengue shock syndrome [DSS]). While initial infections are often mild or asymptomatic, subsequent infections tend to be worse. DHF, a more-severe disease presentation, progresses through three phases: *Febrile Phase:* Symptoms include fever, headache, myalgia, arthralgia, rash, petechiae, easy bruisability, epistaxis, mucosal bleeding, and a positive tourniquet test. Children often present with nausea and vomiting. Symptoms are similar to DF. *Critical Phase:* Characterized by gastrointestinal (GI) hemorrhage and plasma leakage into the chest and peritoneal cavities, occurring after the fever breaks. Abdominal pain, ascites, and dyspnea can occur. DSS can occur in this phase unless aggressive fluid resuscitation is initiated. *Recovery Phase:* Patients will begin to feel better as capillary leakage stops and fluids begin to be reabsorbed. Bradycardia and a rash described as "white islands in a sea of red" may be observed.
Diagnostic Testing:	Labs will reveal leukopenia and thrombocytopenia. Hepatitis is common. Increased hematocrit and decreased albumin indicate capillary leakage and impending shock. IgM and IgG serology and polymerase chain (PCR) testing is available.
Treatments:	Supportive. Acetaminophen can be used as an antipyretic, and NSAIDs should be avoided secondary to thrombocytopenia. IV fluids and blood products may be indicated if the disease progresses to the critical phase.
Prevention:	Vaccines are currently being developed. Avoid mosquitos.

Dengue Fever

(Breakbone Fever)

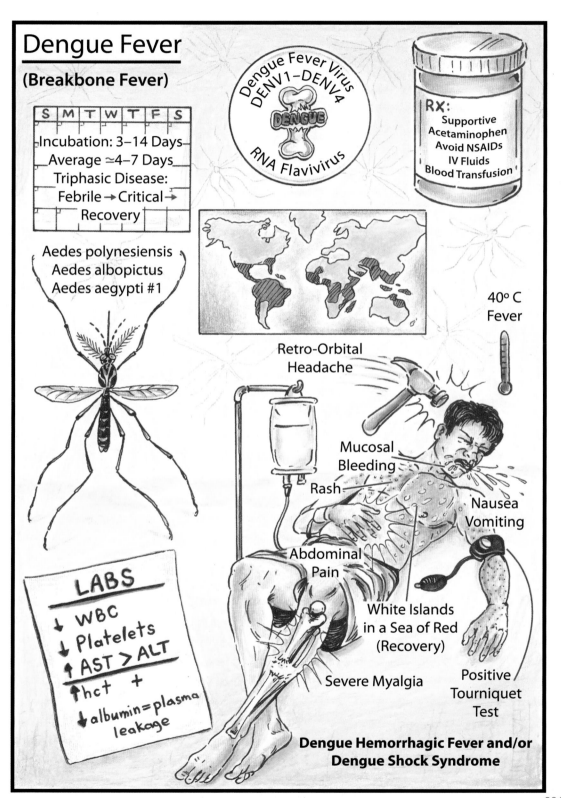

S	M	T	W	T	F	S

Incubation: 3–14 Days
Average ≃4–7 Days
Triphasic Disease:
Febrile → Critical →
Recovery

Dengue Fever Virus
DENV1–DENV4
DENGUE
RNA Flavivirus

RX:
Supportive
Acetaminophen
Avoid NSAIDs
IV Fluids
Blood Transfusion

Aedes polynesiensis
Aedes albopictus
Aedes aegypti #1

40° C
Fever

Retro-Orbital
Headache

Mucosal
Bleeding

Rash

Nausea
Vomiting

Abdominal
Pain

White Islands
in a Sea of Red
(Recovery)

Severe Myalgia

Positive
Tourniquet
Test

LABS

↓ WBC
↓ Platelets
↑ AST > ALT
↑ hct +
↓ albumin = plasma
leakage

**Dengue Hemorrhagic Fever and/or
Dengue Shock Syndrome**

Disease Name: **Yellow Fever**

Causative Agent: Yellow fever virus (YFV)

Vectors: *Aedes* spp. and *Haemagogus* spp.

Reservoir: Humans and nonhuman primates

Incubation: 3–6 days

Geographic Regions Affected: Sub-Saharan Africa, Central and South America. Approximately 90% of all cases occur in Africa.

Description: Yellow fever is an acute febrile mosquito-born viral illness. It is named after the jaundice that occurs during the toxic phase of the illness.

Signs and Symptoms: Many cases are asymptomatic. Mild illness may be limited to fever and headache, whereas moderate disease is characterized by fever, chills, malaise, headache, myalgia, backache, nausea, and vomiting. Symptoms typically last for 3–4 days before resolving. In approximately 15% of symptomatic cases, patients will progress to a more toxic phase of the disease characterized by recurrence of fever, chills, jaundice, liver failure, mucosal bleeding, hematemesis, melena, delirium, renal failure, and shock. Mortality from the toxic phase is high, ranging between 20% and 50%. Surviving the illness confers lifetime immunity.

Diagnostic Testing: Presumptive diagnosis is made based on travel history and signs and symptoms. Labs will reveal elevated AST/ALT, prolonged PT and PTT, thrombocytopenia, and an increased direct bilirubin with a relatively normal alkaline phosphatase. Yellow fever–specific IgM and IgG levels can help confirm the diagnosis, but it is important to note there may be some cross-reactivity with other flaviviruses. Since viremia only lasts for about 3 days, polymerase chain reaction (PCR) testing is of limited value unless obtained early in the course of illness.

Treatments: Supportive. Acetaminophen can be used as an antipyretic, but NSAIDs should be avoided given bleeding risks.

Prevention: Avoid mosquitos. A single subcutaneous (SQ) dose of live-attenuated yellow fever vaccine is indicated for those traveling to or living in at-risk areas or when proof of vaccination is required to enter a specific country.

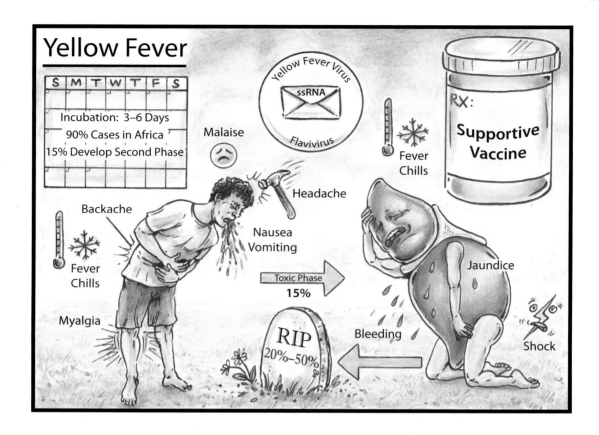

Yellow Fever

S	M	T	W	T	F	S
Incubation: 3–6 Days						
90% Cases in Africa						
15% Develop Second Phase						

Yellow Fever Virus
ssRNA
Flavivirus

Malaise

Headache

Fever Chills

RX:
Supportive Vaccine

Backache

Nausea Vomiting

Fever Chills

Myalgia

Toxic Phase
15%

Jaundice

RIP
20%–50%

Bleeding

Shock

Disease Name: Malaria

Causative Agents: *Plasmodium* spp.—*P. vivax, P. falciparum, P. malariae, P. ovale*

Lifecycle: Malaria is contracted by the bite of an infected female *Anopheles* mosquito during feeding. *Liver Stage*: Sporozoites are injected and migrate through the circulatory system and infect hepatocytes in the liver. Here multinucleated schizonts form. *P. vivax* and *P. ovale* form hypnozoites which can remain dormant or form schizonts. Hepatic schizonts ultimately rupture, releasing merozoites capable of infecting red blood cells. *Blood Stage*: Merozoites infect blood cells and develop into trophozoites and blood cell schizonts or gametocytes. Infected blood cells will rupture, releasing merozoites capable of infecting other red cells or male and female gametocytes capable of being ingested by mosquitos. Sexual reproduction occurs in the mosquito's midgut, and mature sporozoites migrate to the mosquito's salivary gland, ready to infect another human at the next feeding.

Vector: *Anopheles* spp.

Incubation: 7–30 days. Incubation periods are shorter for *P. falciparum* and longer for *P. malariae*. Partial immunity or ineffective malaria prophylaxis may delay symptoms for weeks or months. Also, both *P. vivax* and *P. ovale* can create dormant liver-stage parasites, delaying disease presentation or relapse months or years after treatment.

Geographic Regions Affected: Tropical and subtropical regions. The highest rates of transmission are found in sub-Saharan Africa and New Guinea. Malaria transmission does not occur at high altitude, during cold seasons, in deserts, or in areas with effective mosquito eradication programs.

Description: Malaria is a mosquito-borne febrile illness caused by the *Plasmodium* protozoa. Symptoms of the disease are associated with the rupture and release of merozoites during the blood stage of the infection. Classically paroxysms of chills, fevers, and diaphoresis occur, every second day "tertian fever" from *P. vivax, P. falciparum*, and *P. ovale*, and every third day "quartan fever" from *P. malariae*. Young children and pregnant women are at greater risk for significant disease. *P. falciparum* typically causes more severe malaria infections.

Signs and Symptoms: In *uncomplicated malaria*, patients can present with paroxysmal fever, chills, malaise, arthralgia, myalgia, headache, diaphoresis, tachycardia, tachypnea, abdominal pain, splenomegaly, nausea, and vomiting. In *severe malaria*, patients can develop altered mental status (AMS), seizures, shock, adult respiratory distress syndrome (ARDS), metabolic acidosis, hemoglobinuria, renal failure, hypoglycemia, hepatic failure, coagulopathy, and severe anemia.

Diagnostic Testing: Malaria should be suspected in patients with febrile illness and recent travel to a region where malaria is endemic. Labs may reveal anemia, thrombocytopenia, elevated AST/ALT, elevated bilirubin, and elevated BUN/creatinine. Thick and thin blood smears should be obtained to detect parasites (thick) and identify the species (thin). Blood smears can be obtained every 8 hours for several days if malaria is suspected.

Treatments: Treatment is tailored to the *Plasmodium* spp., severity of illness, pregnancy status, and drug susceptibility based on geographic region of infection. Current Centers for Disease Control and Prevention (CDC) guidelines should be consulted prior to selecting a treatment regimen. Uncomplicated malaria can be treated with: atovaquone/proguanil, artemether/lumefantrine, quinine sulfate plus doxycycline, or mefloquine (mefloquine can cause neuropsychiatric reactions). If chloroquine resistance is not an issue, uncomplicated malaria can be treated with chloroquine phosphate or hydroxychloroquine. *P. vivax* and *P. ovale* require a longer duration of treatment with primaquine to eradicate liver hypnozoites. Primaquine can cause hemolytic anemia in G6PD-deficient patients and cannot be used during pregnancy. Severe malaria should be treated with IV quinidine gluconate plus doxycycline or clindamycin.

Prevention: Avoid mosquitos. Malarial prophylaxis is indicated for travelers to endemic regions and recommendations often vary between the WHO and the CDC. The species of *Plasmodium* and presence/absence of chloroquine resistance are factors to consider when considering prophylaxis. Medications are typically started 1 day to 2 weeks before travel and continued up to 4 weeks after return. The CDC website can be referenced for country-specific recommendations.

Malaria

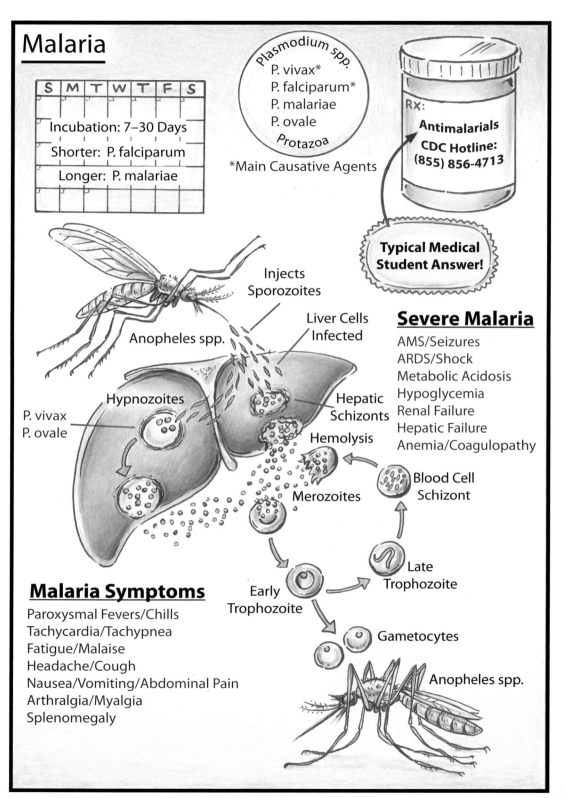

S	M	T	W	T	F	S

Incubation: 7–30 Days

Shorter: P. falciparum

Longer: P. malariae

Plasmodium spp.
P. vivax*
P. falciparum*
P. malariae
P. ovale
Protozoa

*Main Causative Agents

RX:
Antimalarials
CDC Hotline:
(855) 856-4713

Typical Medical Student Answer!

Injects Sporozoites

Anopheles spp.

Liver Cells Infected

Hypnozoites

P. vivax
P. ovale

Hepatic Schizonts

Hemolysis

Merozoites

Blood Cell Schizont

Early Trophozoite

Late Trophozoite

Gametocytes

Anopheles spp.

Severe Malaria

AMS/Seizures
ARDS/Shock
Metabolic Acidosis
Hypoglycemia
Renal Failure
Hepatic Failure
Anemia/Coagulopathy

Malaria Symptoms

Paroxysmal Fevers/Chills
Tachycardia/Tachypnea
Fatigue/Malaise
Headache/Cough
Nausea/Vomiting/Abdominal Pain
Arthralgia/Myalgia
Splenomegaly

Disease Name: **Mosquito-Borne Encephalitis**

Culex spp.

Western Equine Encephalitis
- Causative Agent: Western equine encephalitis virus (WEEV)—Togaviridae
- Vector: *Culex tarsalis*—Encephalitis mosquito
- Region: North and South America—Most cases occur in rural areas West of the Mississippi.
- Incubation: 5–10 days
- Symptoms: Most infections are asymptomatic. Those who become ill develop fever, headache, nausea, and vomiting. Encephalitis occurs in 0.1% of infections and is more common in children. Mortality in neuroinvasive disease ranges between 3% and 7% and is higher in children. Neurologic sequelae in survivors are rare and mostly affect younger children.
- Treatment: Supportive.

West Nile Virus
- Causative Agent: West Nile virus (WNV)—Flaviviridae
- Vector: *Culex* spp.
- Region: Global—First U.S. case was in 1999.
- Incubation: 2–14 days, Average: 2–6 days
- Symptoms: About 70% to 80% of infections are asymptomatic. Those who become ill develop fever, headache, fatigue, myalgia, arthralgia, transient maculopapular rash, nausea, and vomiting. Progression to encephalitis occurs in <1% of symptomatic patients. Patients may develop a "polio-like" acute flaccid paralysis. Mortality for neuroinvasive disease is about 20%, and neurologic sequelae have been reported in up to 50% of survivors.
- Treatment: Supportive.

Japanese Encephalitis
- Causative Agent: Japanese encephalitis virus (JEV)—Flaviviridae
- Vector: *Culex* spp.—*Culex tritaeniorhynchus*
- Region: Asia and Western Pacific Countries—Most common near farms and after heavy rainfall
- Incubation: 5–15 days
- Symptoms: Most infections are asymptomatic or mild causing fever and headache. Children <15 years old are most commonly affected in endemic areas. Less than 1% of patients develop neuroinvasive disease, which has a mortality of 20% to 30%. In those who survive, 30-50% will have neurologic sequelae.
- Treatment: Supportive. Vaccination to prevent illness.

Saint Louis Encephalitis
- Causative Agent: Saint Louis encephalitis virus (SLEV)—Flaviviradae
- Vector: *Culex* spp. – *C. pipiens* and *C. quinquefasciatus*
- Region: North and South America—Eastern and Central U.S. states
- Incubation: 5–15 days
- Symptoms: Almost all cases are asymptomatic. Those who become ill develop fever, headache, dizziness, malaise, nausea, and vomiting. Progression to encephalitis is much more common in older adults than children. Mortality in neuroinvasive disease ranges between 5% and 15% and increases with age.
- Treatment: Supportive.

Murray Valley Encephalitis

- Causative Agent: Murray Valley encephalitis virus (MVEV)—Flaviviradae
- Vector: *Culex annulirostris*—Common banded mosquito
- Region: Australia and New Guinea—Most common after heavy rainfalls
- Incubation: 5–28 days, Average: 7–12 days
- Symptoms: Almost all infections (99.9%) are asymptomatic. Those who become ill develop fever, headache, fatigue, nausea, and vomiting. Encephalitis is uncommon (0.1% overall). Mortality for neuroinvasive cases ranges between 15% and 30% with 30% to 50% of survivors exhibiting neurologic sequela.
- Treatment: Supportive.

Venezuela Equine Encephalitis

- Causative Agent: Venezuela equine encephalitis virus (VEEV)—Togaviridae
- Vector: *Culex* spp.
- Region: Central and South America
- Incubation: 1–6 days
- Symptoms: Those who become ill develop fever, headache, fatigue, nausea, and vomiting. Encephalitis occurs in <0.5% of adults and <4% of children. Mortality and neurologic sequela are rare.
- Treatment: Supportive.

Aedes **spp.**
La Crosse Encephalitis

- Causative Agent: La Crosse virus (LACV)—Bunyaviridae
- Vector: *Aedes triseriatus*—Eastern treehole mosquito
- Region: Upper Midwestern, mid-Atlantic, and Southern U.S.
- Incubation: 5–15 days
- Symptoms: Most infections are asymptomatic. Those who become ill develop fever, headache, fatigue, nausea, and vomiting. Encephalitis is rare and most commonly occurs in children <16 years old. AMS, seizures, and coma can occur with neuroinvasive disease. Mortality in neuroinvasive disease is <1% with neurologic sequela reported in about 10% of survivors.
- Treatment: Supportive.

Culiseta **spp.**
Eastern Equine Encephalitis

- Causative Agent: Eastern equine encephalitis virus (EEEV)—Togaviridae
- Vector: *Culiseta melanura*—Black-tailed mosquito
- Region: North, Central, South America and Caribbean—Most U.S. cases occur in Atlantic and Gulf Coast states.
- Incubation: 4–10 days
- Symptoms: Fever, headache, nausea, and vomiting. Encephalitis occurs in 2% to 6% of infections and progresses from altered mental status (AMS) to seizures and coma. Mortality in neuroinvasive cases is about 30%, making EEE the most severe mosquito-borne illness in the United States. Most survivors will have neurologic sequelae.
- Treatment: Supportive.

Infected Animal Blood,
Culex **and** ***Aedes*** **spp.**

Rift Valley Fever

- Causative Agent: Rift Valley fever virus (RVFV)—Bunyaviridae (Phlebovirus)
- Vector: Blood or body fluids from infected livestock (most common), *Culex tritaeniorhynchus, Aedes vexans*
- Region: Sub-Saharan Africa
- Incubation: 2–6 days
- Symptoms: Most cases are asymptomatic or cause mild febrile illness with malaise, weakness, dizziness, backache, and mild hepatitis. In 10% of cases more-severe illness such as ocular disease with a potential for blindness, encephalitis, (<1%) or hemorrhagic fever (<1%) occurs.
- Treatment: Supportive.

Mosquito-Borne Encephalitis

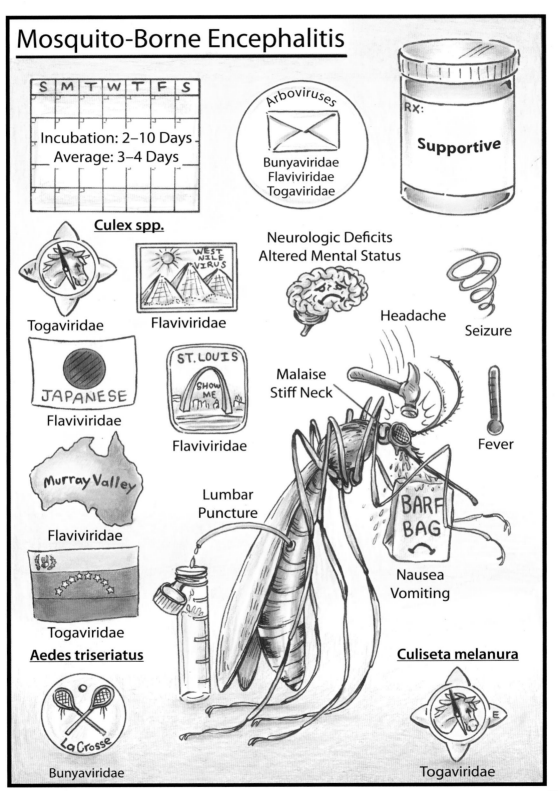

S	M	T	W	T	F	S

Incubation: 2–10 Days
Average: 3–4 Days

Arboviruses
Bunyaviridae
Flaviviridae
Togaviridae

RX:
Supportive

Culex spp.

Togaviridae

WEST NILE VIRUS
Flaviviridae

Neurologic Deficits
Altered Mental Status

Headache

Seizure

JAPANESE
Flaviviridae

ST. LOUIS
SHOW ME MO
Flaviviridae

Malaise
Stiff Neck

Fever

Murray Valley
Flaviviridae

Lumbar
Puncture

BARF BAG

Nausea
Vomiting

Togaviridae

Aedes triseriatus

Culiseta melanura

La Crosse
Bunyaviridae

Togaviridae

Disease Name: **Chikungunya**

Causative Agent:	Chikungunya virus (CHIKV)
Vectors:	*Aedes* spp.—Specifically, *A. aegypti* and *A. albopictus*.
Reservoir:	Human and nonhuman primates. The World Health Organization (WHO) reports that some nonprimates, birds, rodents, and small mammals may serve as reservoirs.
Incubation:	2–12 days; Average: 3–7 days
Geographic Regions Affected:	Tropical and subtropical regions are high-risk areas, as well as any region that may support the *Aedes* spp. mosquito. In late 2013, local transmission of chikungunya was identified in several Caribbean countries and territories. The disease has since spread to South America.
Description:	Chikungunya is an acute febrile mosquito-borne viral illness characterized by high fever and polyarthralgia.
Signs and Symptoms:	The majority (80%) of those infected will be symptomatic. Chikungunya should be suspected patients with recent travel to endemic regions and presenting with high fever and polyarthralgia.
	Fever can be biphasic. Arthralgia is typically bilateral and symmetric, predominantly affecting the peripheral joints of the hands, feet, wrists, and ankles. Knees, elbows, and shoulders can also be involved, while hips are often spared. Myalgia, headache, malaise, conjunctivitis, and nausea can also occur. A transient (3–4 day) maculopapular rash affecting the face, trunk, and extremities is present in 40%–50% of cases. Unlike with dengue, hemorrhage is very rare. Guillian-Barré syndrome may occur as a post-infectious complication. Patients may develop chronic polyarthritis, with as many as 20% still complaining of arthralgia 1 year after the initial infection.
Diagnostic Testing:	Serum can be tested for the virus, viral nucleic acid, or chikungunya-specific IgM. According to the Centers for Disease Control and Prevention (CDC), the virus can be detected for 3 days, and viral RNA for 8 days, and IgM should be elevated within 1 week of symptom onset. IgG elevates within 2 weeks of infection. Since the diseases have similar presentations, testing for Zika and dengue should also be considered. More detailed information is available on the CDC website.
Treatments:	Supportive
Prevention:	Avoid mosquitos.
Pearls:	Post-chikungunya polyarthritis can mimic rheumatoid arthritis (RA). Careful history and diagnostic testing can help distinguish the two. Chikungunya IgG should remain elevated for years after initial infection.

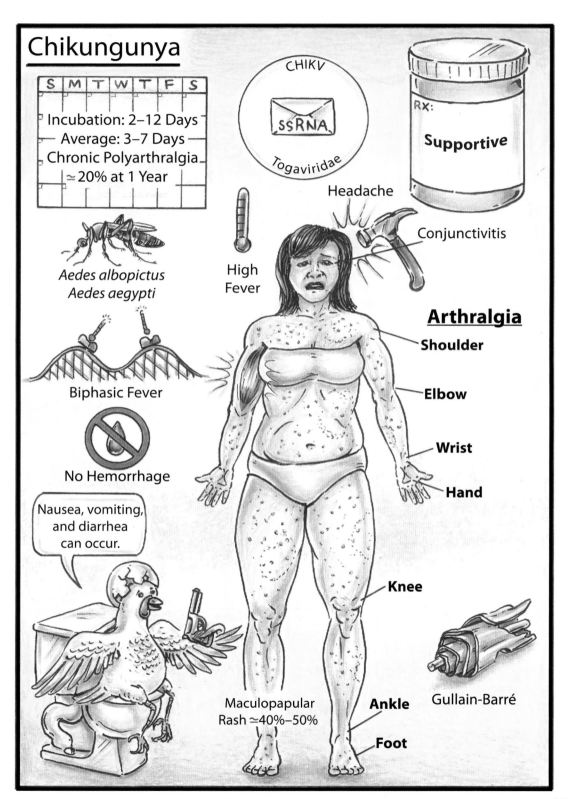

Chikungunya

Incubation: 2–12 Days
Average: 3–7 Days
Chronic Polyarthralgia
≃20% at 1 Year

CHIKV
SSRNA
Togaviridae

RX:
Supportive

Aedes albopictus
Aedes aegypti

High Fever

Biphasic Fever

No Hemorrhage

Nausea, vomiting, and diarrhea can occur.

Headache

Conjunctivitis

Arthralgia
Shoulder

Elbow

Wrist

Hand

Knee

Maculopapular Rash ≃40%–50%

Ankle

Foot

Gullain-Barré

PART 10

RAT-, FLEA-, LOUSE-, AND CHIGGER-BORNE ILLNESSES

Disease Name: Hemorrhagic Fever with Renal Syndrome

Synonyms: HFRS, epidemic hemorrhagic fever, Korean hemorrhagic fever, Manchurian hemorrhagic fever

Causative Agents: Hantaviruses of the Bunyaviridae family: Hantaan River virus (HTNV), Saaremaa virus (SAAV), Seoul virus (SEOV), Puumala virus (PUUV), and Dobrava virus (DOBV)

Transmission: Aerosolized virus from infected rodent excreta, saliva, and urine.

Reservoir: Striped field mouse for Saaremaa (SAAV) and Hantaan viruses (HTNV); Norway rat for Seoul virus (SEOV); bank vole for Puumala virus (PUUV); yellow-necked field mouse for Dobrava virus (DOBV)

Incubation Period: 1–8 weeks; Average: 1–2 weeks

Geographic Regions Affected: Saaremaa virus in Central Europe and Scandinavia; Hantaan virus in East Asia; Seoul virus worldwide; Puumala virus in Scandinavia, Western Europe, and Western Russia; and Dobrava virus in the Balkans.

Peak Incidence: Spring and fall peaks for Saaremaa and Hantaan viruses due to mouse breeding seasons and human agricultural practices.

Description: Hemorrhagic fever with renal syndrome (HFRS) is a viral zoonotic infection caused by exposure to aerosolized excreta, urine, or saliva from infected rodents. The infection has been divided into five clinical phases: febrile, hypotensive, oliguric, diuretic, and convalescent.

Signs and Symptoms: *Febrile*: Flu-like symptoms predominate, including fever, chills, headache, malaise, nausea, vomiting, diarrhea, cough, and abdominal and back pain. Conjunctivitis, blurred vision, and a petechial rash are often present. *Hypotensive*: Severe capillary leak syndrome, edema, hypotension, tachycardia, and thrombocytopenia. *Oliguric*: Characterized by renal failure with proteinuria. *Diuretic*: Diuresis and polyuria, up to several liters per day. *Convalescent*: The recovery phase, which can be lengthy.

Diagnostic Testing: Recognition of exposure to infected rodents is key. Labs will reveal thrombocytopenia, leukocytosis with a shift to the left including immature myeloid cells and atypical lymphocytes. Serology, polymerase chain reaction (PCR), and immunohistochemical testing can be performed to confirm the diagnosis.

Treatments: Treatment is supportive. Ribavirin may have some benefit if given early. Hemodialysis may be necessary. Complete recovery may take weeks or months.

Pearls: Human-to-human transmission is extremely rare. Infection is prevented by rodent control. Hantaan and Dobrava virus infections usually cause severe symptoms, while Seoul and Saaremaa virus infections are usually more moderate. Puumala virus infections are mild and often asymptomatic.

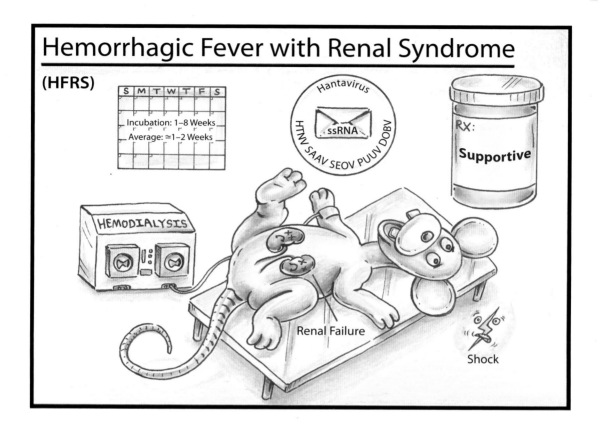

Disease Name: **Hantavirus Pulmonary Syndrome**

Synonym: Hantavirus cardiopulmonary syndrome

Causative Agents: American Hantaviruses of the Bunyaviridae family: Sin Nombre virus (SNV); New York virus (NYV); Bayou virus (BAYV); Black Creek Canal virus (BCCV); Andes virus (ANDV).

Transmission: Aerosolized virus from infected rodent excreta, saliva, and urine

Reservoir: Deer mouse *(Peromyscus maniculatus)* for Sin Nombre virus (SNV); white-footed mouse *(Peromyscus leucopus)* for New York virus (NYV); cotton rat *(Sigmodon hispidus)* for Black Creek Canal virus (BCCV); rice rat *(Oryzomys palustris)* for Bayou virus (BAYV); long-tailed rice rat *(Oligoryzomys longicaudatus)* for Andes virus (ANDV)

Incubation Period: 1–4 weeks

Geographic Regions Affected: United States and Canada (Sin Nombre virus); Northeastern United States (New York Hantavirus); Southeastern United States (Bayou Hantavirus); Florida (Black Creek Canal Hantavirus); South America (Andes Hantavirus).

Peak Incidence: Can occur throughout the year, but peaks in summer and fall.

Description: Hantavirus pulmonary syndrome (HPS) is a viral zoonotic infection caused by exposure to aerosolized excreta, urine, or saliva from infected rodents. The infection has been divided into three distinct clinical phases: prodromal, cardiopulmonary, and convalescent.

Signs and Symptoms: *Prodromal*: Flu-like symptoms including fever, headache, myalgia, nausea, vomiting, and diarrhea. Respiratory symptoms are minimal and the prodromal symptoms may be mistaken as gastroenteritis. The duration of symptoms lasts 3–5 days. *Cardiopulmonary*: Severe dyspnea, nonproductive cough, pulmonary edema, and circulatory collapse occur. Mechanical ventilation is often required. This phase lasts only 24–48 hours. *Convalescent*: The recovery phase, which begins with the onset of massive diuresis.

Diagnostic Testing: Recognition of exposure to infected rodents is key. Labs will reveal leukocytosis with left shift and atypical lymphocytes, coagulopathy, thrombocytopenia, elevated liver enzymes, renal failure, and proteinuria. Serology, polymerase chain reaction (PCR), and immunohistochemical testing can be performed to confirm the diagnosis.

Treatments: Treatment is supportive. Ribavirin may have some benefit if given early. Endotracheal intubation with mechanical ventilation and extracorporeal membrane oxygenation may be necessary.

Pearls: Early treatment in an intensive care unit may be life-saving. Rodent infestation in and around homes in rural areas is the primary risk for Hantavirus exposure. The disease is maximal in high rodent years. The Andes Hantavirus can cause person-to-person transmission.

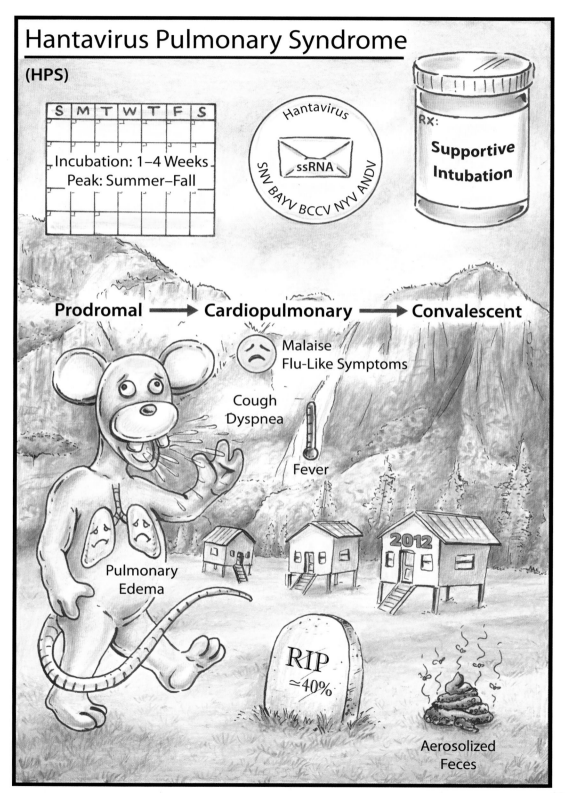

Hantavirus Pulmonary Syndrome

(HPS)

Incubation: 1–4 Weeks
Peak: Summer–Fall

Hantavirus
ssRNA
SNV BAYV BCCV NYV ANDV

RX:
Supportive
Intubation

Prodromal → **Cardiopulmonary** → **Convalescent**

Malaise
Flu-Like Symptoms

Cough
Dyspnea

Fever

Pulmonary
Edema

2012

RIP
≈40%

Aerosolized
Feces

Disease Name: **Plague**

Synonyms:	Plague, Black Death, The Great Plague
Causative Agent:	*Yersinia pestis*
Vector:	Rat flea *(Xenopsylla cheopis)*
Reservoir:	Rats, mice, many rodents, foxes, coyotes, wild cats
Incubation Period:	2–6 days
Geographic Regions Affected:	Southwestern United States, South America, Africa, and Asia

Peak Incidence: In the mid-1300s *Yersinia pestis* was responsible for The Black Death, a global pandemic spread by flea-infested rats traveling along trade routes throughout the known world. Plague has become endemic in certain rural regions such as the Southwestern United States.

Description: Plague is a zoonotic disease of rodents that is transmitted to humans by the bites of infected fleas. There are three clinical forms: bubonic, septicemic, and pneumonic, depending on the route of infection. *Bubonic plague* is the most common form, caused by the bite of an infected flea. *Y. pestis* enters at the bite site and travels through the lymphatic system to the nearest lymph node, where it replicates and causes painful lymphadenopathy (bubo). These bubos can ulcerate and become open sores. *Septicemic plague* occurs when the infection enters the bloodstream, either directly from flea bites or secondary to advanced bubonic plague. *Pneumonic plague* is classified as either primary or secondary. Primary pneumonic plague is caused by the inhalation of aerosolized droplets from another person with pneumonic plague, while secondary pneumonic plague occurs when bubonic plague spreads to the lungs in advanced disease.

Signs and Symptoms: *Bubonic plague* is characterized by high fever, chills, weakness, fatigue, and headache associated with the rapid formation of tender bubo(s). Over time, the bubo(s) may ulcerate and become suppurative. Patients may develop hypotension, shock, and disseminated intravascular coagulation (DIC). Blood clots can block small arterioles and cause acral gangrene, thought to give rise to the term "Black Death." *Septicemic plague* is characterized by the sudden onset of febrile illness without bubo formation. Nausea, vomiting, and diarrhea can occur. Hypotension and shock develop quickly, and mortality rates are high. *Pneumonic plague* is characterized by fever, cough, dyspnea, and hemoptysis. Lobar consolidation is often present.

Diagnostic Testing: Labs will reveal an elevated white blood cell count (WBC), predominantly immature neutrophils. Increased BUN/creatinine, elevated liver enzymes, and thrombocytopenia can occur. Blood cultures are often positive. Diagnosis is confirmed by the identification of *Y. pestis* in a sample of fluid from a bubo, blood, or sputum. Serology can be obtained, and rapid diagnostic test kits exist in some countries.

Treatments: Streptomycin and gentamicin are considered first-line agents. Doxycycline, ciprofloxacin, and chloramphenicol are also effective treatment options. Doxycycline or ciprofloxacin can be used as postexposure prophylaxis. A vaccine is available for laboratory and field workers.

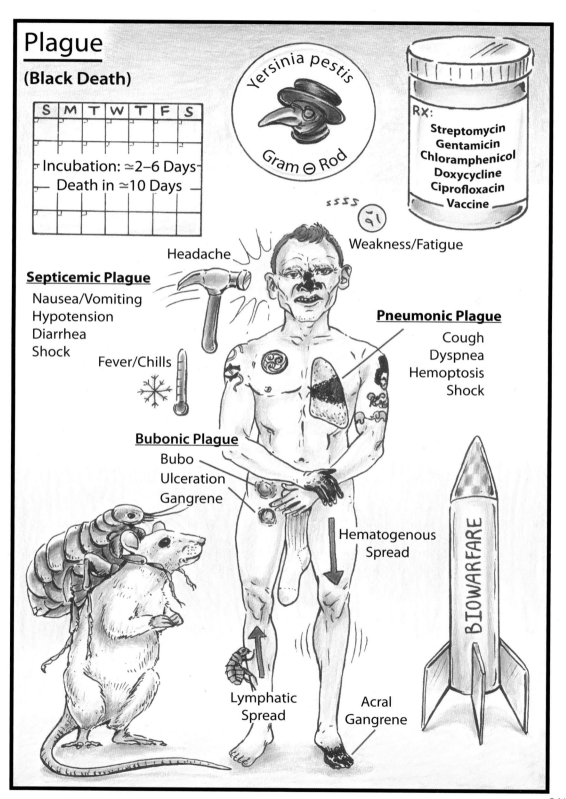

Plague
(Black Death)

Incubation: ≃2–6 Days
Death in ≃10 Days

Yersinia pestis
Gram ⊖ Rod

RX:
Streptomycin
Gentamicin
Chloramphenicol
Doxycycline
Ciprofloxacin
Vaccine

Weakness/Fatigue

Headache

Septicemic Plague
Nausea/Vomiting
Hypotension
Diarrhea
Shock

Fever/Chills

Pneumonic Plague
Cough
Dyspnea
Hemoptosis
Shock

Bubonic Plague
Bubo
Ulceration
Gangrene

Hematogenous
Spread

Lymphatic
Spread

Acral
Gangrene

BIOWARFARE

Disease Name: Leptospirosis

Causative Agent: *Leptospira* spp.

Reservoir: Rodents, small mammals, domestic animals, and livestock can harbor chronic renal leptospirosis and excrete bacteria in their urine throughout their lifetime.

Incubation: 4–14 days

Geographic Regions Affected: Worldwide. Endemic in tropical climates with infectious peaks after periods of heavy rainfall.

Description: Leptospirosis is a zoonosis caused by exposure to infectious urine from reservoir animals. Indirect contact with urine via contaminated soil or water is the most common mode of transmission. The disease presents as a mild self-limiting infection but can progress to a severe life-threatening illness in 10% of patients.

Signs and Symptoms: *Mild Disease*: High fever, chills, headache, myalgia, abdominal pain, nausea, vomiting, diarrhea, and conjunctivitis. *Severe Disease*: Characterized by renal failure, hepatic failure, jaundice, meningitis, myocarditis, cardiac arrhythmia or collapse, and/or pneumonia with pulmonary hemorrhage.

Diagnostic Testing: Diagnosis is based on a high index of suspicion. IgM and IgG serology can be obtained, and rapid diagnostic tests are available in some countries. Positive serological tests can be confirmed with microscopic agglutination testing (MAT).

Treatments: *Mild Disease*: Oral doxycycline and amoxicillin are effective treatments. Azithromycin can be used in lieu of doxycycline and has fewer side effects. *Severe Disease*: Intravenous (IV) penicillin G or ceftriaxone is required for the treatment of severe disease. Penicillin can cause Jarisch-Herxheimer reaction. While corticosteroids may have some benefit in the treatment of severe leptospirosis, further research is required.

Prevention: Chemoprophylaxis with oral doxycycline 200 mg weekly can be considered for people with a high risk of exposure to leptospirosis.

Pearls: There is an urban legend that leptospirosis has been contracted by a person drinking from an unwashed soda can contaminated with dried rat urine.

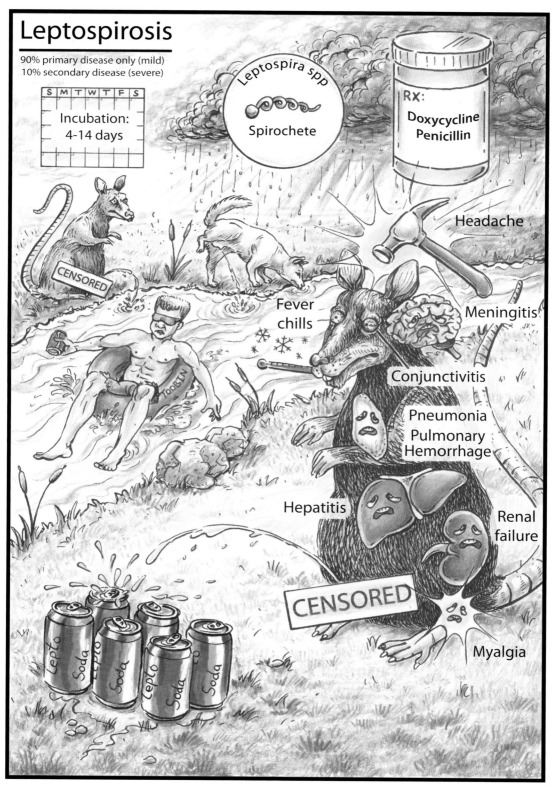

Disease Name: **Rat-Bite Fever**

Synonyms:	Streptobacillary Rat-bite fever (RBF) (North America), spirillary RBF or Sodoku (Asia), Haverhill fever (when contracted via ingestion of contaminated food or water)
Causative Agents:	RBF is caused by two different bacteria: *Streptobacillus moniloformis* in North America and *Spirillum minus* in Asia. These bacteria are part of the normal respiratory flora in rodents.
Reservoir:	Rats predominantly, but mice, gerbils, and ferrets can also serve as reservoirs.
Incubation:	Streptobacillary: 2–10 days; Spirillary: 2–4 weeks
Geographic Regions Affected:	Streptobacillary RBF has been documented on most continents, but is predominant in North America. Spirillary RBF is predominantly found in Asia.
Description:	RBF is a zoonosis caused by the bite of an infected rodent or through the consumption of bacterially contaminated food or water.
Signs and Symptoms:	*Streptobacillary RBF:* Short incubation followed by fever, chills, headache, nausea, and vomiting. A maculopapular rash occurs on the extremities 2–4 days after fever onset and about 50% of patients will develop polyarthritis. The bite site is typically well healed and without regional lymphadenopathy. *Spirillary RBF:* Longer incubation followed by fever, chills, and ulceration at the bite site with associated lymphangitis and lymphadenopathy. Arthritis is uncommon and a red-brown macular rash is common on the face, trunk, and extremities. *Haverhill Fever:* Fever, chills, rigors, prostration, myalgia, arthralgia, rash, and severe nausea and vomiting. Mortality for untreated infections is about 10%.
Diagnostic Testing:	Rat-bite fever should be suspected in patients with rash, fever, and arthritis with known exposure to rats or other reservoir animals. Labs will show leukocytosis with a shift to the left and mild to moderate anemia. *S. moniloformis* is difficult to culture and may be identified on Gram stain as a gram-negative pleomorphic rod. *S. minus* cannot be cultured and requires darkfield microscopy or differential staining. A false positive for syphilis occurs in 25% of cases for *S. moniloformis* and 50% for *S. minus*.
Treatments:	Effective treatment options include amoxicillin/clavulnante or doxycycline.
Prevention:	Avoid rats, specifically in the wild. Proper handling of domestic rodents to avoid biting behaviors. Handwashing after animal handling and cleaning cages. Rat bites should be treated prophylactically with antibiotics.

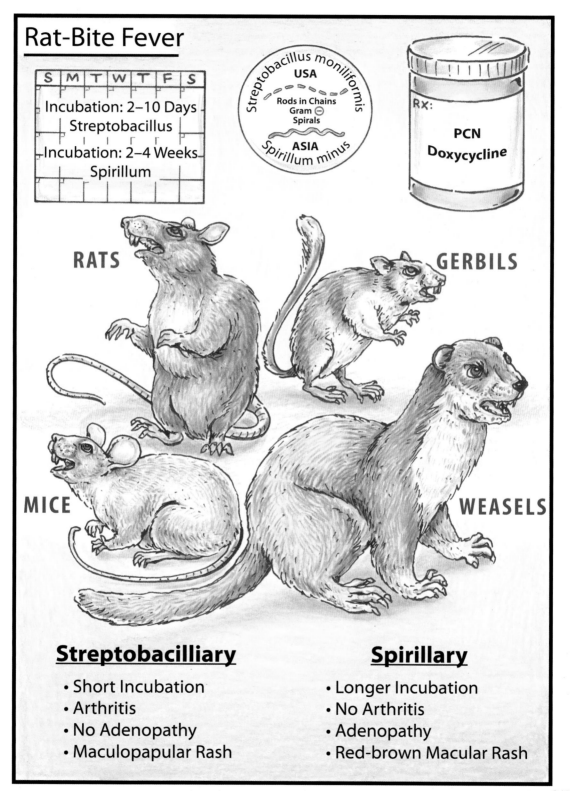

Rat-Bite Fever

S	M	T	W	T	F	S

Incubation: 2–10 Days
Streptobacillus
Incubation: 2–4 Weeks
Spirillum

Streptobacillus moniliformis
USA
Rods in Chains
Gram ⊖
Spirals
ASIA
Spirillum minus

RX:
PCN
Doxycycline

RATS

GERBILS

MICE

WEASELS

Streptobacilliary

- Short Incubation
- Arthritis
- No Adenopathy
- Maculopapular Rash

Spirillary

- Longer Incubation
- No Arthritis
- Adenopathy
- Red-brown Macular Rash

Disease Name:	**Trench Fever**

Synonyms:	Shin bone fever, urban trench fever, 5-day fever, Quintan fever
Causative Agent:	*Bartonella quintana*
Vector:	Human Body Louse *(Pediculus humanus corporis)*
Reservoir:	Humans
Incubation:	3–38 days; Average: 12–25 days
Geographic Regions Affected:	Worldwide
Description:	Trench fever is a zoonotic bacterial infection transmitted via the body louse classically presenting as a 5-day relapsing fever with associated headache, dizziness, and shin pain. The disease was most common during WWI trench warfare with fewer cases reported during WWII. "Urban trench fever" has been reported in homeless populations.
Signs and Symptoms:	After a relatively long incubation period, patients present with fever, retro-orbital headache, malaise, dizziness, arthralgia, myalgia, splenomegaly, shin pain, and truncal rash. Fever can be an isolated episode, last for 4–5 days, present as several episodes of 4–5 days of relapsing fever, or can be persistent for 2–6 weeks' duration. Contemporary *B. quintana* infections are more common in the homeless and HIV/AIDS population and can present as "urban trench fever," bacteremia with or without endocarditis, bacillary angiomatosis, and/or peliosis hepatitis.
Diagnostic Testing:	Trench fever should be suspected in homeless individuals or persons with known exposure to the body louse presenting with shin pain and relapsing fevers. Serology and blood cultures should be obtained. The bacteria are difficult to culture. Polymerase chain reaction (PCR), cultures, and immunohistochemical testing should be performed when endocarditis and/or bacillary angiomatosis is suspected.
Treatments:	Effective treatment for patients without endocarditis requires doxycycline daily for 4 weeks and gentamycin daily for 2 weeks. Asymptomatic infections can be treated with oral doxycycline for 15 days. If bacillary angiomatosis or peliosis hepatitis is present in patients with AIDS: doxycycline, erythromycin, or azithromycin should be used for at least 3 months. Endocarditis requires more frequent dosing of gentamycin and a 6-week duration of doxycycline. Ceftriaxone or another third-generation cephalosporin may be added for the treatment of endocarditis.
Prevention:	Hygiene and avoidance of lice. Patients with pediculosis can be treated with ivermectin and their clothing and bedding should be washed in hot water and/or treated with insecticides.

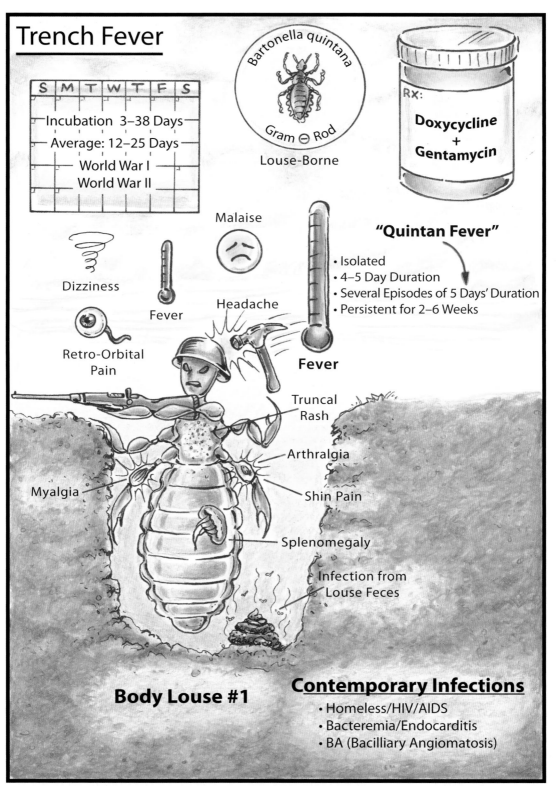

Trench Fever

S	M	T	W	T	F	S

Incubation 3–38 Days
Average: 12–25 Days
World War I
World War II

Bartonella quintana
Gram ⊖ Rod
Louse-Borne

RX:
Doxycycline + Gentamycin

Dizziness

Malaise

Fever

Retro-Orbital Pain

Headache

"Quintan Fever"
• Isolated
• 4–5 Day Duration
• Several Episodes of 5 Days' Duration
• Persistent for 2–6 Weeks

Fever

Truncal Rash

Arthralgia

Myalgia

Shin Pain

Splenomegaly

Infection from Louse Feces

Body Louse #1

Contemporary Infections
• Homeless/HIV/AIDS
• Bacteremia/Endocarditis
• BA (Bacilliary Angiomatosis)

Disease Name: **Scrub Typhus**

Causative Agent:	*Orientia tsutsugamushi*
Vector:	Chiggers (Trombiculid mites)
Reservoir:	Small rodents
Incubation:	7–10 days
Geographic Regions Affected:	Asia Pacific Rim. Peaks in summer and autumn. Higher incidence in farmers, given increased exposure to scrub brushes and thus, chiggers.
Description:	Scrub typhus is a zoonotic rickettsial-like infection spread by mites (chiggers) common to farmers in the Pacific Rim exposed to scrub brushes. The geography, clinical picture, presence of regional lymphadenopathy, and eschars assist in the diagnosis.
Signs and Symptoms:	The disease may have a mild prodrome or can occur abruptly. Symptoms can include fever, chills, headache, diffuse myalgia, and malaise; fever can persist for up to 2 weeks. Regional lymphadenopathy and characteristic eschars may be identified at the bite sites and about 50% of patients develop a nonpruritic macular/maculopapular centrifugal rash that begins on the abdomen and spreads to the face and extremities. Nausea, vomiting, diarrhea, hepatosplenomegaly, cough, and relative bradycardia can also occur. The disease may cause multisystemic organ dysfunction and spontaneous abortion in pregnancy.
Diagnostic Testing:	The disease is often diagnosed and treated based on clinical suspicion. Serology is the most commonly used lab test, and polymerase chain reaction (PCR) testing can be performed on blood, eschar, or lymph node biopsy. A fourfold increase in IgG in convalescence is confirmatory.
Treatments:	Effective treatment options include doxycycline twice daily or chloramphenicol four times a day for 1 week. Azithromycin can be used in pregnancy or doxycycline resistance. Alternatively, rifampin can be added to doxycycline if doxycycline resistance is suspected.
Prevention:	Avoid chiggers and use insect repellants like DEET when traveling in rural areas of endemic countries.

Scrub Typhus

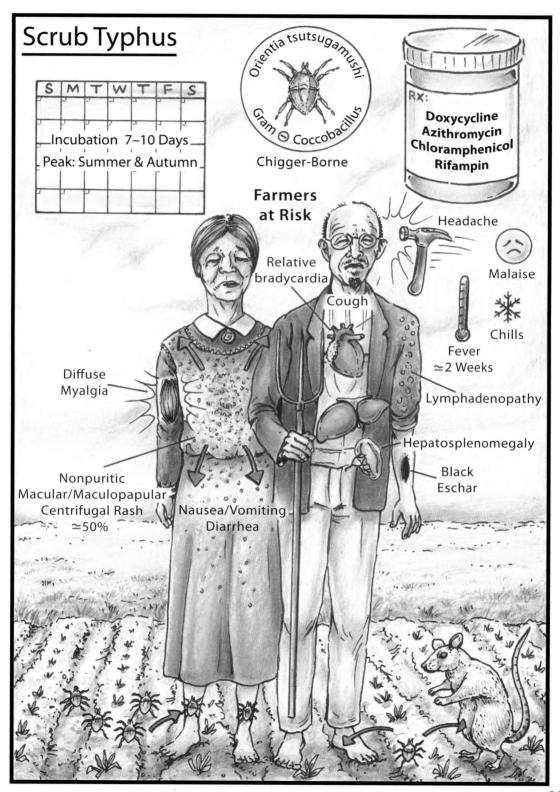

S	M	T	W	T	F	S

Incubation 7–10 Days
Peak: Summer & Autumn

Orientia tsutsugamushi
Gram ⊖ Coccobacillus
Chigger-Borne

RX:
Doxycycline
Azithromycin
Chloramphenicol
Rifampin

Farmers at Risk

Headache
Malaise
Chills
Fever ≃2 Weeks

Relative bradycardia
Cough
Lymphadenopathy
Hepatosplenomegaly
Black Eschar

Diffuse Myalgia

Nonpuritic Macular/Maculopapular Centrifugal Rash ≃50%

Nausea/Vomiting Diarrhea

Disease Name: **Epidemic Typhus**

Synonyms:	Louse-borne typhus, jail fever
Causative Agent:	*Rickettsia prowazekii*
Vector:	Human Body and Head Louse (*Pediculus humanus corporis* and *capitis*)
Reservoir:	Humans. The flying squirrel is a potential animal reservoir.
Incubation:	5–23 days; Average: 10–14 days
Geographic Regions Affected:	Can occur worldwide; however, most recent cases have occurred in Burundi, Rwanda, and Ethiopia.
Description:	Epidemic typhus is a zoonosis transmitted via the human body or head louse. Recent cases in the United States have implicated the flying squirrel as a potential animal reservoir.
Signs and Symptoms:	*Acute*: High fever, chills, headache, confusion, myalgia, cough, dyspnea, tachypnea, arthralgia, nausea, and abdominal pain occur early in the illness followed by the appearance of a dark macular/maculopapular, centrifugal rash that spares the face, palms, and soles. The rash occurs in 64% of individuals after several days of illness. If untreated, mortality is around 40%. *Brill-Zinsser Disease*: After years or decades, individuals with a previous infection and weakened immune system may have a recrudescence of disease. This occurs in the elderly and mimics the initial infection, although milder and with a fainter rash. Severe symptoms and death are rare.
Diagnostic Testing:	Labs may reveal thrombocytopenia, hyponatremia, hypocalcemia, hypoalbuminemia, and elevated liver enzymes. WBC can be normal, elevated, or decreased. Polymerase chain reaction (PCR) testing can confirm the diagnosis acutely, while serology mostly confirms the diagnosis in retrospect. A fourfold increase in IgG in convalescence is confirmatory.
Treatments:	Effective treatment options include doxycycline twice daily for 1 week or chloramphenicol four times a day for 5 days.
Prevention:	Avoid flying squirrels. Delousing humans, bedding, and clothing can reduce the transmission of *P. humanus*. A weekly dose of 200 mg oral doxycycline can be used as chemoprophylaxis if there is a high likelihood of exposure.
Pearls:	Crowding, overpopulation, war, and famine are all linked to an increased incidence of epidemic typhus.

Epidemic Typhus

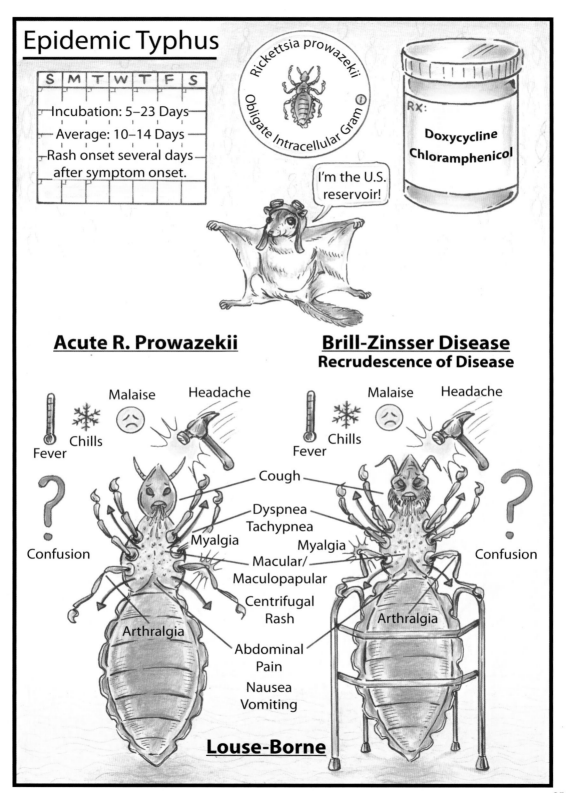

S	M	T	W	T	F	S
Incubation: 5–23 Days						
Average: 10–14 Days						
Rash onset several days after symptom onset.						

Rickettsia prowazekii
Obligate Intracellular Gram ⊕

RX:
Doxycycline
Chloramphenicol

I'm the U.S. reservoir!

Acute R. Prowazekii

Fever — Chills — Malaise — Headache
Confusion
Myalgia
Arthralgia

Brill-Zinsser Disease
Recrudescence of Disease

Fever — Chills — Malaise — Headache
Confusion
Myalgia
Arthralgia

Cough
Dyspnea
Tachypnea
Macular/ Maculopapular
Centrifugal Rash
Abdominal Pain
Nausea
Vomiting

Louse-Borne

Disease Name: **Endemic Typhus**

Synonyms:	Murine typhus, flea-borne typhus
Causative Agent:	*Rickettsia typhi*
Vector:	Rat Flea *(Xenopsylla cheopis);* less commonly, cat and mouse fleas serve as vectors.
Reservoir:	Rats
Incubation:	1–2 weeks
Geographic Regions Affected:	Worldwide. U.S. cases have been reported in Texas, California, and Hawaii.
Description:	Endemic typhus is a zoonosis transmitted to humans by fleas from infected rats.
Signs and Symptoms:	Fever, chills, headache, and myalgia occur early in the illness followed by the appearance of a faint, maculopapular, centrifugal rash that spares the palms and soles. The rash occurs in 20% to 50% of individuals after several days of illness. Nausea, vomiting, diarrhea, and abdominal pain may occur and is more common in children. Severe disease can cause cough and dyspnea, liver dysfunction, acute kidney injury, and/or splenomegaly with rupture.
Diagnostic Testing:	Labs may reveal thrombocytopenia, hyponatremia, hypoalbuminemia, and increased liver enzymes. WBC can be normal, elevated, or decreased. Anemia may be present. The disease is often diagnosed and treated based on clinical suspicion, as serology mostly confirms the disease in retrospect.
Treatments:	Effective treatment options include doxycycline twice daily for 1 week or chloramphenicol four times a day for 5 days.
Prevention:	Rodent control to reduce the number of hosts. Proper flea control measures for domestic pets, specifically cats.
Pearls:	A clinical disease picture similar to endemic typhus has been found to be caused by *Rickettsia felis*, carried by cat fleas, with opossums and cats serving as potential reservoirs.

Endemic Typhus

(Murine Typhus)

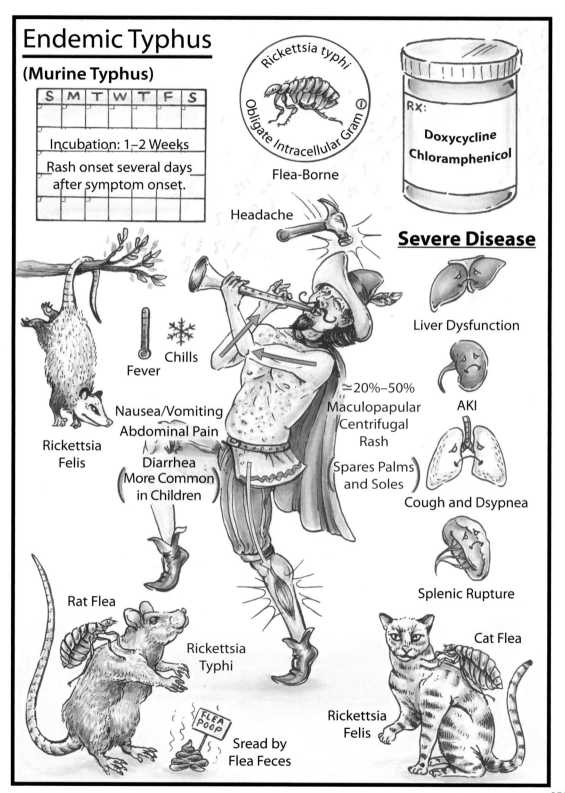

S	M	T	W	T	F	S

Incubation: 1–2 Weeks

Rash onset several days after symptom onset.

Rickettsia typhi
Obligate Intracellular Gram ⊖

Flea-Borne

RX:
Doxycycline
Chloramphenicol

Headache

Severe Disease

Fever

Chills

Liver Dysfunction

Nausea/Vomiting
Abdominal Pain

≈20%–50%
Maculopapular
Centrifugal
Rash

AKI

Rickettsia
Felis

Diarrhea
(More Common
in Children)

Spares Palms
and Soles

Cough and Dsypnea

Splenic Rupture

Rat Flea

Rickettsia
Typhi

Cat Flea

FLEA
POOP

Rickettsia
Felis

Sread by
Flea Feces

Disease Name: **Arenaviridae**

Lymphocytic Choriomeningitis:

- Causative Agent: Lymphocytic choriomeningitis virus (LCMV)
- Vector: Urine from *Mus musculus*—house mouse
- Region: Worldwide. The Centers for Disease Control and Prevention (CDC) estimates that 5% of U.S. house mice carry the LCMV virus.
- Incubation: 8–13 days
- Symptoms: LCM is a biphasic febrile disease, with the second stage thought to be related to the host immune response. Initial symptoms include fever, malaise, headache, myalgia, nausea, and vomiting. In some individuals, a second phase of illness with fever, meningitis, encephalitis, or meningoencephalitis occurs. Acute hydrocephalus can occur in the second phase. The overall mortality is low. Some patients have developed postinfectious myocarditis, orchitis, and/or arthritis.
- Diagnosis: Lumbar puncture (LP) will reveal an increased opening pressure, increased CSF proteins, and a large number of lymphocytes.
- Treatment: Supportive.

Viral Hemorrhagic Fevers:

Viral hemorrhagic fevers caused by the Arenaviruses are thought to be transmitted to humans via the excreta of rodents. Lassa is the best understood of these infections and early treatment with ribavirin is thought to have some benefit.

Disease	Virus	Vector	Distribution	Discovered
Argentine HF	Junin Virus	Drylands Vesper Mouse	Argentina	1958
Bolivian HF	Machupo Virus	Large Vesper Mouse	Bolivia	1963
Brazilian HF	Sabia Virus	Unknown Rodent (?)	Brazil	1993
Chapare HF	Chapare Virus	Unknown Rodent (?)	Bolivia	2008
Lassa HF	Lassa Virus	Multimammate Rat	West Africa	1969
Lujo HF	Lujo Virus	Unknown Rodent (?)	South Africa	2008
Venezuelan HF	Guanarito Virus	Short-tailed Cane Mouse	Venezuela	1989

Arenaviridae

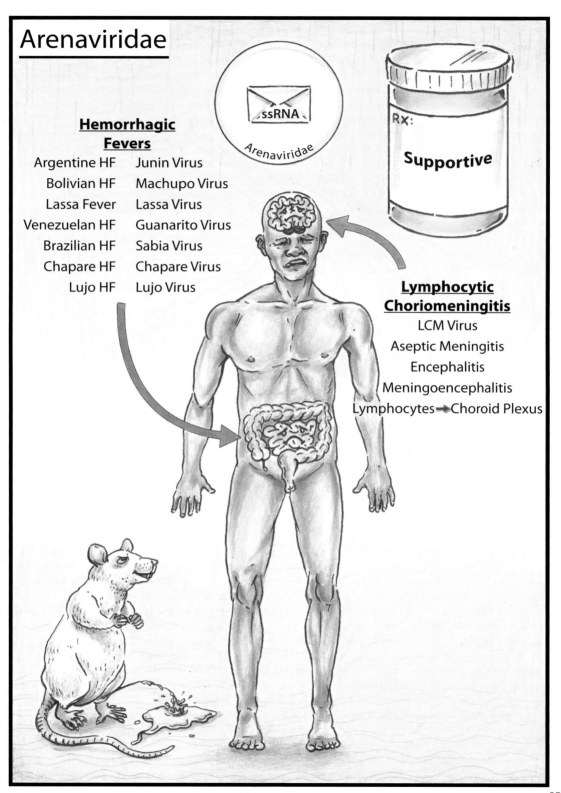

Hemorrhagic Fevers

Argentine HF	Junin Virus
Bolivian HF	Machupo Virus
Lassa Fever	Lassa Virus
Venezuelan HF	Guanarito Virus
Brazilian HF	Sabia Virus
Chapare HF	Chapare Virus
Lujo HF	Lujo Virus

ssRNA
Arenaviridae

RX:
Supportive

Lymphocytic Choriomeningitis

LCM Virus

Aseptic Meningitis

Encephalitis

Meningoencephalitis

Lymphocytes → Choroid Plexus

PART 11

OROPHARYNGEAL INFECTIONS

Disease Name: **Peritonsillar Abscess**

Synonym: Quinsy

Causative Agents: Aerobic bacteria: *Streptococcus, Staphylococcus, Haemophilus*
Anaerobic bacteria: *Fusobacterium, Peptostreptococcus, Prevotella, Bacteroides*

Incubation: Variable—Patients usually present a few days after initial symptom onset.

Geographic Regions Affected: Worldwide

Description: Peritonsillar abscess (PTA) is a common soft tissue abscess encountered in clinical practice that occurs either spontaneously or as the result of untreated tonsillitis.

Signs and Symptoms: Symptoms are often progressive and begin as odynophagia and sore throat on the ipsilateral (same) side of the infection. Fever, malaise, worsening pain, and ipsilateral lymphadenopathy and neck pain occur next, as well as halitosis and muffled "hot potato voice." Significant illness can present with trismus and/or drooling. Complications can include Lemierre syndrome, a thrombophlebitis of the internal jugular vein, most commonly from anaerobic *Fusobacterium*.

Diagnostic Testing: PTA is often a visual diagnosis. Inspection of the oropharynx will reveal erythema and swelling of the peritonsillar area and uvular deviation toward the unaffected side. If trismus is present, a soft-tissue CT of the neck with IV contrast can be obtained to evaluate for PTA and rule out other types of soft tissue abscesses/deep space infections. Gram stain and wound cultures can be obtained during drainage or aspiration of the abscess. Peripheral labs would likely reveal a leukocytosis and elevated C-reactive protein (CRP).

Treatments: Needle aspiration or incision and drainage are often performed at the bedside by the EM physician or ENT. Appropriate antibiotics following drainage include penicillin with or without metronidazole or clindamycin in cases of penicillin allergy. Amoxicillin with clavulanic acid is often a good antibiotic choice for outpatient management.

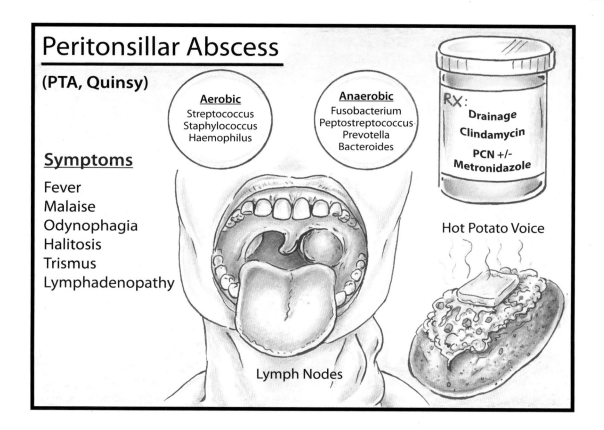

Peritonsillar Abscess

(PTA, Quinsy)

Aerobic
Streptococcus
Staphylococcus
Haemophilus

Anaerobic
Fusobacterium
Peptostreptococcus
Prevotella
Bacteroides

RX:
Drainage
Clindamycin
PCN +/-
Metronidazole

Symptoms

Fever
Malaise
Odynophagia
Halitosis
Trismus
Lymphadenopathy

Hot Potato Voice

Lymph Nodes

Disease Name: Diphtheria

Causative Agent: *Corynebacterium diphtheriae*

Incubation: 2–5 days

Geographic Regions Affected: Worldwide. The disease is extremely rare in the United States secondary to vaccinations.

Description: Diphtheria is a vaccine-preventable, bacterial infection of the respiratory tract caused by *C. diphtheriae*, a gram-positive, pleomorphic, toxin-producing bacteria. Disease can occur anywhere from the nasopharynx to the tracheobronchial tree, with the tonsils and oropharynx (tonsillopharyngeal) the most common sites of infection. Diphtheria is known for its characteristic gray pseudomembrane.

Signs and Symptoms: Some patients may become asymptomatic carriers after exposure.

Tonsillopharyngeal diphtheria: Symptoms are often progressive and begin as odynophagia, pharyngeal erythema, and sore throat. Low-grade fever, chills, malaise, fatigue, worsening pain, and lymphadenopathy follow. A characteristic gray pseudomembrane comprised of white blood cells, fibrin, and dead tissue often forms. This membrane can potentially spread through the respiratory tract, causing more significant symptoms.

Nasal diphtheria: Involvement of the nasopharynx is characterized by nasal congestion and mucopurulent, bloody nasal discharge.

Laryngeal diphtheria: If the pseudomembrane extends down into the larynx, "diphtheritic croup" can occur, potentially causing respiratory compromise. These patients will have a barking cough, stridor, hoarseness, significant neck swelling (bull neck), and may become hypoxic and cyanotic. In addition to localized disease, diphtheria toxin may spread hematogenously and cause damage to the cardiac, renal, and/or nervous systems.

Diagnostic Testing: Nasopharyngeal and oropharyngeal cultures should be obtained and plated on Loffler or Tindale media. Gram stain may reveal gram-positive rods in "Chinese character" distribution. Polymerase chain reaction (PCR) and enzyme-linked immunosorbent assay (ELISA) antigen tests can be used to detect diphtheria toxin.

Treatments: Patients should be put on isolation. Antibiotics and horse serum-based antitoxin are the mainstay of treatment. Antibiotic choices include erythromycin or penicillin for 14 days. Patients are not infectious after 48 hours of antibiotic therapy. The diphtheria antitoxin can be obtained from the Centers for Disease Control and Prevention (CDC) and dosing is based on stage and severity of illness.

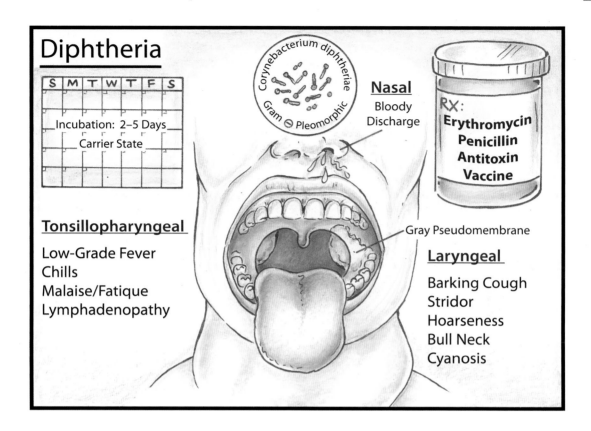

Diphtheria

S	M	T	W	T	F	S
		Incubation: 2–5 Days				
		Carrier State				

Corynebacterium diphtheriae
Gram ⊖ Pleomorphic

Nasal
Bloody Discharge

RX:
**Erythromycin
Penicillin
Antitoxin
Vaccine**

Tonsillopharyngeal

Low-Grade Fever
Chills
Malaise/Fatique
Lymphadenopathy

Gray Pseudomembrane

Laryngeal

Barking Cough
Stridor
Hoarseness
Bull Neck
Cyanosis

Disease Name: **Herpangina**

Causative Agents: ssRNA enteroviruses: Coxsackievirus A is the most common culprit. The disease can also be caused by Coxsackievirus B, Enterovirus 71, and Echovirus.

Incubation: Approximately 4 days

Geographic Regions Affected: Worldwide

Description: Herpangina is a viral disease of infants, children, and young adults characterized by fever and oropharyngeal blister formation. The disease is more common in the summer and occasionally affects adults.

Signs and Symptoms: Symptom onset is acute and consists of fever, anorexia, malaise, sore throat, headache, and neck pain. Within 2 days of symptom onset, a viral enanthem appears on the tonsillar pillars, uvula, soft palate, and posterior pharynx. Lesions may also appear on the hard palate and tongue. The enanthem typically consists of several (5–10) red papules that progress to vesicles before ulcerating. Ulcers tend to be less than 5 mm in size and heal over the course of a week.

Diagnostic Testing: Herpangina tends to be a visual diagnosis.

Treatments: Supportive. Acetaminophen and/or ibuprofen can be given for pain. Infants unable to tolerate oral feeding secondary to pain may need intravenous fluids. "Magic Mouthwash" or a lidocaine swish, gargle, and spit may be used in older patients.

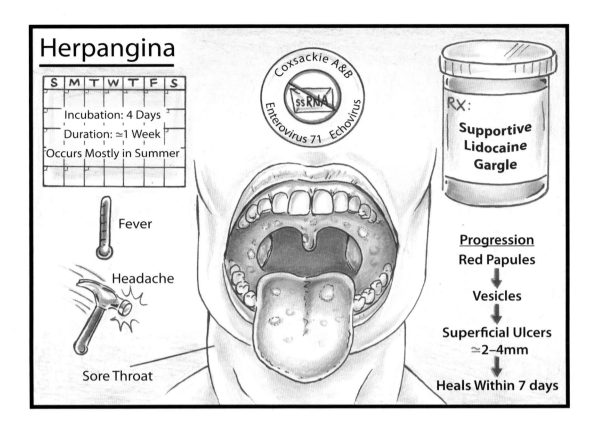

Herpangina

S	M	T	W	T	F	S
	Incubation: 4 Days					
	Duration: ≃1 Week					
	Occurs Mostly in Summer					

Fever

Headache

Sore Throat

Coxsackie A&B
Enterovirus 71   Echovirus
ssRNA

RX:
**Supportive
Lidocaine
Gargle**

Progression
Red Papules
⬇
Vesicles
⬇
Superficial Ulcers
≃2–4mm
⬇
Heals Within 7 days

Disease Name: **Thrush**

Synonyms:	Oropharyngeal candidiasis, candidal stomatitis
Causative Agent:	*Candida albicans*
Incubation:	Varied
Geographic Regions Affected:	Worldwide

Description:

Candidiasis can affect various mucous membranes, including those of the oropharynx, esophagus, and vagina. Oral candidiasis presents in one of two forms: pseudomembranous and atrophic. Thrush refers to pseudomembranous oropharyngeal candidiasis and is common in infants, patients using inhaled corticosteroids, and those with compromised immune systems (AIDS, immunosuppressants, chemotherapy, etc.) Atrophic or erythematous candidiasis lacks a pseudomembrane and is more common in older adults who wear dentures. Antibiotic use is associated with vulvovaginal candidiasis and esophageal candidiasis is associated with HIV/AIDS.

Signs and Symptoms:

While most cases of thrush are asymptomatic, patients may complain of decreased taste or mild irritation secondary to the pseudomembrane. Atrophic candidiasis can make it painful to denture wearers. HIV/AIDS patients with thrush complaining of pain with swallowing (odynophagia) should be screened for esophageal candidiasis.

Diagnostic Testing:

Usually a visual diagnosis. The pseudomembrane can be easily scraped off using a tongue depressor and will cause some mild bleeding. Samples can be sent for KOH preparation and microscopic examination.

Treatments:

Nystatin swish and swallow four times a day is the classic treatment. Clotrimazole troches placed in the buccal surface of the mouth and allowed to dissolve five times a day are more effective than nystatin. In cases of failed response to topical treatments, oral fluconazole can be prescribed.

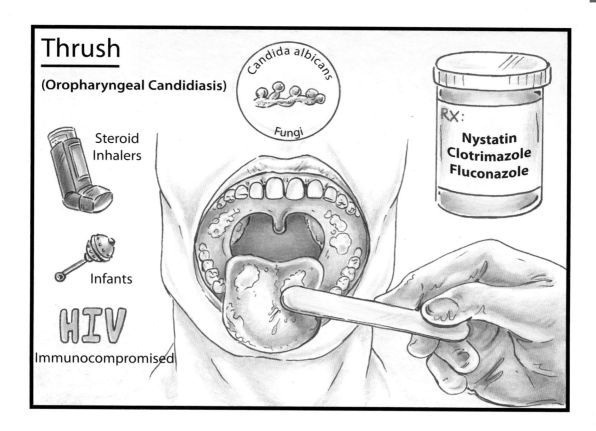

Disease Name: Streptococcal Pharyngitis

Synonym:	Strep throat
Causative Agent:	Group A *Streptococcus* (GAS), AKA: *Streptococcus pyogenes*
Incubation:	Approximately 2–5 days
Geographic Regions Affected:	Worldwide
Description:	Strep throat is the most common form of bacterial pharyngitis and peaks in late winter and early spring. Complications of strep throat can include rheumatic fever, poststreptococcal glomerulonephritis, and peritonsillar abscess.
Signs and Symptoms:	Symptom onset is acute and may consist of fever, anorexia, malaise, sore throat, headache, abdominal pain, nausea, and vomiting. On examination, patients may have enlarged tonsils with or without exudate, pharyngeal erythema, oral petechiae, and enlarged, tender cervical lymphadenopathy. Some patients may develop a scarlatiniform rash. Cough is notably absent.
Diagnostic Testing:	Rapid Strep Test (RADT: Rapid Antigen Detection Test) and throat culture are both readily available, the latter being the gold standard.
Treatments:	The purpose of treatment is to lessen disease severity, reduce transmission, and decrease the likelihood of complications like rheumatic fever. Penicillins, amoxicillin, and cephalosporins are effective treatments. Erythromycin, clindamycin, or macrolides can be used in those patients with penicillin allergies.
Modified Centor Criteria:	The Modified Centor Criteria can be applied to estimate the likelihood of strep pharyngitis. Points are added or subtracted based on risk factors to create a total score ranging from −1 to 5. The higher the score, the more likely the patient has strep pharyngitis.

Criteria	
Fever > 38°	+1
Exudate	+1
Tender Nodes	+1
Absent Cough	+1
Age 3–14	+1
Age 15–44	0
Age ≥45	−1

Interpretation	
Total Points	**Strep Probability (%)**
0	1–2.5
1	5–10
2	11–17
3	28–35
≥4	51–53

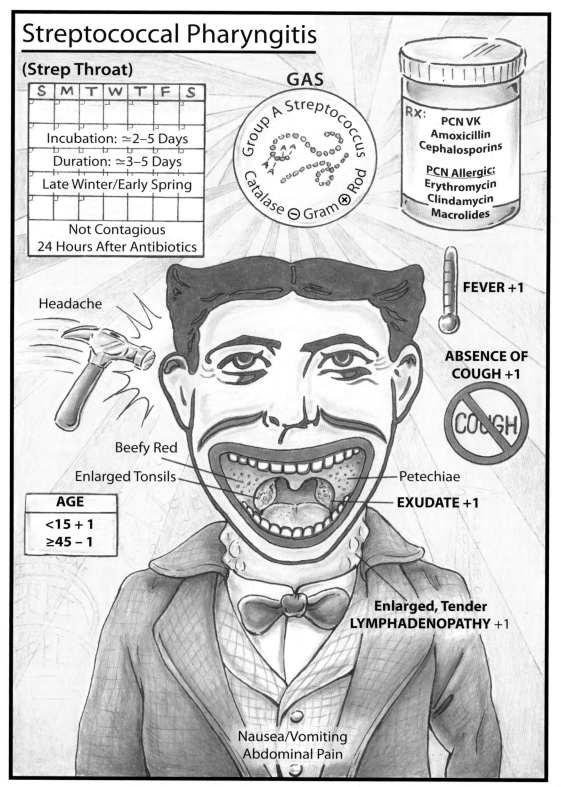

Streptococcal Pharyngitis

(Strep Throat)

S	M	T	W	T	F	S
	Incubation: ≃2–5 Days					
	Duration: ≃3–5 Days					
	Late Winter/Early Spring					
	Not Contagious					
	24 Hours After Antibiotics					

GAS
Group A Streptococcus
Catalase ⊖ Gram ⊗ Rod

RX:
PCN VK
Amoxicillin
Cephalosporins

PCN Allergic:
Erythromycin
Clindamycin
Macrolides

FEVER +1

ABSENCE OF COUGH +1

Headache

Beefy Red

Enlarged Tonsils

Petechiae

EXUDATE +1

AGE
<15 + 1
≥45 − 1

Enlarged, Tender LYMPHADENOPATHY +1

Nausea/Vomiting
Abdominal Pain

PART 12

VIRAL

Disease Name: **Ebola**

Synonyms:	Ebola hemorrhagic fever, Ebola virus disease
Causative Agent:	Ebola virus
Reservoir:	Fruit bats
Incubation:	2–21 days; Average: 8–10 days
Geographic Regions Affected:	West and Central Africa

Description: Ebola is viral hemorrhagic fever disease of humans and primates with a high mortality. Bats are thought to serve as the animal reservoir and humans initially get infected by consuming bushmeat (bats, gorillas, chimpanzees, shrews, and duikers). Once infected, human-to-human transmission occurs via contact with infectious blood or bodily fluids including mucus, feces, vomit, saliva, breastmilk, semen, and possibly sweat. Blood, vomit, and feces are the most infectious fluids. Dead bodies may also be infectious, exposing those who prepare and touch the body during burial ceremonies to risk of infection.

Signs and Symptoms: Initial symptoms are flu-like and include fever, chills, malaise, weakness, headache, and myalgia. Next, patients develop nausea, vomiting, watery diarrhea, abdominal pain, and a maculopapular rash. Severe disease can cause renal failure, transaminitis, disseminated intravascular coagulation (DIC), and hemorrhage. Signs of hemorrhage include hematochezia, petechiae, bruising, mucosal bleeding, and hematemesis.

Diagnostic Testing: ELISA, IgM/IgG, virus isolation, immunohistochemistry, and polymerase chain reaction (PCR) tests are available to confirm the diagnosis.

Treatment: Supportive. Experimental treatments and vaccines are being pursued.

Pearls: There are five species of the Ebola virus genus: Zaire ebolavirus (ZEBOV), Bundibugyo ebolavirus (BDBV), Tai Forest ebolavirus (TAFV), Sudan ebolavirus (SUDV), and Reston ebolavirus (RESTV). Ebola viruses are closely related to the Marburg virus, another filovirus that causes outbreaks of viral hemorrhagic fever.

Ebola

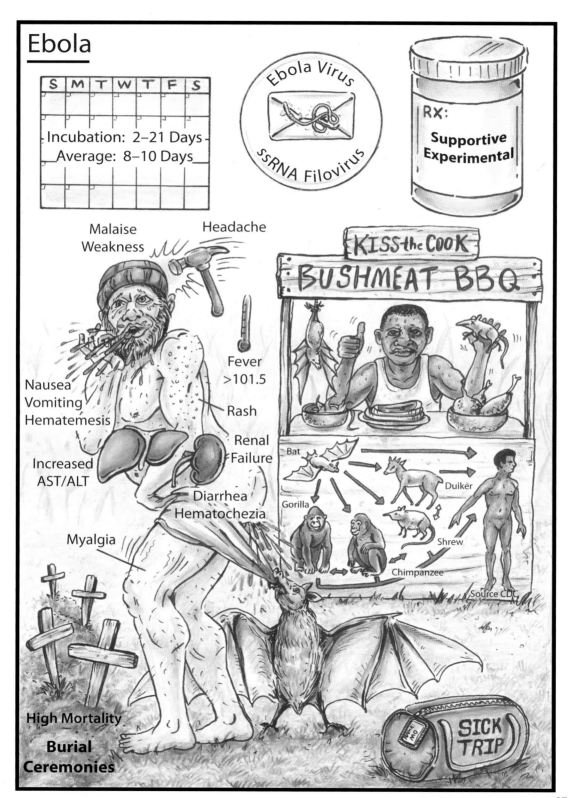

Incubation: 2–21 Days
Average: 8–10 Days

Ebola Virus
ssRNA Filovirus

RX: **Supportive Experimental**

Malaise Weakness
Headache
Fever >101.5
Nausea Vomiting Hematemesis
Rash
Increased AST/ALT
Renal Failure
Diarrhea Hematochezia
Myalgia
High Mortality
Burial Ceremonies

KISS the COOK
BUSHMEAT BBQ

Bat
Gorilla
Duiker
Shrew
Chimpanzee
Source CDC

SICK TRIP

Disease Name: **Rabies**

Synonym:	Hydrophobia
Causative Agent:	Rabies virus
Reservoirs:	Bats, raccoons, skunks, and foxes in the United States; dogs in developing nations.
Incubation:	About 1–3 months for most cases. Onset can be delayed for years!
Geographic Regions Affected:	Worldwide; highest incidence in Asia and Africa.
Description:	Rabies is a fatal viral zoonosis transmitted from the saliva of infected animals to humans. After a relatively long incubation period, patients develop an encephalopathy followed by death. The disease can have one of two presentations, either encephalopathic (furious rabies) or paralytic (dumb rabies). Encephalopathic rabies is the classic and more common presentation, notable for hydrophobia (fear of water) and spasms of the pharynx that occur when the patient attempts to drink water.
Signs and Symptoms:	Prodromal symptoms may include fever, headache, malaise, nausea, vomiting, and pain or paresthesia at the site of the bite. When the virus spreads to the central nervous system, patients will exhibit one of two clinical presentations of the disease. *Furious Rabies*: This is the most common presentation (70%) and includes the classic findings of hydrophobia, insomnia, confusion, paranoia, anxiety, agitation, and hallucinations progressing to coma and death. *Paralytic Rabies*: Presents in 30% of patients and is associated with an ascending flaccid paralysis, fever, confusion, coma, and death.
Diagnostic Testing:	Direct immunofluorescent staining of skin biopsy specimen, polymerase chain reaction (PCR) testing of saliva or skin biopsy, and/or detection of anti-rabies virus antibodies in serum or cerebral spinal fluid (CSF).
Treatments:	Supportive. Most patients die within 10 days of the onset of coma. There is a vaccination series to prevent rabies given as either a preexposure or postexposure prophylaxis. Preexposure vaccinations are given on days 0, 7, and 21 or 28 and are recommended for veterinarians, rabies researchers, and some travelers. Postexposure vaccinations are given on days 0, 3, 7, and 14, with immunocompromised patients getting a fifth dose on day 28. In addition to vaccination, postexposure prophylaxis includes weight-based rabies immune globulin on day 0, with half the dose administered as close to the wound as possible. Those who have received the preexposure vaccination series do not need immune globulin and should be given booster shots of the vaccine at days 0 and 3. Proper handwashing and cleaning of any bite wounds with iodine can help reduce transmission of rabies.

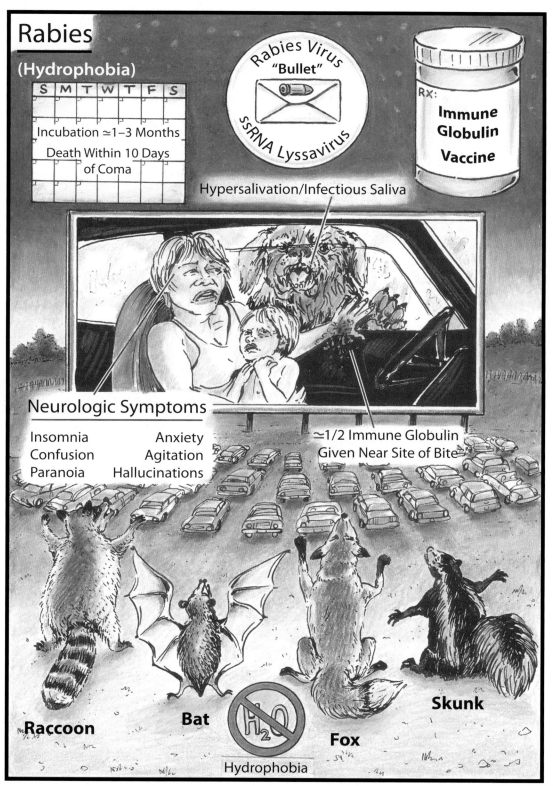

Rabies

(Hydrophobia)

S	M	T	W	T	F	S

Incubation ≃1–3 Months

Death Within 10 Days of Coma

Rabies Virus "Bullet"

ssRNA Lyssavirus

RX: **Immune Globulin Vaccine**

Hypersalivation/Infectious Saliva

Neurologic Symptoms

Insomnia	Anxiety
Confusion	Agitation
Paranoia	Hallucinations

≃1/2 Immune Globulin Given Near Site of Bite

Raccoon

Bat

H₂O — Hydrophobia

Fox

Skunk

273

Disease Name: AIDS: Opportunistic Infections

We have summarized the most common opportunistic infections associated with HIV/AIDS and have organized them based on organ system and CD4 counts. With HIV infections, it is important to remember that an individual's viral load indicates how infectious they are to others and their CD4 count indicates how healthy their immune system is. The CD4 counts we have selected indicate when the patient is at a higher risk for infection and/or when prophylactic treatment should be initiated.

Any CD4 Count

Tuberculosis: Patients with HIV are at higher risk of tuberculosis (TB) infection and should be screened with purified protein derivative (PPD) regardless of CD4 counts. Latent TB should be treated to prevent potential reactivation to active TB.

Oral Candidiasis: Thrush can occur at any time in HIV-positive individuals, although it is less common with CD4 counts ≥500. Incidence increases as CD4 counts become lower (≤200), and recurrent infections are often a sign of HIV disease progression. Treatment options include oral fluconazole daily for 1–2 weeks, nystatin swish and swallow 4–5 times a day for 1–2 weeks, or clotrimazole troches 4–5 times a day for 1–2 weeks.

Kaposi Sarcoma: Kaposi sarcoma (KS) is an AIDS-defining illness that can occur with any CD4 count, although is more common when CD4 counts drop below 250. The cancer is caused by human herpes virus 8 (HHV-8) and typically presents as red, purple, brown, or black papular lesions on the skin or mucous membranes. KS and bacillary angiomatosis (BA) may have similar appearances.

CD4 Count ≤250

Coccidioidomycosis: HIV-infected individuals residing in endemic regions are at greater risk of infection when CD4 counts drop below 250. Patients with CD4 counts <250 should be screened serologically (IgM/IgG) once or twice a year and positive results may indicate active disease. Asymptomatic patients with positive serological findings should be treated with daily fluconazole until CD4 counts rise to >250.

CD4 Count ≤200

Bacterial Pneumonia: HIV-positive individuals can acquire bacterial pneumonia at any time; however, risk increases with lower CD4 counts. HIV-positive individuals with CD4 counts ≤200 should be vaccinated against *Streptococcus pneumoniae* using the *23*-valent polysaccharide pneumococcal vaccine once every 5 years.

Pneumocystis Pneumonia: Pneumocystis pneumonia is an AIDS-defining illness caused by the yeast-like fungus *Pneumocystis jirovecii*. Symptoms of infection include fever, chills, nonproductive cough, chest pain, and dyspnea. Diagnosis should be suspected in susceptible individuals with the above symptoms, especially in those with lower CD4 counts. Chest x-ray can be normal early in the course of disease, but often reveals bilateral, ground-glass, interstitial infiltrates in a butterfly pattern. Diagnosis is confirmed via sputum sample or broncheoalveolar lavage. Prophylaxis with TMP/SMX should be initiated in patients with CD4 counts ≤200. Sulfa allergic patients can take dapsone, dapsone and pyrimethamine with leucovorin, aerosolized pentamidine, or atovaquone as alternatives to TMP/SMX. TMP/SMX is the preferred treatment of active disease, with prednisone added for more severe illness.

Isosporiasis: Isosporiasis (AKA: Cystoisosporiasis) is a watery, nonbloody, diarrheal illness caused by a protozoal infection with *Cystoisospora belli*. The disease is more common in subtropical and tropical regions, such as the Caribbean and Central and South America. In the immunocompromised, diarrheal illness can be quite severe. Infections lasting longer than 1 month are considered chronic and serve as an AIDS-defining illness. Diagnosis is made with stool ova and parasite (O&P) studies. Acute infections should be treated with TMP/SMX. Pyrimethamine with leucovorin or ciprofloxacin as a single agent are alternatives to TMP/SMX in sulfa-allergic patients. Patients will require chronic antibiotic maintenance therapy until CD4 counts rise to ≥200 and then for at least 6 months thereafter.

CD4 Count ≤150

Histoplasmosis: Individuals living in hyperendemic areas with CD4 counts ≤150 should start primary prophylaxis against histoplasmosis using itraconazole 200 mg by mouth daily. Prophylaxis can be discontinued if CD4 counts rise and stay above 150 for at least 6 months. If patients develop active disease, the preferred treatment for moderate to severe disseminated histoplasmosis is intravenous (IV) amphotericin B for at least 2 weeks followed by daily itraconazole maintenance for at least 12 months.

CD4 Count ≤100

Esophageal Candidiasis: Candidal infections of the esophagus tend to present with concurrent oropharyngeal candidiasis, but not always. Symptoms of esophageal involvement include retrosternal chest pain and pain with swallowing (odynophagia). While oropharyngeal candidiasis can occur anytime during HIV infection, incidence increases with CD4 counts ≤200. Esophageal candidiasis is more likely with CD4 counts ≤100. Diagnosis of esophageal candidiasis is often made based on symptoms and can be confirmed with EGD. Treatment requires systemic antifungals and patients will often have symptomatic improvement within a few days of initiating treatment. Preferred treatments include fluconazole (oral or intravenous) or itraconazole (oral) for 2–3 weeks.

Toxoplasmosis: *Toxoplasma gondii* is an intracellular protozoa capable of causing encephalitis in individuals with low CD4 counts, typically ≤50. Primary infection is often asymptomatic and is acquired through the ingestion of cysts in undercooked meat or oocysts commonly found in cat feces and litter boxes. Since the vast majority of disease occurs via the reactivation of tissue cysts in immunocompromised hosts, prophylaxis is indicated for patients with CD4 counts ≤100 and previous exposure to toxoplasmosis (IgG positive). TMP/SMX is the preferred prophylactic agent. Dapsone, dapsone and pyrimethamine with leucovorin, atovaquone, or atovaquone and pyrimethamine with leucovorin are alternatives to TMP/SMX in sulfa-allergic patients. Toxoplasmosis encephalitis can present as a new focal neurologic deficit, such as hemiparesis or speech deficit, seizure, or coma. Other symptoms can include fever, headache, and altered mental status. CT or MRI classically reveals multiple ring-enhancing lesions. The diagnosis can be confirmed via lumbar puncture and polymerase chain reaction (PCR) testing of cerebral spinal fluid (CSF) for toxoplasmosis. Preferred treatment is pyrimethamine and sulfadiazine with leucovorin.

Cryptococcus: *Cryptococcus neoformans* is a yeast that causes disseminated disease in HIV/AIDS patients with low CD4 counts. It often presents as subacute meningoencephalitis or meningitis with symptoms including fever, malaise, and headache, often without photophobia and meningismus. Diagnosis is confirmed with lumbar puncture and CSF analysis. Opening pressure is often elevated. Cryptococcal antigen (CrAg) testing can be performed on both serum and CSF. CSF microscopy using India ink staining will often show encapsulated, budding yeast. Various treatment regimens exist and utilize amphotericin B, flucytosine, fluconazole, and/or combinations thereof.

Cryptosporidiosis: Cryptosporidiosis is a watery, non-bloody, diarrheal illness caused by a protozoal infection of the small bowel mucosa. Severity of illness correlates to immune system health. Immune-competent patients may be asymptomatic or have a mild diarrheal illness, while immunocompromised patients may present with fever, abdominal pain, and profuse diarrhea. Individuals with CD4 counts ≤100 are more likely to have severe symptoms and prolonged infections. Treatment focuses on improving CD4 counts with antiretroviral therapy (ART). Nitazoxanide or paromomycin may be added as an adjunctive treatment.

Microsporidiosis: Microsporidia are ubiquitous, water-borne protozoa capable of causing gastrointestinal (GI) illness and diarrhea in immunocompromised hosts. Risk of infection increases when CD4 counts drop to ≤100. Treatment is focused on raising CD4 counts to ≥100 using antiretroviral therapy (ART), after which diarrhea typically resolves.

CD4 Count ≤50

Cytomegalovirus Infections: Cytomegalovirus (CMV) can cause localized or disseminated disease in individuals with HIV/AIDS, typically not until CD4 counts drop to ≤50. HIV/AIDS-associated CMV infections include retinitis, esophagitis, colitis, and encephalitis. CMV retinitis is the most common presentation of CMV infection. The symptoms are often unilateral (two thirds of cases) and include vision changes, peripheral vision loss, scotomata, and/or floaters. Patients should be seen by an ophthalmologist for dilated fundoscopy to confirm the diagnosis. CMV esophagitis can present with chest pain, odynophagia, and nausea. Endoscopy (EGD) will reveal ulcerations and the distal esophagus and biopsies can be obtained to confirm the diagnosis. Symptoms of CMV colitis include abdominal pain, anorexia, weight loss, and bloody diarrhea. Colonoscopy will reveal mucosal ulcers and is required to confirm the diagnosis. Encephalitis from CMV can present as fever, headache, and confusion, often without focal neurologic deficits. Diagnosis is made with neuroimaging and lumbar puncture confirming the presence of CMV virus in the cerebral spinal fluid (CSF) using polymerase chain reaction (PCR) testing. Medications used in the treatment of CMV infections include ganciclovir, valganciclovir, and foscarnet.

Mycobacterium Avian Complex: Mycobacterium avian complex (MAC) infections are caused by either *Mycobacterium avium* or *M. intracellulare* and present as either localized or disseminated disease. Localized disease often presents as lymphadenitis with fever, while disseminated disease presents as fever with abdominal pain and diarrhea. If a disseminated MAC infection is suspected, mycobacterial blood cultures should be obtained. Blood cultures in localized disease will be negative. Primary prophylaxis against MAC should be started for individuals without active MAC infections and CD4 counts ≤50. Preferred agents for prophylaxis include azithromycin or clarithromycin; rifabutin can be used as an alternative option. Treatment for active infections consists of azithromycin or clarithromycin plus ethambutol with or without rifabutin.

Bacillary Angiomatosis: BA is the cutaneous manifestation of *Bartonella henselae* or *B. quintana* and presents as red or purplish, nonblanching papules or nodules in HIV-infected individuals. It can appear similar to KS and may require a biopsy for definitive diagnosis. Treatment is with erythromycin, doxycycline, or azithromycin.

AIDS: Opportunistic Infections

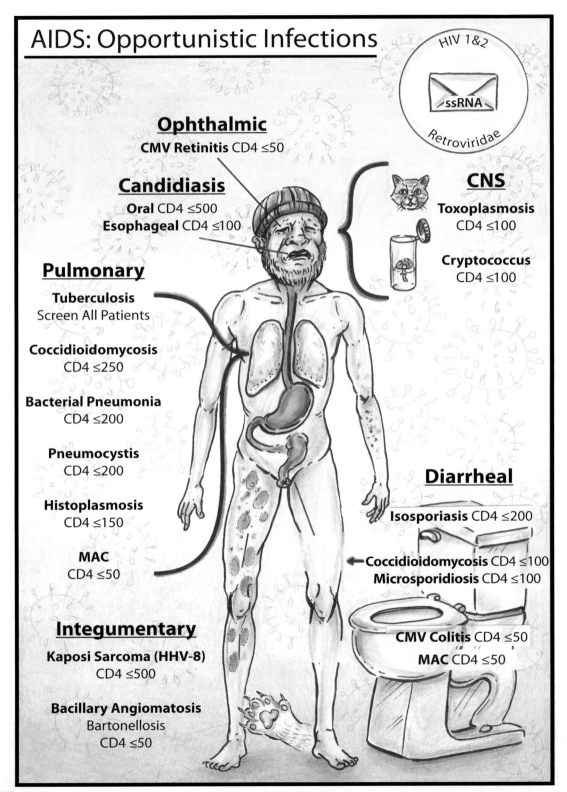

HIV 1&2
ssRNA
Retroviridae

Ophthalmic
CMV Retinitis CD4 ≤50

Candidiasis
Oral CD4 ≤500
Esophageal CD4 ≤100

CNS
Toxoplasmosis
CD4 ≤100

Cryptococcus
CD4 ≤100

Pulmonary

Tuberculosis
Screen All Patients

Coccidioidomycosis
CD4 ≤250

Bacterial Pneumonia
CD4 ≤200

Pneumocystis
CD4 ≤200

Histoplasmosis
CD4 ≤150

MAC
CD4 ≤50

Diarrheal

Isosporiasis CD4 ≤200

Coccidioidomycosis CD4 ≤100
Microsporidiosis CD4 ≤100

CMV Colitis CD4 ≤50
MAC CD4 ≤50

Integumentary

Kaposi Sarcoma (HHV-8)
CD4 ≤500

Bacillary Angiomatosis
Bartonellosis
CD4 ≤50

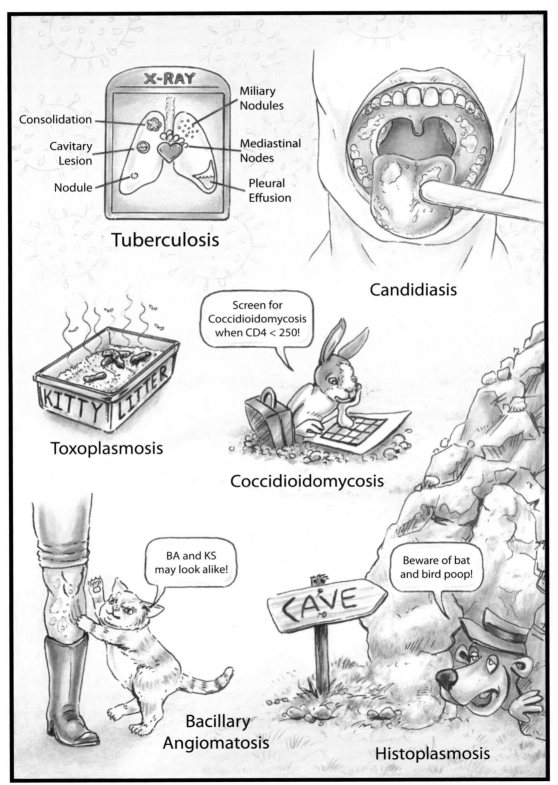

Disease Name: **Smallpox**

Causative Agent:	Variola virus
Incubation:	7–17 days; Average: 10–12 days
Geographic Regions Affected:	Eradicated globally in 1980

Description: Smallpox is a highly contagious, vaccine-preventable viral disease that was eradicated from the globe in 1980. The disease was caused by one of two strains of the Variola virus, either major or minor. Variola major is the more severe of the two, which causes a higher fever, a more significant rash, and a mortality rate up to 50%. Variola minor is less severe and carries a mortality rate of <1%. Smallpox is still studied for historical purposes and as a potential agent of bioterrorism.

Signs and Symptoms: The classic presentation of smallpox follows several phases and includes a prodrome consisting of fever, malaise, headache, myalgia, prostration, abdominal pain, nausea, vomiting, and diarrhea. Next, an enanthem appears in the mouth and on the tongue, followed by an exanthem starting on the face that spreads in a descending, centrifugal pattern. All lesions will be at the same stage as the rash progresses from macules, to papules, to vesicles, to pustules, to scabs. Patients are most contagious early in the enanthem phase of illness and are no longer contagious once all of the scabs have crusted over and fallen off. It takes about 3 weeks for the rash to progress from start to finish.

Diagnostic Testing: Polymerase chain reaction (PCR) testing of lesions and/or blood and serum as per guidelines from the Centers for Disease Control and Prevention (CDC).

Treatments: Supportive. Patient should be placed in airborne infection isolation room. The CDC should be contacted for all suspected cases of smallpox.

Pearls: The below chart is helpful in distinguishing smallpox for chickenpox.

	Smallpox	Chickenpox
Fever	2–4 Days Before Rash	At Time of Rash
Pox Progression	Slow	Rapid
Pox Stages	Same	Different
Pruritus	Doesn't Itch	Itch
Pox Depth	Deep	Superficial
Pox on Trunk	Less	More
Pox on Extremities	More	Less
Pox on Palms/Soles	More	Less

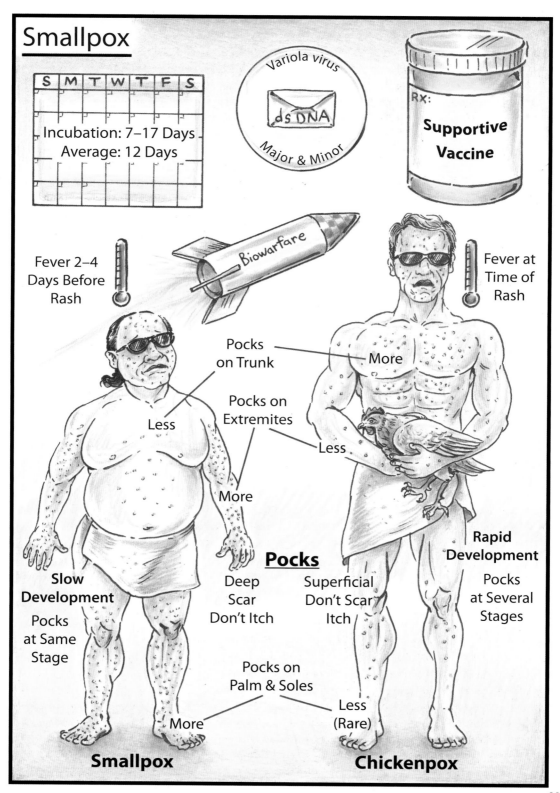

Smallpox

S	M	T	W	T	F	S

Incubation: 7–17 Days
Average: 12 Days

Variola virus
ds DNA
Major & Minor

RX:
Supportive Vaccine

Biowarfare

Fever 2–4 Days Before Rash

Fever at Time of Rash

Pocks on Trunk — **More**

Pocks on Extremites — **Less**

Less

More

Rapid Development
Pocks at Several Stages

Slow Development
Pocks at Same Stage

Pocks

Deep Scar Don't Itch

Superficial Don't Scar Itch

Pocks on Palm & Soles
More — Less (Rare)

Smallpox

Chickenpox

Disease Name: Mononucleosis

Synonyms: Infectious mononucleosis, mono, glandular fever, the kissing disease

Causative Agents: Epstein-Barr virus (EBV), AKA: human herpesvirus 4 (HHV-4)

Incubation: 4–6 weeks

Geographic Regions Affected: Worldwide

Description: Mononucleosis is a viral disease primarily of adolescents and young adults characterized by fever, pharyngitis, lymphadenopathy, and extreme fatigue. Mononucleosis is known as the kissing disease because the virus is transmitted via oral secretions and can shed into the saliva for several months after initial infection. The disease may also be spread sexually. When EBV infection occurs in early childhood, it is often asymptomatic and subclinical.

Signs and Symptoms: A mild prodrome of headache, malaise, and fatigue may precede the classic triad of high fever, pharyngitis, and lymphadenopathy. Extreme fatigue is common and may last for months, even after the other symptoms have resolved. Lymphadenopathy is symmetric and typically involves the posterior cervical chain. Pharyngitis with exudative tonsillitis is common and is often mistaken for strep throat. If ampicillin or amoxicillin is prescribed for presumed strep throat, a diffuse maculopapular rash often occurs. Hepatitis and splenomegaly are common. Splenic rupture can potentially occur and contact sports should be avoided for at least 3–4 weeks.

Diagnostic Testing: Labs will reveal lymphocytosis with ≥50% lymphocytes on peripheral smear, with ≥10% atypical in appearance. Liver enzymes (ALT/AST) are often elevated and self-limiting. Patients with mononucleosis will produce heterophile antibodies, which will cause a positive Monospot test. IgM and IgG antibody testing can also be obtained, as well as EBV DNA polymerase chain reaction (PCR) testing. Clinical presentation with characteristic CBC findings and a positive Monospot are often sufficient to make the diagnosis.

Treatments: Supportive.

Pearls: Acute cytomegalovirus (CMV) infection can have a clinical presentation similar to infectious mononucleosis. In both cases, the illnesses are self-limiting and treatment is supportive. IgM and IgG antibodies to CMV can be obtained to distinguish it from EBV infection.

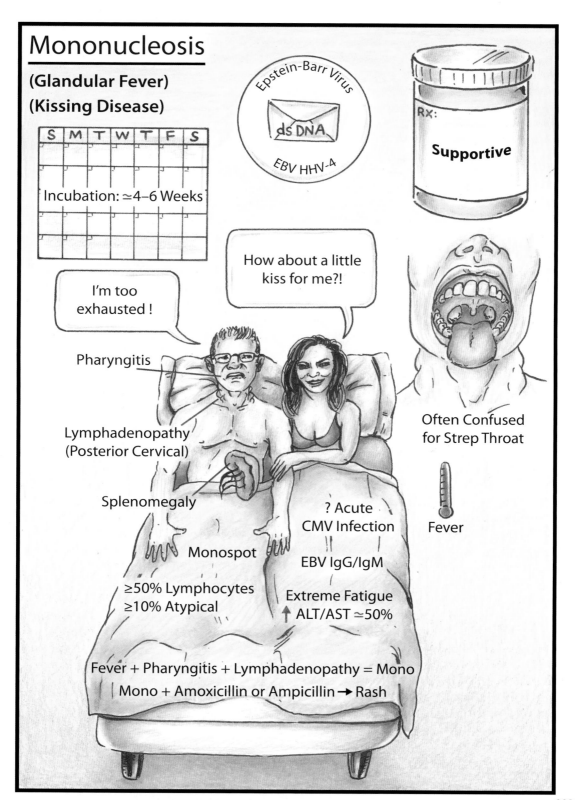

Mononucleosis

(Glandular Fever)
(Kissing Disease)

Incubation: ≃4–6 Weeks

Epstein-Barr Virus
ds DNA
EBV HHV-4

RX:
Supportive

I'm too exhausted!

How about a little kiss for me?!

Often Confused for Strep Throat

Pharyngitis

Lymphadenopathy (Posterior Cervical)

Splenomegaly

? Acute CMV Infection

EBV IgG/IgM

Fever

Monospot

≥50% Lymphocytes
≥10% Atypical

Extreme Fatigue
↑ ALT/AST ≃50%

Fever + Pharyngitis + Lymphadenopathy = Mono
Mono + Amoxicillin or Ampicillin → Rash

Disease Name: **Polio**

Synonym:	Poliomyelitis
Causative Agent:	Poliovirus, serotypes 1–3
Incubation:	Non-paralytic: 3–6 days; Paralytic: 7–21 days
Geographic Regions Affected:	Africa and Asia

Description: Poliomyelitis is a vaccine-preventable viral disease caused by one of three strains of poliovirus, a member of the enterovirus family. Due to widespread global vaccination efforts, the disease has largely been eradicated from the developed world, with some wild strain polio infections still occurring in Africa and Asia.

Signs and Symptoms: Most cases of polio ($\approx$72%) are asymptomatic. Symptomatic infections without central nervous system (CNS) involvement ($\approx$24%) are limited to several days of fever, malaise, headache, fatigue, sore throat, nausea, and vomiting. These mild infections do not involve the CNS and are referred to as "abortive polio." When there is CNS involvement (1%–5% of cases), patients develop an aseptic meningitis several days after the initial illness. Those patients who make a full recovery from the aseptic meningitis phase are said to have had non-paralytic polio. In a small percentage of patients with CNS involvement, there will be selective destruction of motor neurons, resulting in paralytic polio.

Overall, paralytic polio occurs in <1% of all infections and presents as spinal, bulbospinal, or bulbar disease. Spinal polio is the most common form of paralytic polio and causes an asymmetric weakness of the extremities, affecting the lower extremities more commonly than the upper extremities. Deep tendon reflexes will be diminished, while sensation remains intact. Bulbar polio is the least common form of paralytic polio and can present as dysphagia, dysarthria, dyspnea, and/or pooling of oral secretions. Bulbospinal polio combines aspects of both bulbar and spinal polio.

Diagnostic Testing: Polio is often suspected and diagnosed based on clinical presentation. Patients presenting with signs and symptoms of meningitis should undergo lumbar puncture. Polymerase chain reaction (PCR) testing can be performed on cerebral spinal fluid (CSF) to confirm the diagnosis. Serology can also be obtained, comparing acute and convalescent titers.

Treatments: Supportive.

Pearls: Post-polio syndrome (PPS) is a noncontagious condition that can affect adult survivors of polio 15–40 years after their initial infection. Symptoms include fatigue, arthralgia, muscle weakness, and atrophy, occurring in a slow and progressive fashion marked by long periods of stability.

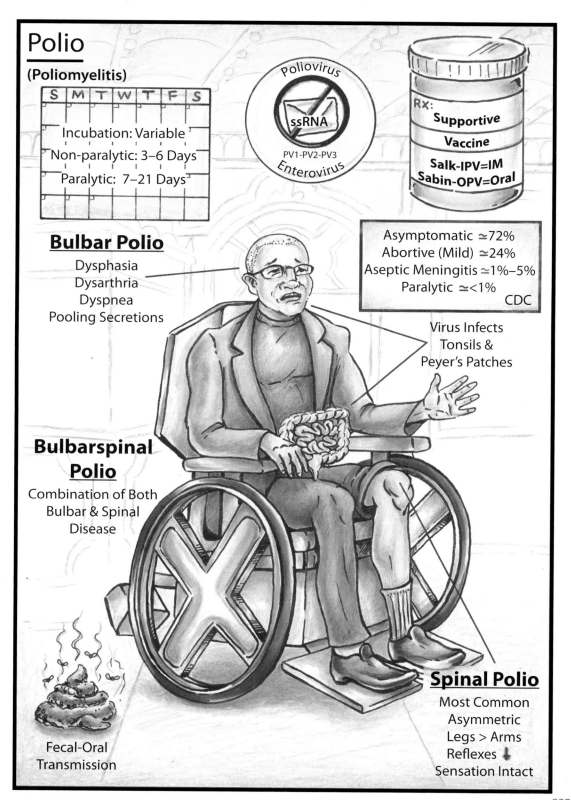

Polio

(Poliomyelitis)

S	M	T	W	T	F	S

Incubation: Variable

Non-paralytic: 3–6 Days

Paralytic: 7–21 Days

Poliovirus

ssRNA

PV1-PV2-PV3

Enterovirus

RX:
Supportive
Vaccine
Salk-IPV=IM
Sabin-OPV=Oral

Bulbar Polio

Dysphasia
Dysarthria
Dyspnea
Pooling Secretions

Asymptomatic ≃72%
Abortive (Mild) ≃24%
Aseptic Meningitis ≃1%–5%
Paralytic ≃<1%
CDC

Virus Infects
Tonsils &
Peyer's Patches

Bulbarspinal Polio

Combination of Both
Bulbar & Spinal
Disease

Fecal-Oral
Transmission

Spinal Polio

Most Common
Asymmetric
Legs > Arms
Reflexes ↓
Sensation Intact

PART 13

PARASITES AND PRIONS

Disease Name: **Chagas Disease**

Synonym:	American trypanosomiasis
Causative Agent:	*Trypanosoma cruzi*
Vector:	Triatomine bugs, also known as reduviid bugs, kissing bugs, blood suckers
Reservoir:	Many small and large mammals. In the United States, opossums, raccoons, armadillos, and rodents are common reservoirs.
Incubation:	1–2 weeks
Geographic Regions Affected:	Endemic in Mexico and Central and South America. States in the southern United States are potentially at risk (time will tell).
Description:	Chagas disease is a tropical parasitic zoonosis caused by the flagellated protozoa *T. cruzi* transmitted to humans via the feces of various Reduviid "kissing bugs." Chagas disease can also be transmitted congenitally, via blood transfusion, organ transplantation, or via consumption of food or water contaminated with bug feces. The disease has acute, intermediate, and chronic phases.
Signs and Symptoms:	*Acute Phase*: Often mild or asymptomatic, but can include fever, malaise, edema, lymphadenopathy, and hepatosplenomegaly. A chagoma is an acute sign of infection consisting of localized erythema and edema where the parasites have entered the skin. Romaña sign is the more classic sign of acute infection and consists of painless palpebral edema and conjunctivitis 1–2 weeks after the parasites have entered through the conjunctiva of the involved eye. Once the signs and symptoms of acute infection have resolved, patients enter an intermediate (latent/asymptomatic) phase that may evolve into chronic disease years or decades later. *Chronic Phase*: About one third of patients will ultimately show signs and symptoms of chronic disease, which include dilated cardiomyopathy, megaesophagus, achalasia, megacolon, and neuritis.
Diagnostic Testing:	Signs, symptoms, and history of travel or residence in an endemic region are important when considering the diagnosis. Blood smears may reveal the presence of parasites, but only in the acute phase of the disease. Chronic disease is diagnosed with serology.
Treatments:	Effective treatments include either benznidazole or nifurtimox.
Pearls:	Treatment in the United States is only available through the Centers for Disease Control and Prevention (CDC). There is a consensus that treatment is beneficial for acute infections, congenital infections, and chronic infections in children. The treatment of adults with chronic infections is considered on a case-by-case basis.

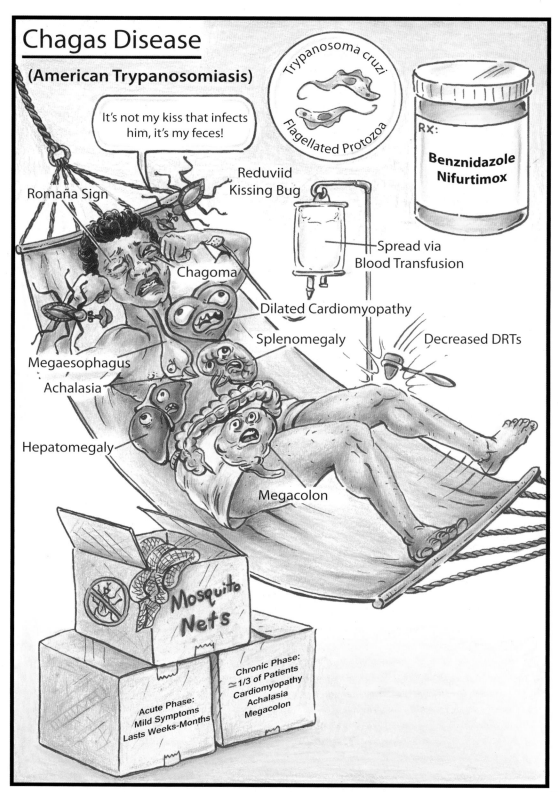

Disease Name: African Sleeping Sickness

Synonym: Human African trypanosomiasis (HAT)

Causative Agent: *Trypanosoma brucei gambiense* (West African trypanosomiasis)
Trypanosoma brucei rhodesiense (East African trypanosomiasis)

Vector: Tsetse fly

Reservoir: West African trypanosomiasis: Humans
East African trypanosomiasis: Cattle and antelope

Geographic Regions Affected: West African trypanosomiasis: tropical rainforests in Central and West Africa;
East African trypanosomiasis: savannas and wooded areas in Central, South, and
East Africa.

Description: Human African trypanosomiasis is a parasitic zoonosis caused by flagellated protozoa
T. brucei transmitted to humans via the bite of the Tsetse fly. "African sleeping sickness"
is broken down into two specific entities based on trypanosome subspecies, clinical
course, and principle regions affected. West African trypanosomiasis *(Tb. gambiense)*
has a more protracted course of illness over several months to years and accounts for
about 95% of all cases. In contrast, East African trypanosomiasis *(Tb. rhodesiense)*
progresses very rapidly over several months and accounts for less than 5% of all
cases.

Signs and Symptoms: Locally, a small chancre may develop within 1–2 weeks at the site of initial infection.
Systemically, the disease progresses through two stages. *Stage 1*: The hemolymphatic stage
is characterized by flu-like symptoms, headache, malaise, arthralgia, intermittent fever,
and progressive lymphadenopathy. Winterbottom sign (characteristic lymphadenopathy
seen at the back of the neck) is typical for West African trypanosomiasis and may be
seen at this time. *Stage 2*: The neurologic phase occurs when the parasites penetrate the
blood-brain barrier and is characterized by mood disturbances, insomnia, daytime
somnolence, Parkinson-like symptoms, tremors, ataxia, and various other neurologic
disturbances. Stage 2 illness will progress to coma and death if left untreated.

Diagnostic Testing: Signs, symptoms, and history of travel or residence in an endemic region are
important when considering the diagnosis. Tourists exploring game parks are more
likely to be exposed to East African trypanosomiasis. Microscopy of centrifuged
blood, cerebral spinal fluid (CSF), chancre fluid, and/or lymph node aspirate.
Presence of parasites in CSF confirms stage 2 disease. There are some commercially
available serologic tests.

Treatments: Choice of agent is determined by trypanosome subspecies and stage of disease. Stage
2 disease requires pharmaceutics that can penetrate the blood-brain barrier, all of
which tend to have greater side effects. Medications for each respective stage include
Stage 1: Pentamidine or suramin. *Stage 2*: Eflornithine or melarsoprol or nifurtimox.

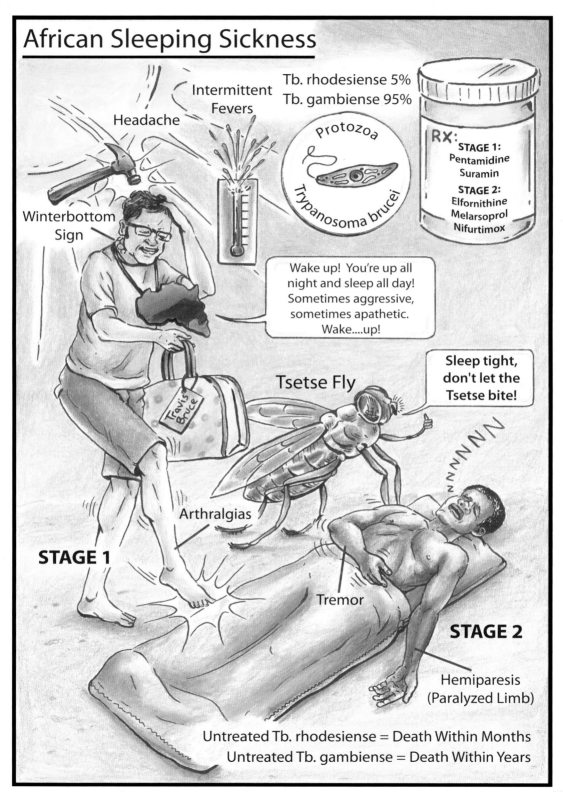

Disease Name: **Pediculosis**

Synonyms:	Lice, head lice, body lice
Causative Agents:	*Pediculus humanus capitis* (head) and *Pediculosis humanus humanus* (body)
Lifecycle:	The adult head louse is infectious and passed from human to human by close contact, including the sharing of headbands, hats, combs, and towels. Adult females lay and attach eggs (nits) to hair shafts close to the scalp. These eggs hatch after 1 week and release nymphs that go through three molts before becoming adults. Adults are about 2–3 mm long and live for about 30 days. Since head lice need frequent blood meals to survive, they can only live off of humans for 2 days.
	The body louse is very similar to the head louse with a few exceptions. Body lice are a bit larger (3–4 mm long), live and lay eggs within the seams of clothing or bedding, and only migrate onto the human to feed. They can live away from a person for longer (5–7 days) and their eggs take 1–2 weeks to hatch.
Incubation:	Variable. It takes several days for head lice to show symptoms and typically longer for body lice.
Geographic Regions Affected:	Worldwide
Description:	Head and body lice are topical ectoparasites that feed on human blood. Head lice live and lay eggs on hairs of the head near the scalp, whereas body lice live and lay their eggs in clothing. Head lice are more common in young children and are often transmitted in school via close contact or during sleepovers. Body lice are common in homeless populations, colder climates, and conditions of overcrowding.
Signs and Symptoms:	The saliva of the louse causes intense itching.
Diagnostic Testing:	Diagnosis is made via the visualization of nits (eggs) or lice attached to hair shafts near the scalp (head lice) or within the seams of clothing (body lice). A magnifying glass and/or Wood lamp are often helpful in making the diagnosis.
Treatments:	For head lice: permethrin, malathion, spinosad, or ivermectin can be used. For body lice, topical or oral medication is not indicated for the patient. However, clothing and bedding should be discarded and if not possible, thoroughly washed in hot water and treated with malathion or permethrin powder.
Pearls:	Chronic body lice infestation and subsequent bites can cause thickening and hyperpigmentation of the skin, particularly around the waistline. This condition is known as Vagabond disease. Body lice are also known to transmit epidemic typhus, trench fever, and louse-borne relapsing fever.

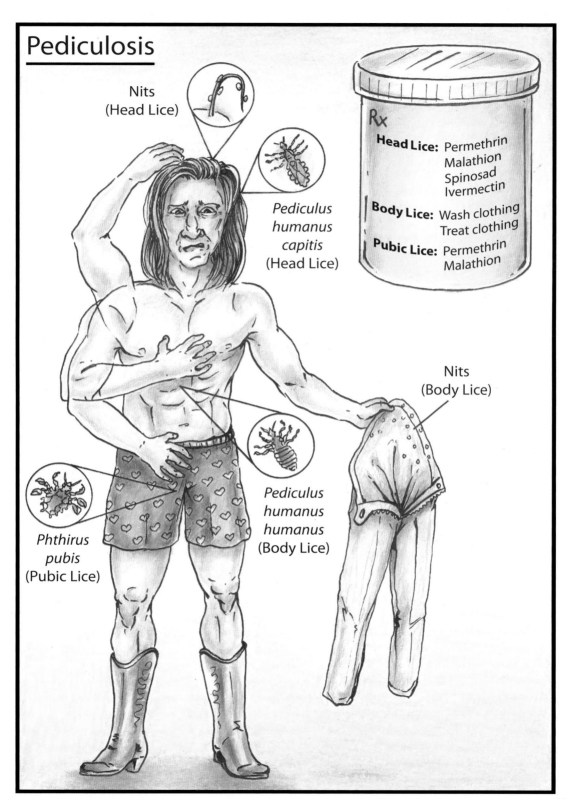

Pediculosis

Nits
(Head Lice)

Pediculus humanus capitis
(Head Lice)

Rx

Head Lice: Permethrin
Malathion
Spinosad
Ivermectin

Body Lice: Wash clothing
Treat clothing

Pubic Lice: Permethrin
Malathion

Nits
(Body Lice)

Pediculus humanus humanus
(Body Lice)

Phthirus pubis
(Pubic Lice)

Disease Name: **Naegleriasis**

Synonyms:	Primary amoebic meningoencephalitis (PAM), "brain eating amoeba"
Causative Agent:	*Naegleria fowleri*
Incubation:	1–7 days; Average: 5 days
Geographic Regions Affected:	Worldwide

Description: PAM is an extremely rare and highly fatal type of meningoencephalitis caused by the *N. fowleri* amebae. These amoebas live freely in warm bodies of freshwater and can cause PAM if they are inhaled nasally and penetrate the cribriform plate, thus gaining exposure to the brain and meninges. In most cases, there is a history of recreational exposure to bodies of warm freshwater preceding illness by several days.

Signs and Symptoms: Symptom onset is acute and similar to bacterial meningitis. Fever, headache, meningeal signs and symptoms, photophobia, neck stiffness, nausea, vomiting, altered mental status, and seizures can occur. The disease progresses rapidly, causing increased intracranial pressure and is often fatal.

Diagnostic Testing: Lumbar puncture is obligatory to make the diagnosis and often reveals an increased opening pressure. Cerebral spinal fluid (CSF) will reveal a neutrophil-predominant leukocytosis, erythrocytosis, decreased glucose, and increased protein. Gram stain, bacterial cultures, and tests for viral causes of meningitis will be negative. Amoebas may be seen on a wet mount prepared from centrifuged CSF.

Treatments: Given the rarity of the disease, there is no single established treatment protocol, and Infectious Disease specialists and the Centers for Disease Control and Prevention (CDC) should be consulted. Some treatment regimens call for amphotericin B, fluconazole, rifampin, and miltefosine. The CDC should be contacted for guidance regarding miltefosine, an anti-leishmanial drug that has had benefit against *N. fowleri* and other amoeba species.

Pearls: Amoeba is the correct term for a singular organism and amoebas or amebae is plural. PAM is fortunately quite rare, but often reported on in U.S. media outlets in the summer months given its high fatality rate. *N. fowleri* can survive comfortably in some hot springs and is occasionally found in some regional tap water systems. Infections in the United States are more common in the summer months (swimming and water sports) and in the southern states.

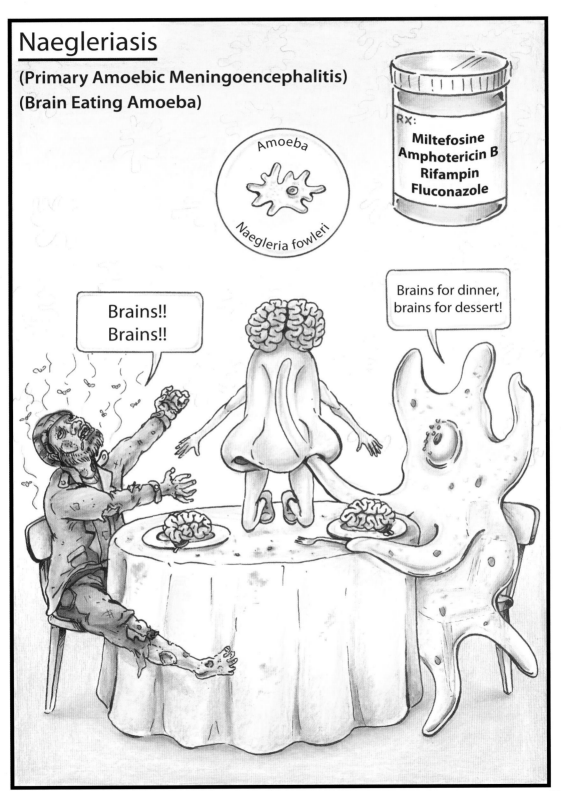

Disease Name: Prion Diseases: Transmissible Spongiform Encephalopathies

Transmissible spongiform encephalopathies (TSEs) are unique infections caused by abnormally folded, heat-stable, protease-resistant proteins known as prions. When introduced into a healthy person or animal, prions will encourage native proteins to take on abnormal folding patterns and cause disease over time. Prion diseases affect both humans and animals and are thought to be acquired (cannibalism or contaminated instruments) or caused by inherited (familial) or spontaneous genetic mutations. The diseases have extremely long incubation periods followed by chronic, progressive neurodegeneration. Bovine spongiform encephalopathy (BSE) or "Mad cow disease" is the best-known TSE and caused an epidemic in the United Kingdom starting in the mid-1980s.

Kuru: Kuru is a human prion disease endemic to the Fore people of Papua New Guinea and was associated with cannibalism. The disease has a long incubation period (averaging 10+ years) and causes progressive neurodegeneration, cerebellar ataxia, and myoclonus. As the disease progresses, patients lose the ability to ambulate and develop dysphagia. Unable to eat, people would ultimately die from severe malnutrition.

Creutzfeldt-Jakob Disease: Creutzfeldt-Jakob disease (CJD) is a human prion spongiform encephalopathy characterized by rapidly progressive dementia, myoclonus, ataxia, and Parkinson-like symptoms. CJD is the most common human prion disease and can occur spontaneously (via spontaneous genetic mutation), iatrogenically (unsterilized surgical instruments), or through familial transmission (inherited genetic mutation). Symptoms of CJD from spontaneous mutations tend to manifest themselves in patients around age 60.

variant Creutzfeldt-Jakob Disease: vCJD is considered the manifestation of BSE in humans and occurs when prions from infected cows are ingested. It is distinguished from CJD by a younger age of onset and slower disease progression.

Gerstmann-Straussler-Scheinker: Gerstmann-Straussler-Scheinker (GSS) is an inherited human prion disease characterized by dementia and progressive cerebellar ataxia. The disease begins to manifest symptoms in affected individuals in their mid-40s and typically results in death within 5 years of symptom onset.

Fatal Familial Insomnia: Fatal familial insomnia is typically an inherited human prion disease, although some sporadic cases have been reported. Symptoms of the disease tend to manifest themselves in the mid-50s and include insomnia, mental status changes, confusion, and hallucinations. Over time, motor symptoms including cerebellar ataxia and Parkinson-like symptoms occur. Death typically occurs within 3 years of symptom onset.

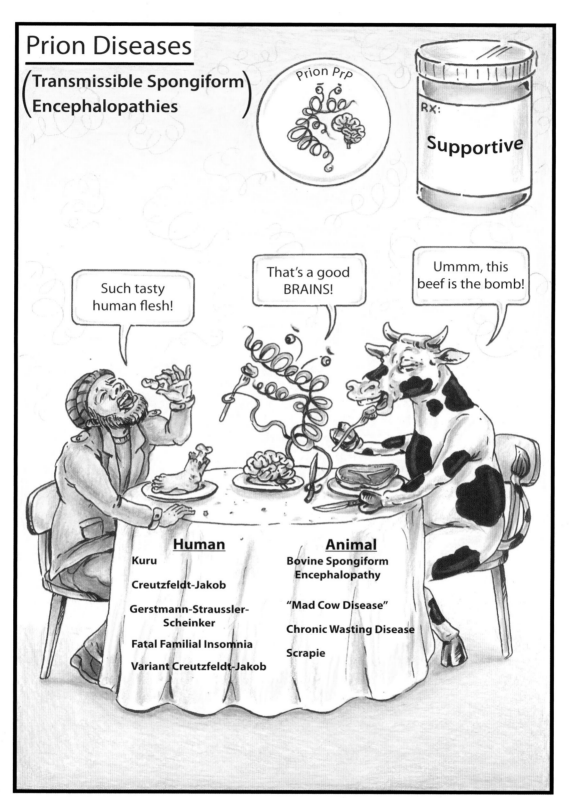

PART 14

BACTERIAL

Disease Name: **Anthrax**

Synonym:	Woolsorter disease
Causative Agent:	*Bacillus anthracis*
Reservoir:	Domestic sheep, cattle, and goats
Incubation:	GI and cutaneous: 1–7 days; Injection: 1–4 days; Inhalation: 1 day–2 weeks
Geographic Regions Affected:	Worldwide, rare in the United States and Canada

Description: Anthrax is a human bacterial zoonosis caused by the gram-positive, rod-shaped, spore-forming *Bacillus anthracis*. It can present in one of several forms: cutaneous, inhalation, gastrointestinal (GI), injection, and meningeal. Cutaneous anthrax is by far the most common (>95% of cases). The disease can be contracted by exposure to spores in animal hides, like those used in traditional drums. Anthrax spores have been used as an agent of bioterrorism.

Signs and Symptoms: *Cutaneous*: Subcutaneous inoculation of bacterial spores result in local tissue infection with edema, regional lymphadenopathy, and the formation of a characteristic black eschar. *Inhalation*: The inhalation of spores leads to a biphasic illness characterized by a prodrome of fever, chills, malaise, cough, chest pain, and flu-like symptoms, followed by the fulminant phase with severe dyspnea, hypoxia, pulmonary edema, acute respiratory distress syndrome (ARDS), shock, and death. Pleural effusions and a widened mediastinum secondary to lymphadenopathy on chest x-ray are characteristic for inhalation anthrax. *Gastrointestinal*: The consumption of undercooked, anthrax-infected meat can cause GI disease. The infected parts of the GI tract will develop edema, inflammation, and ulcerations, and patients will present with nausea, vomiting, abdominal pain, diarrhea, and possibly, GI hemorrhage. *Injection Anthrax*: Outbreaks have occurred in IV drug users injecting heroin. Cutaneous ulcers were typically absent and hematogenous spread was common. *Meningeal*: Hematogenous spread of anthrax can cause hemorrhagic meningitis.

Diagnostic Testing: Gram stain, cultures, polymerase chain reaction (PCR) testing, and serology can be obtained. Histopathology and immunohistochemistry testing can be performed on submitted tissue specimens, specifically for those obtained when testing for cutaneous anthrax.

Treatments: Vaccination is available. Ciprofloxacin or doxycycline can be used as prophylaxis after potential exposure and to treat cutaneous anthrax. Inhalation anthrax requires intravenous (IV) ciprofloxacin and linezolid; other treatment options are available. An immune globulin also exists.

Pearls: It is illegal to import goat-skin drums from Haiti, given their association with anthrax.

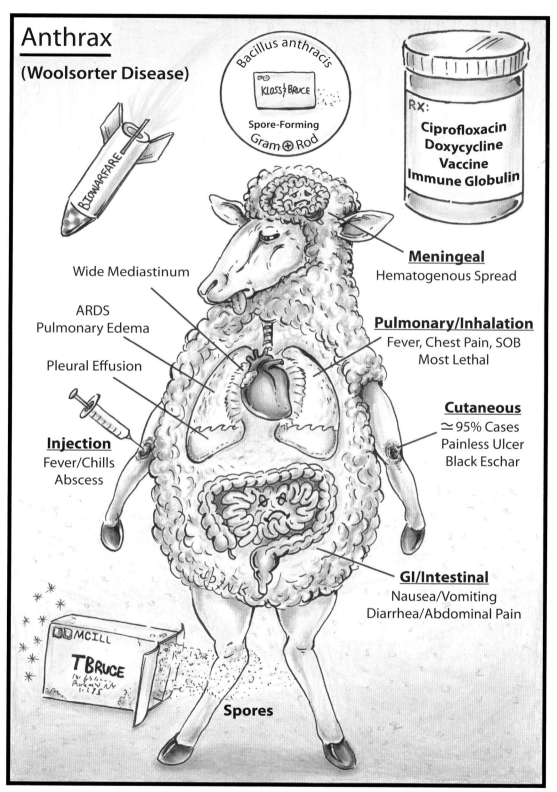

Anthrax
(Woolsorter Disease)

Bacillus anthracis
KLOSS & BRUCE
Spore-Forming
Gram ⊕ Rod

BIOWARFARE

RX:
**Ciprofloxacin
Doxycycline
Vaccine
Immune Globulin**

Meningeal
Hematogenous Spread

Wide Mediastinum

ARDS
Pulmonary Edema

Pleural Effusion

Pulmonary/Inhalation
Fever, Chest Pain, SOB
Most Lethal

Cutaneous
≃ 95% Cases
Painless Ulcer
Black Eschar

Injection
Fever/Chills
Abscess

GI/Intestinal
Nausea/Vomiting
Diarrhea/Abdominal Pain

MCILL
T BRUCE

Spores

Disease Name: **Botulism**

Causative Agent: *Clostridium botulinum*—botulism toxin

Incubation: Food-borne: 6 hours to 10 days; Average: 12-36 hours
Wound: 4-14 days
Infant: Unknown

Geographic Regions Affected: Worldwide.

Description: Botulism is a rare paralytic illness caused by the toxin produced by the gram-positive, spore-forming, bacillus-shaped, obligate anaerobic bacteria *C. botulinum*. Botulism most commonly occurs as the result of the ingestion of preformed toxin (foodborne) or spores (infant). In infant botulism, the spores colonize the GI tract and produce toxin. Other, less common causes of botulism occur secondary to wound infection (typically from intramuscular or intravenous drug use), spore inhalation, or iatrogenically (cosmetic Botox).

Signs and Symptoms: *Food-borne Botulism*: Acute onset bilateral facial palsy and descending weakness in the absence of fever. Sensation and neurologic status remain intact. Blurry vision, bradycardia, and GI symptoms such as nausea, vomiting, diarrhea, and abdominal pain may be present. *Infant Botulism*: Also known as "floppy baby syndrome." Infant may have weak cry, poor feeding, drooling, weakness, and constipation in the absence of fever. *Wound Botulism*: Similar presentation to food-borne botulism, but without GI symptoms. The patient is still exposed to the circulating toxin from the wound, but their GI tract is spared exposure. Fever may be present, secondary to the wound infection.

Diagnostic Testing: Patient history, clinical presentation, and electromyogram (EMG) testing suggest the diagnosis. Infant botulism is confirmed via the isolation of infectious spores and botulin toxin in stool samples. Food-borne botulism in adults is confirmed via the detection of botulin toxin in serum, stool, vomitus, or suspect food specimens. Patients with wound botulism would have detectable toxin in their serum, but not stool (no GI tract involvement).

Treatments: Supportive. Intubation and mechanical ventilation as indicated. A horse-serum based antitoxin is available for adults and children 12 months or older and a human-derived botulism immune globulin is available for infants <12 months of age. Poison Control can be contacted at 1-800-222-1222 for guidance on how to obtain and dose these treatments. Antibiotics should be prescribed for wound botulism, but would have no effect of infant or food-borne botulism.

Prevention: Use caution with home canning. Discard dented or bulging cans. Do not feed children less than 1 year of age honey, as it may contain botulism spores.

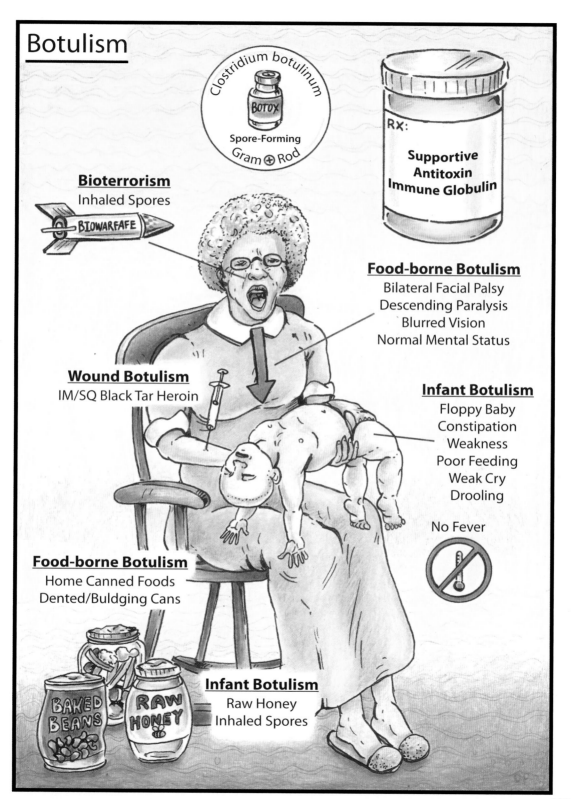

Botulism

Clostridium botulinum
BOTOX
Spore-Forming
Gram ⊕ Rod

RX:
**Supportive
Antitoxin
Immune Globulin**

Bioterrorism
Inhaled Spores
BIOWARFAFE

Food-borne Botulism
Bilateral Facial Palsy
Descending Paralysis
Blurred Vision
Normal Mental Status

Wound Botulism
IM/SQ Black Tar Heroin

Infant Botulism
Floppy Baby
Constipation
Weakness
Poor Feeding
Weak Cry
Drooling

No Fever

Food-borne Botulism
Home Canned Foods
Dented/Buldging Cans

BAKED BEANS
RAW HONEY

Infant Botulism
Raw Honey
Inhaled Spores

Disease Name: **Brucellosis**

Synonyms:	Mediterranean fever, Malta fever, undulant fever
Causative Agents:	*Brucella* spp.
Reservoir:	Sheep: *B. melitensis*; Swine: *B. suis*; Cattle: *B. abortus*; Dogs: *B. canis*
Incubation:	5 days–5 months; Average: 1–4 weeks
Geographic Regions Affected:	Worldwide. More common in the Mediterranean Basin, the Middle East, Eastern Europe, Asia, Africa, Central and South America.
Description:	Brucellosis is a human bacterial zoonosis caused by gram-negative, intracellular, coccobacilli members of the *Brucella* spp. The disease is transmitted to humans via exposure to infectious bodily fluids from animals or food products such as raw milk or unpasteurized cheese. Brucellosis can be acute or chronic, localized or systemic, and the disease has a wide range of clinical presentations from asymptomatic to fulminant. Infection during pregnancy may result in abortion. Fever may be undulant (wax and wane).
Signs and Symptoms:	Systemic illness has nonspecific symptoms including fever, malaise, weakness, fatigue, headache, dizziness, myalgia, arthralgia, and night sweats. Localized infections can occur almost anywhere, with bone and joint involvement the most common. Examples of localized infection include sacroiliitis, epididymo-orchitis, pneumonia, hepatitis, endocarditis, uveitis, dermatitis, and meningitis. Symptoms of localized infection are dependent on affected organ system. Brucellosis is considered chronic when symptoms last for more than a year. Disease may reoccur or relapse if antibiotics are discontinued prematurely.
Diagnostic Testing:	Culture, serology, and polymerase chain reaction (PCR) testing. Since *Brucella* is difficult to grow, the laboratory should be alerted when specimens are submitted for culture.
Treatments:	Nonfocal, uncomplicated brucellosis can be treated with gentamycin daily for 7 days combined with doxycycline twice daily for 6 weeks or rifampin daily combined with doxycycline twice daily for 6 weeks. Alternative regimens include the combination of ciprofloxacin with doxycycline or rifampin. Specific treatment regimens exist for localized infection (spondylitis, sacroiliitis, endocarditis, and meningitis) and for infections during pregnancy.
Prevention:	Avoid raw milk and unpasteurized cheese.
Pearls:	Grandpa Kloss was a dairy worker in New Jersey, loved to drink raw buttermilk to quell his peptic ulcer disease, and subsequently developed brucellosis "undulant fever" as a result.

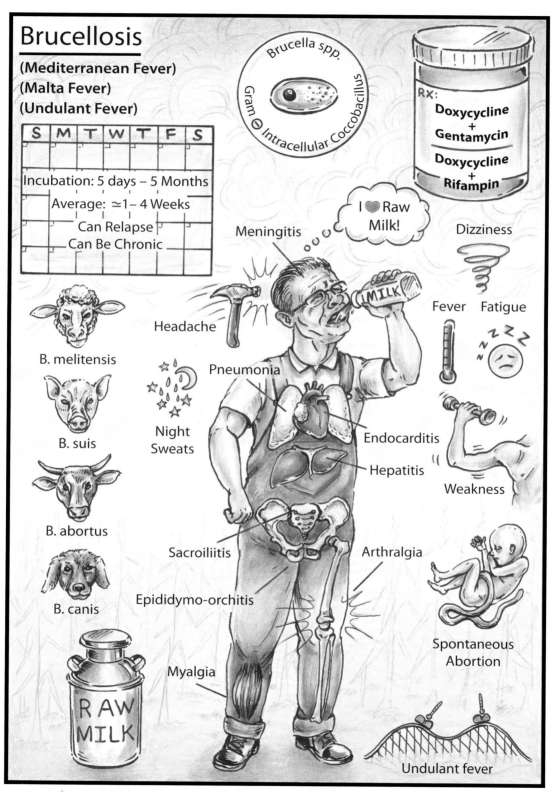

Brucellosis

(Mediterranean Fever)
(Malta Fever)
(Undulant Fever)

Brucella spp.
Gram ⊖ Intracellular Coccobacillus

RX:
Doxycycline
+
Gentamycin

Doxycycline
+
Rifampin

S	M	T	W	T	F	S

Incubation: 5 days – 5 Months
Average: ≃1– 4 Weeks
Can Relapse
Can Be Chronic

I ♥ Raw Milk!

Meningitis

Dizziness

Fever   Fatigue

Headache

B. melitensis

B. suis

B. abortus

B. canis

Night Sweats

Pneumonia

Endocarditis

Hepatitis

Weakness

Sacroiliitis

Arthralgia

Epididymo-orchitis

Spontaneous Abortion

Myalgia

RAW MILK

Undulant fever

Disease Name: **Typhoid Fever**

Synonym: Enteric fever

Causative Agent: *Salmonella enterica* serotype Typhi

Reservoir: Humans—Bacteria tend to colonize in the gallbladder in chronic carriers.

Incubation: 6–30 days; Average: 10–14 days

Geographic Regions Affected: Worldwide—Most common in developing nations. The vast majority of U.S. cases have been linked to travel to endemic countries (about 75%–80%).

Description: Typhoid fever is systemic bacterial illness characterized by abdominal pain and fever caused by the gram-negative, flagellated, rod-shaped bacteria *Salmonella enterica* serotype Typhi. Paratyphoid, a similar illness, is caused by *S. enterica* serotype Paratyphi A, B, or C.

Signs and Symptoms: Typhoid classically goes through several phases, each lasting about a week. Symptoms during the first week include progressive fever, chills, malaise, relative bradycardia, headache, and cough. In the second week of illness, severe fatigue, abdominal pain, delirium, and a characteristic rash consisting of salmon-colored "rose spots" appear on the chest and abdomen. Constipation or diarrhea can also occur, as well as hepatosplenomegaly. In the third week of illness, severe complications such as encephalitis and gastrointestinal (GI) hemorrhage or perforation can occur. Convalescence typically begins after the third week of illness and it may take several months for the patient to fully recover.

Diagnostic Testing: Culture and serological testing. Cultures can be obtained from blood, stool, duodenal aspirates, vomitus, rose spots, and bone marrow. Multiple sets of blood cultures increase the likelihood of detection.

Treatments: Ciprofloxacin or levofloxacin can be used for treatment of cases of typhoid fever that were not acquired in Asia. Given increasing resistances to fluoroquinolones in Asia, ceftriaxone or azithromycin should be used for infections linked to that region. Azithromycin can be used in children. Dexamethasone is indicated as an adjunct in cases of severe infection.

Prevention: Oral and intramuscular (IM) typhoid vaccines are available in the U.S. for travelers to endemic areas.

Pearls: Typhoid Mary, AKA Mary Mallon, was the first person in the United States identified as an asymptomatic carrier of *S. enterica* serotype Typhi. She worked as a cook in upper-class homes and is presumed to have infected more than 50 people. After outbreaks of typhoid occurred in her place of employment, she would quit and move on, often changing her name and inadvertently infecting others. She spent the last years of her life under forced quarantine.

Typhoid Fever

(Enteric Fever)

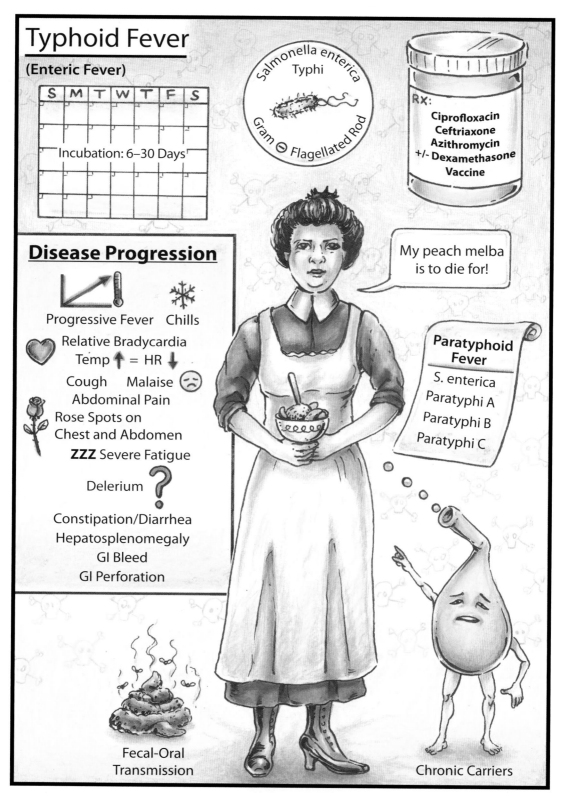

Incubation: 6–30 Days

Salmonella enterica Typhi
Gram ⊖ Flagellated Rod

RX:
**Ciprofloxacin
Ceftriaxone
Azithromycin
+/- Dexamethasone
Vaccine**

Disease Progression

Progressive Fever   Chills

Relative Bradycardia
Temp ↑ = HR ↓

Cough   Malaise

Abdominal Pain

Rose Spots on
Chest and Abdomen

ZZZ Severe Fatigue

Delerium ?

Constipation/Diarrhea
Hepatosplenomegaly
GI Bleed
GI Perforation

My peach melba
is to die for!

**Paratyphoid
Fever**

S. enterica
Paratyphi A
Paratyphi B
Paratyphi C

Fecal-Oral
Transmission

Chronic Carriers

Disease Name: **Cat Scratch Fever**

Synonym:	Cat scratch disease
Causative Agent:	*Bartonella henselae*
Vector:	Cat flea (*Ctenocephalides felis*)—Fleas transmit the bacteria between cats.
Reservoir:	Cats are the natural reservoir, with kittens more likely to carry the bacteria.
Incubation:	1–2 weeks
Geographic Regions Affected:	Worldwide
Description:	Cat scratch disease is a gram-negative bacterial zoonosis caused by *B. henselae*. It gets transmitted to cats by infected fleas. Humans can become infected through the bite or scratch of an infected cat or from direct exposure to infected cat fleas. The disease is characterized by a primary papule or pustule at the site of inoculation followed by the development of ipsilateral regional lymphadenopathy.
Signs and Symptoms:	In the vast majority of cases, a small papule or nodule forms at the inoculation site followed by the development of ipsilateral regional lymphadenopathy. Patients may also present with low-grade fever, malaise, and headache. Arthralgia, myalgia, and arthritis can also occur. Meningitis, osteomyelitis, and endocarditis can occur, but are rare. Ocular manifestations can include *parinaud oculoglandular syndrome*, a granulomatous conjunctivitis with preauricular lymphadenopathy. Immunocompromised (HIV +/AIDS) patients are at risk of developing *peliosis hepatis* and/or *bacillary angiomatosis* (BA).
Diagnostic Testing:	Labs may reveal mild leukocytosis, predominantly neutrophils, and an elevated erythrocyte sedimentation rate (ESR). IgM and IgG antibodies can be obtained.
Treatments:	Azithromycin is the first-line antibiotic. Alternatives include rifampin, TMP/SMX, ciprofloxacin, and doxycycline.
Prevention:	Flea control for cats, hand washing after contact with cats or cat feces, and keeping cats indoors to limit exposure to fleas.
Pearls:	Bacillary angiomatosis (BA) may be mistaken for Kaposi sarcoma and vice versa.

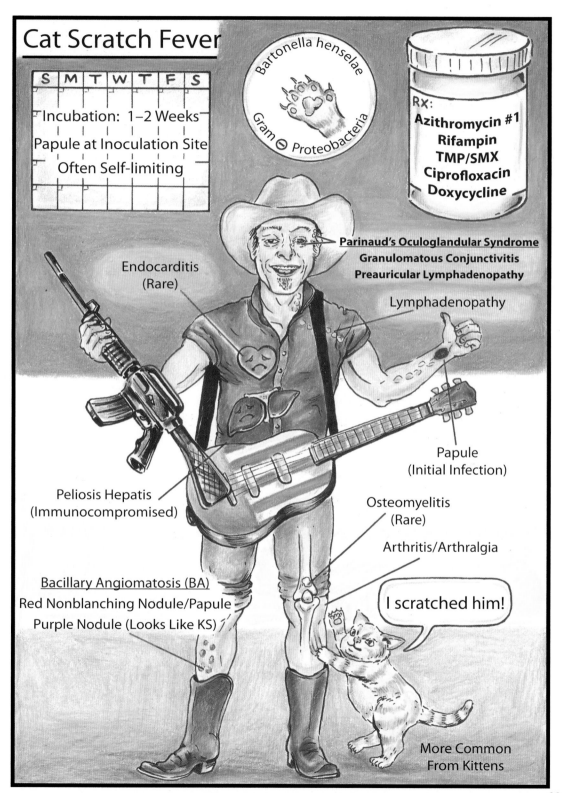

Disease Name: **Leprosy**

Synonym:	Hansen disease
Causative Agent:	*Mycobacterium leprae*
Reservoir:	Armadillos
Incubation:	9 months–20 years; Average: 5 years
Geographic Regions Affected:	India, Brazil, and Indonesia have the highest incidence.
Description:	Leprosy is an infection of the skin, nasal mucosa, and cutaneous nerves caused by the slow-growing, gram-positive, intracellular bacteria *M. leprae*. There are several ways to categorize leprosy, with the World Health Organization's (WHO) classification being the simplest. The WHO classifies the disease as paucibacillary (tubercular) when there are five or fewer skin lesions or multibacillary (lepromatous) when there are six or more lesions. Multibacillary leprosy is a more severe presentation found in patients with a weaker immune response to the infection. Despite long-held historical beliefs, leprosy is not very contagious.
Signs and Symptoms:	Cutaneous skin lesions, neuromas, and sensory loss are hallmarks of the disease. Hypopigmented skin patches, decreased sensation, paresthesias, muscle weakness, thickened earlobes, loss of eyebrows and eyelashes, nasal perforation, saddle nose, and corneal scaring leading to blindness can occur. Diminished sensation can lead to burns or wounds on the palms and soles. In more severe disease, auto-amputation of digits, peroneal, tibial, and ulnar neuropathy may be seen.
Diagnostic Testing:	Skin biopsies and polymerase chain reaction (PCR) testing can be performed to confirm the diagnosis.
Treatments:	Dapsone was used for many years as a single agent to treat leprosy until resistance emerged. Multidrug therapy is now required, often for 6–12 months or longer. There are two current treatment protocols, one put forth by the World Health Organization (WHO) and another by the National Hansen's Disease Program. According to the WHO protocol, paucibacillary leprosy is treated with dapsone and rifampicin for 6 months and multibacillary leprosy is treated with dapsone, rifampicin, and clofazimine for 12 months.
Pearls:	The bacteria that carries leprosy reproduces at cooler temperatures, thus disease is limited to the skin and cutaneous nerves in humans. Since armadillos have a lower core body temperature than most mammals, they serve well as a natural reservoir. *M. leprae*, like the mycobacterium that causes tuberculosis (TB), has a waxy outer layer.

Leprosy
(Hansen Disease)

S	M	T	W	T	F	S

Incubation: 9 Months – 20 Years

Average: ≃5 Years

Mycobacterium leprae
Gram ⊕ Rod
Intracellular Plemorphic

RX:
Dapsone
Rifampicin
Clofazimine

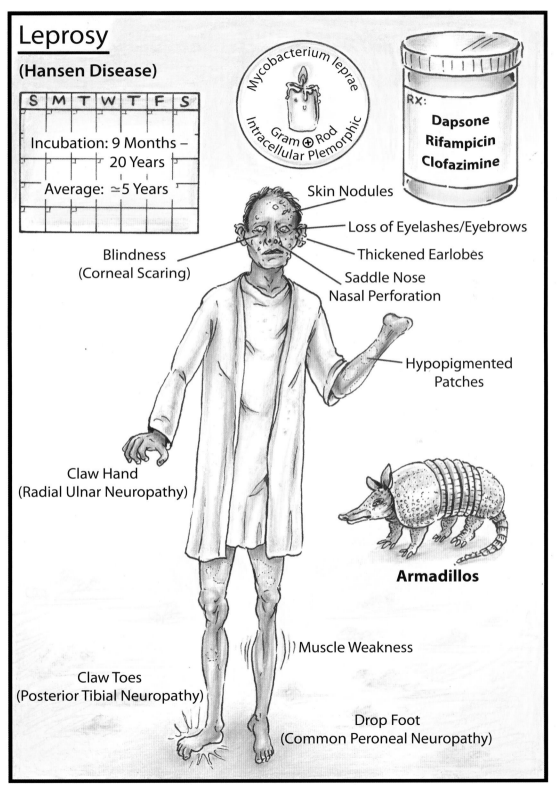

Skin Nodules

Loss of Eyelashes/Eyebrows

Thickened Earlobes

Saddle Nose
Nasal Perforation

Blindness
(Corneal Scaring)

Hypopigmented
Patches

Claw Hand
(Radial Ulnar Neuropathy)

Armadillos

Muscle Weakness

Claw Toes
(Posterior Tibial Neuropathy)

Drop Foot
(Common Peroneal Neuropathy)

Disease Name: Infective Endocarditis

Causative Agents: Staphylococci and streptococci are the most common culprits causing BE, with *Staphylococcus aureus* and *Streptococcus viridans* taking the lead from each respective genus. Other important bacteria include the HACEK bacteria: *Haemophilus*, *Aggregatibacter*, *Cardiobacterium*, *Eikenella*, and *Kingella*. HACEK bacteria are small, fastidious, gram-negative rods.

Description: Infective endocarditis is an infectious process of the inner lining of the heart, mostly of the heart valves, typically caused by bacteria (bacterial endocarditis [BE]). The disease may have a short incubation period and present acutely (acute BE) or may have a more insidious and indolent course of progression and develop over several weeks (subacute BE).

Risk Factors: Intravenous (IV) drug abuse, poor dentition, valvular heart disease, congenital heart disease, prosthetic heart valves, indwelling lines, pacemakers, past history of infective endocarditis, and chronic hemodialysis.

Signs and Symptoms: Fever is the most common presenting symptom (up to 90%) and is often associated with chills, fatigue, and malaise. A heart murmur is present in up to 85% of patients. Patients may also develop myalgia, arthralgia, splinter hemorrhages, septic emboli, petechiae, splenomegaly, cough, weight loss, and/or glomuleronephritis. Janeway lesions, Osler nodes, and Roth spots are highly suggestive of bacterial endocarditis.

Definitions: Janeway lesions are nontender erythematous macules on the palms and soles. Osler nodes are painful, purplish-red lesions found on the pads of the fingers. Roth spots are retinal hemorrhages with pale centers.

Diagnosis: Bacterial endocarditis should be considered when patients with any of the above risk factors present with fever, heart murmur, and clinical signs and/or symptoms supporting the diagnosis. Blood cultures should be obtained from at least three different sites and an echocardiogram, preferably transesophageal, should be performed looking for valvular vegetations. Labs may show elevated C-reactive protein (CRP), erythrocyte sedimentation rate (ESR), and rheumatoid factor.

Treatments: Empiric treatment should be initiated in acutely ill patients once blood cultures have been obtained. Vancomycin and ceftriaxone or gentamycin are good first-line agents until a more tailored regimen can be provided based on blood culture results. If patients are not acutely ill or in heart failure, treatment can be withheld until blood cultures are resulted. If the initial round of blood cultures is negative in suspect patients, two to three more sets should be drawn prior to the initiation of empiric treatment.

Infective Endocarditis

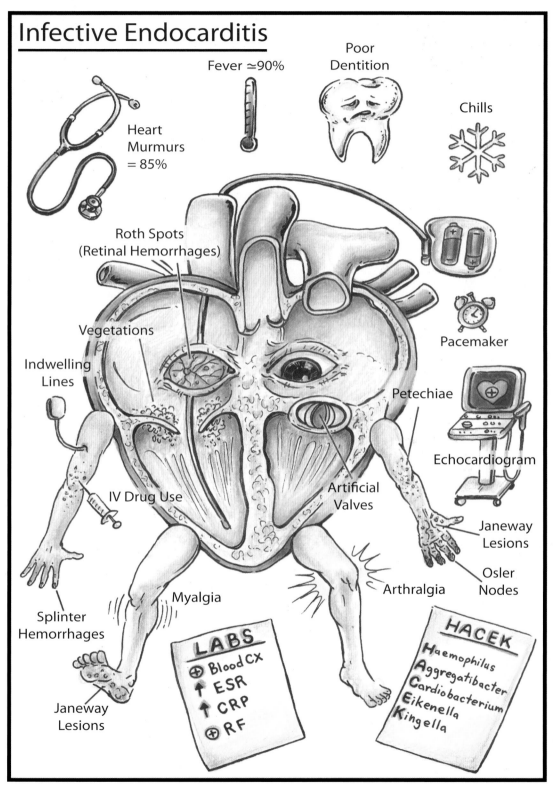

Fever ≃90%

Poor Dentition

Chills

Heart Murmurs = 85%

Roth Spots (Retinal Hemorrhages)

Pacemaker

Vegetations

Indwelling Lines

Petechiae

Echocardiogram

IV Drug Use

Artificial Valves

Janeway Lesions

Osler Nodes

Arthralgia

Splinter Hemorrhages

Myalgia

Janeway Lesions

LABS
⊕ Blood CX
↑ ESR
↑ CRP
⊕ RF

HACEK
Haemophilus
Aggregatibacter
Cardiobacterium
Eikenella
Kingella

Disease Name: **Tetanus**

Synonym:	Lockjaw
Causative Agent:	*Clostridium tetani*
Incubation:	3–21 days; Average: 10 days
Geographic Regions Affected:	Worldwide—More common in developing nations, where mass vaccination with tetanus toxoid is less common.
Description:	Tetanus is an infection characterized by muscle spasms caused by the gram-positive, anaerobic bacteria *C. tetani*. This bacteria is commonly found in soil and manure and creates a toxin that causes muscle spasms. Tetanus can present in one of four forms: (1) generalized, (2) localized/wound tetanus, (3) neonatal tetanus, and (4) cephalic tetanus.
Signs and Symptoms:	*Generalized Tetanus:* This is the most common form of tetanus (about 80%) and often presents as trismus or risus sardonicus with muscle spasms that develop in a descending pattern. Patients may develop sympathetic hyperactivity, laryngospasm, and opisthotonus (clenched fists, flexed arms, arched back, and extended legs). Mortality is around 10%–20%. *Localized Tetanus:* This is a mild form of tetanus with localized muscle spasm in close proximity to the wound. It is more common in partially immunized patients and has a low mortality. *Neonatal Tetanus:* This form of tetanus has the highest mortality and results from the contamination of the infant's umbilical stump with dirt or bacteria-laden matter. Infants first exhibit poor feeding and later progress to full-blown tetanus. *Cephalic Tetanus:* This is the rarest form of the disease, has a short 1–2 day incubation period, and results from a head or neck wound. Unlike the other forms that cause muscle spasm/tetany, cephalic tetanus commonly presents as unilateral facial nerve palsy.
Diagnostic Testing:	Tetanus tends to be a clinical diagnosis based on clinical findings and a history of wound infection in an unvaccinated or undervaccinated patient.
Treatments:	Tetanus immune globulin should be given to sequester unbound toxin and vaccination with tetanus toxoid should be initiated. Wound debridement, wound care, and antibiotic administration should also be performed. Patients may require intubation to secure the airway and provide ventilation. Benzodiazepines and/or neuromuscular blocking agents can be given for muscle spasm.

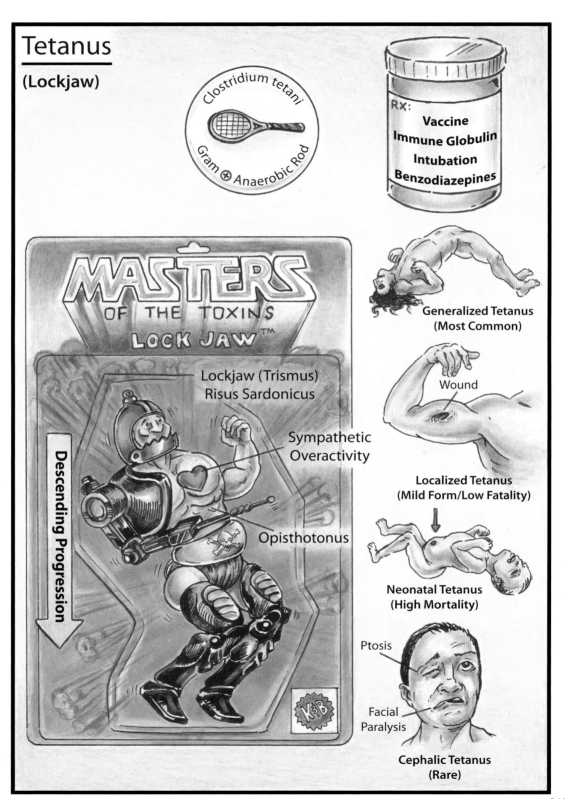

Tetanus
(Lockjaw)

Clostridium tetani
Gram ⊕ Anaerobic Rod

RX:
Vaccine
Immune Globulin
Intubation
Benzodiazepines

MASTERS OF THE TOXINS
LOCK JAW™

Descending Progression

Lockjaw (Trismus)
Risus Sardonicus

Sympathetic Overactivity

Opisthotonus

Generalized Tetanus
(Most Common)

Wound

Localized Tetanus
(Mild Form/Low Fatality)

Neonatal Tetanus
(High Mortality)

Ptosis

Facial Paralysis

Cephalic Tetanus
(Rare)

Disease Name: Listeriosis

Causative Agent:	*Listeria monocytogenes*
Reservoir:	Soil, infected animals and their derived food products
Incubation:	Gastroenteritis: 1–2 days; Invasive disease: ≈30 days
Geographic Regions Affected:	Worldwide
Description:	Listeriosis is a human bacterial infection caused by the gram-positive, rod-shaped, facultative anaerobe *L. monocytogenes*. It can present as a febrile gastroenteritis or as a more severe, invasive illness in pregnant women and the immunocompromised. Pregnant women can pass the bacteria to the fetus, causing septicemia, miscarriage, or stillbirth. Since listeria can be found in paté, raw milk, and young cheeses, pregnant women are encouraged to avoid these foods. There have been several food-borne outbreaks of listeriosis in the United States over the past several years, including one associated with cantaloupes in 2011.
Signs and Symptoms:	*Gastroenteritis*: Fever, nausea, vomiting, diarrhea, headache, and myalgia are common symptoms. *Invasive Disease*: Pregnant women with listeriosis may become bacteremic and develop fever, chills, back pain, myalgia, and other flu-like symptoms. Passage of the bacteria to the fetus in utero may result in premature birth, miscarriage, and/or stillbirth. Infants infected in utero may be born with sepsis or granulomatosis infantiseptica, a severe infection characterized by numerous abscesses throughout the infant's internal organs. Those infants infected at birth via asymptomatic vaginal infections may develop meningitis and/or sepsis. The immunocompromised, including those at extremes of age, are at higher risk of invasive disease and may present with fever, chills, myalgia, sepsis, meningoencephalitis, and/or sepsis. Cutaneous and ocular infections have been occasionally reported in veterinarians and farmers.
Diagnostic Testing:	Positive blood or cerebral spinal fluid (CSF) cultures will confirm the diagnosis.
Treatments:	Ampicillin plus gentamycin is the preferred treatment. TMP/SMX is an alternative.
Pearls:	Mortality rate from invasive disease ranges between 20% and 30%. Listeriosis in pregnancy is most common in the third trimester and often has a mild flu-like presentation with fever, myalgia, and back pain. Blood cultures for febrile pregnant women should be obtained when listeria is suspected and/or there is no other explanation for the febrile illness.

Listeriosis

(Listeria)

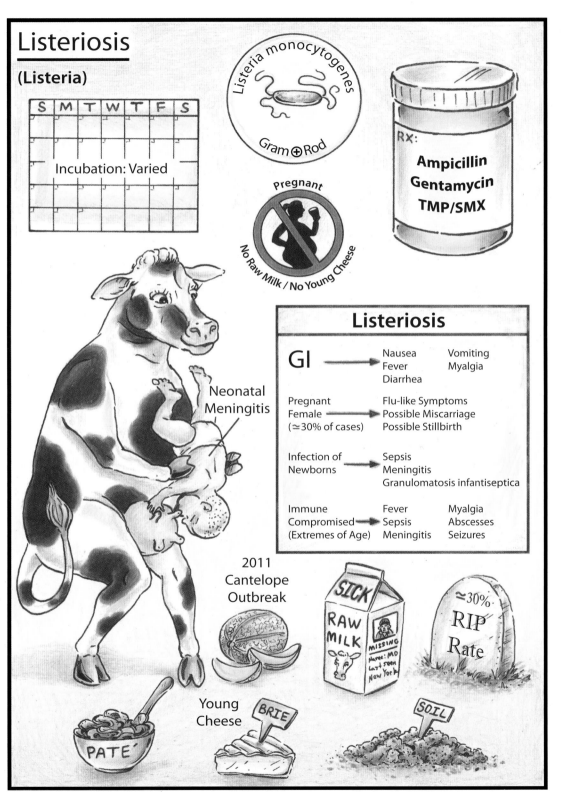

S	M	T	W	T	F	S

Incubation: Varied

Listeria monocytogenes

Gram ⊕ Rod

Pregnant

No Raw Milk / No Young Cheese

RX:

Ampicillin
Gentamycin
TMP/SMX

Neonatal Meningitis

Listeriosis

GI ⟶	Nausea	Vomiting
	Fever	Myalgia
	Diarrhea	
Pregnant Female ⟶ (≃30% of cases)	Flu-like Symptoms	
	Possible Miscarriage	
	Possible Stillbirth	
Infection of Newborns ⟶	Sepsis	
	Meningitis	
	Granulomatosis infantiseptica	
Immune Compromised ⟶ (Extremes of Age)	Fever	Myalgia
	Sepsis	Abscesses
	Meningitis	Seizures

2011 Cantelope Outbreak

SICK RAW MILK

MISSING
Nurse: MD
Last seen
New York

≈30% RIP Rate

PATE

Young Cheese

BRIE

SOIL

Disease Name: Q Fever

Causative Agent: *Coxiella burnetii*

Reservoirs: Domestic sheep, cattle, and goats

Incubation: 2–3 weeks

Geographic Regions Affected: Worldwide

Description: Q fever is a human bacterial zoonosis caused by the gram-negative, obligate intracellular, spore-forming *Coxiella burnetii*. It is carried by sheep, cattle, and goats and can be transmitted to humans through exposure to bacterial spores or infectious bodily fluids. The disease can have one of several presentations, including a mild flu-like illness, pneumonia, hepatitis, or endocarditis. Its spores can be used as an agent of bioterrorism.

Signs and Symptoms: *Flu-like Illness*: This is the most common manifestation and presents as acute fever, chills, malaise, fatigue, headache, and diaphoresis. Fever can last for 2–3 weeks. *Pneumonia*: Patients may develop a mild pneumonia with nonspecific chest x-ray findings. Dyspnea, pleuritic chest pain, and nonproductive cough are common. Arthralgia and myalgia may also occur. *Hepatitis*: Transaminitis, fever, hepatomegaly, and granulomas on liver biopsy are typical findings. Additional gastrointestinal (GI) symptoms can include nausea, vomiting, and, less commonly, diarrhea. *Endocarditis*: Acute or chronic endocarditis can occur, with chronic endocarditis more common in the immunocompromised and those with preexisting valvular abnormalities.

Diagnostic Testing: Polymerase chain reaction (PCR) testing can be performed on blood or serum in the first 2 weeks of infection and prior to antibiotic administration. IgM/IgG levels can be obtained. A fourfold rise of IgG levels in convalescence is confirmatory.

Treatments: Doxycycline is the first-line agent. TMP/SMX can be used in children or pregnant women. Endocarditis is very difficult to treat and requires doxycycline and hydroxychloroquine for 18–36 months or doxycycline and a fluoroquinolone for 2–4 years.

Pearls: Relapse can occur after discontinuation of treatment; if so, treatment should be resumed.

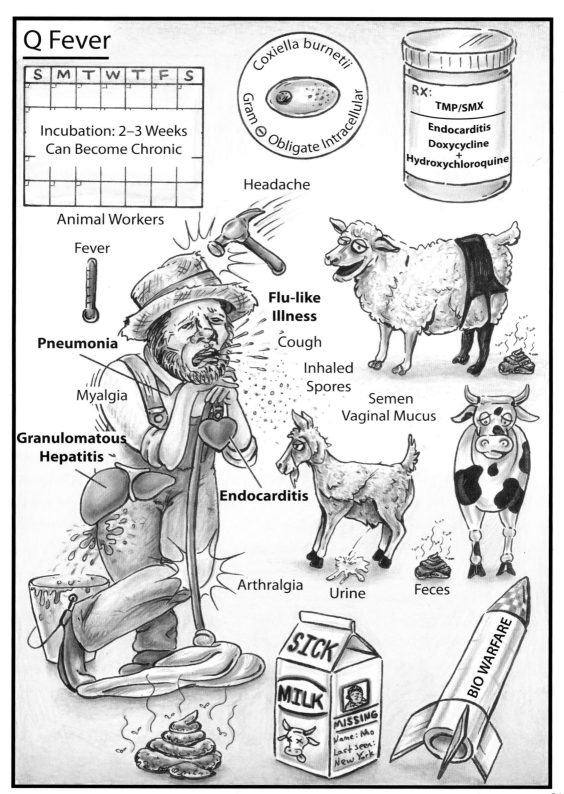

Q Fever

S	M	T	W	T	F	S

Incubation: 2–3 Weeks
Can Become Chronic

Animal Workers

Coxiella burnetii
Gram ⊖ Obligate Intracellular

RX:
TMP/SMX
Endocarditis
Doxycycline
+
Hydroxychloroquine

Headache

Fever

Flu-like Illness

Cough

Pneumonia

Inhaled Spores

Myalgia

Semen
Vaginal Mucus

Granulomatous Hepatitis

Endocarditis

Arthralgia

Urine

Feces

SICK MILK
MISSING
Name: Mo
Last seen:
New York

BIO WARFARE

Disease Name: **Melioidosis**

Synonyms:	Pseudoglanders, Whitmore disease
Causative Agent:	*Burkholderia pseudomallei*
Incubation:	1–21 days; Average: 9 days
Geographic Regions Affected:	Southeast Asia, China, and northern Australia

Description: Melioidosis is an infection caused by the gram-negative, intracellular bacteria *B. pseudomallei*. Since the disease is contracted via direct contact with bacteria found in contaminated water or moist soil, disease incidence is highest during rainy or wet (monsoon) seasons. Infections are categorized as either acute or chronic, with chronic infections defined as those having symptoms lasting for 2 months or longer. While most infections are subclinical, symptomatic disease often presents as pneumonia or cutaneous ulcers or abscesses. Diabetics, alcoholics, renal insufficient, and immunocompromised patients have a higher likelihood of symptomatic disease.

Signs and Symptoms: Symptoms vary based on organ system involved. Pneumonia is the most common disease manifestation and presents as fever, chills, malaise, headache, anorexia, and cough. Cutaneous disease includes skin abscesses and ulcerations. Bacteremia can lead to sepsis, pneumonia, or disseminated disease. Genitourinary infections, osteomyelitis, septic arthritis, parotitis, hepatic abscesses, and splenic abscesses may also occur. Chronic pulmonary infections may mimic tuberculosis (TB).

Diagnostic Testing: Cultures of blood, sputum, urine, and cutaneous ulcers should be obtained. Gram stain and microscopy may reveal the bacteria, which has a bipolar "safety pin" appearance. Serology and polymerase chain reaction (PCR) are of little benefit in diagnosis.

Treatments: Two stages of treatment are required: intravenous antibiotics such as ceftazidime or meropenem are typically given for 10–14 days followed by doxycycline and TMP/SMX orally for 3–6 months.

Pearls: The authors dedicate this illustration to Mike Cadogan, MD, our EM colleague in the great Down Under. Please check out his Life in the Fast Lane Medical Blog. Melioidosis is endemic in northern Australia.

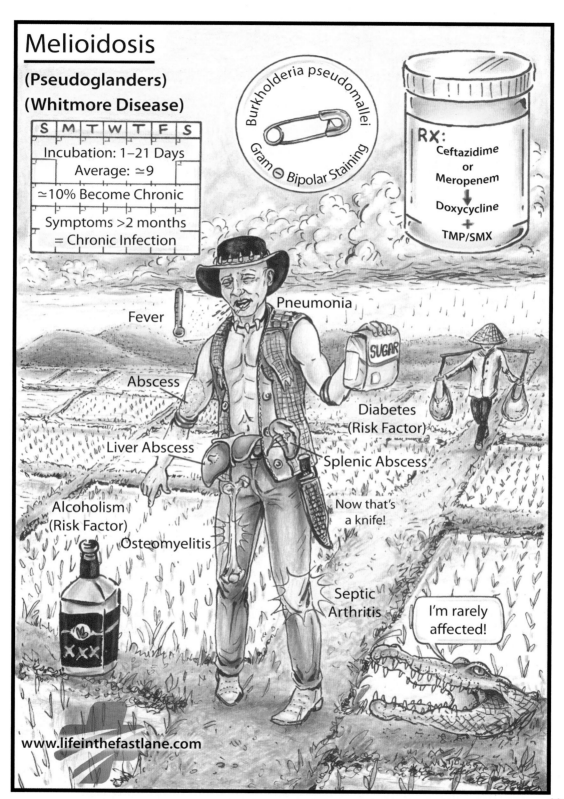

SELECTED READINGS AND REFERENCES

VIRAL HEPATITIS

HEPATITIS A

Averhoff F, Khudyakov Y, Bell BP. Hepatitis A Virus. In: Bennett JE, Dolin R, Blaser MJ, eds. *Principles and Practice of Infectious Diseases*. 8th ed. Philadelphia: Elsevier Saunders; 2015:2095-2112.

Bhamidimarri KR, Martin P. Acute viral hepatitis. In: Schlossberg D, ed. *Clinical Infectious Disease*. 2nd ed. Cambridge, United Kingdom: Cambridge University Press; 2015:287-295.

Gilbert DN, Chambers HF, Eliopoulos GM, eds., et al. *The Sanford Guide to Antimicrobial Therapy*. 46th ed. Sperryville, VA: Antimicrobial Therapy Inc; 2016.

Centers for Disease Control and Prevention (CDC). *Hepatitis A Outbreak Associated with Green Onions at a Restaurant — Monaca, Pennsylvania, 2003*. 2003. Available at: https://www.cdc.gov/mmwr/preview/mmwrhtml/mm5247a5.htm. Accessed October 6, 2017.

Nelson NP. Hepatitis A. In: Brunette GW, ed. *CDC Yellow Book 2018 Health Information for International Travel*. Oxford, United Kingdom: Oxford University Press; 2017: 183-187.

HEPATITIS B & HEPATITIS B SERUM MARKERS

Averhoff F. Hepatitis B. In: Brunette GW, ed. *CDC Yellow Book 2018 Health Information for International Travel*. Oxford, United Kingdom: Oxford University Press; 2017: 187-193.

Freshman ME, Friedman LS. Chronic hepatitis. In: Schlossberg D, ed. *Clinical Infectious Disease*. 2nd ed. Cambridge, United Kingdom: Cambridge University Press; 2015:296-307.

Gilbert DN, Chambers HF, Eliopoulos GM, eds., et al. *The Sanford Guide to Antimicrobial Therapy*. 46th ed. Sperryville, VA: Antimicrobial Therapy Inc; 2016.

Terrault NA, Bzowej NH, Chang KM, Hwang JP, Jonas MM, Murad MH. AASLD guidelines for treatment of chronic hepatitis B. *Hepatology*. 2016;63(1):261-283. doi:10.1002/hep.28156.

Thio LC, Hawkins C. Hepatitis B Virus and Hepatitis Delta Virus. In: Bennett JE, Dolin R, Blaser MJ, eds. *Principles and Practice of Infectious Diseases*. 8th ed. Philadelphia: Elsevier Saunders; 2015:1815-1839.

HEPATITIS C

AASLD/IDSA HCV Guidance Panel. Hepatitis C guidance: AASLD-IDSA recommendations for testing, managing, and treating adults infected with hepatitis C virus. *Hepatology*. 2015;62(3):932-954.

Freshman ME, Friedman LS. Chronic hepatitis. In: Schlossberg D, ed. *Clinical Infectious Disease*. 2nd ed. Cambridge, United Kingdom: Cambridge University Press; 2015: 296-307.

Gilbert DN, Chambers HF, Eliopoulos GM, et al., eds. *The Sanford Guide to Antimicrobial Therapy*. 46th ed. Sperryville, VA: Antimicrobial Therapy Inc; 2016.

Holtzman D. Hepitatis C. In: Brunette GW, ed. *CDC Yellow Book 2018 Health Information for International Travel*. Oxford, United Kingdom: Oxford University Press; 2017: 193-197.

Initial Treatment of HCV Infection | HCV Guidance. Available at: https://www.hcvguidelines.org/treatment-naive. Accessed October 6, 2017.

Ray SC, Thomas DL. Hepatitis C. In: Bennett JE, Dolin R, Blaser MJ, eds. *Principles and Practice of Infectious Diseases*. 8th ed. Philadelphia: Elsevier Saunders; 2015: 1904-1927.

Recommendations for Testing, Managing, and Treating Hepatitis C | HCV Guidance. Available at: https://www.hcvguidelines.org/. Accessed October 6, 2017.

HEPATITIS D

Freshman ME, Friedman LS. Chronic hepatitis. In: Schlossberg D, ed. *Clinical Infectious Disease*. 2nd ed. Cambridge, United Kingdom: Cambridge University Press; 2015:296-307.

Gilbert DN, Chambers HF, Eliopoulos GM, et al., eds. *The Sanford Guide to Antimicrobial Therapy*. 46th ed. Sperryville, VA: Antimicrobial Therapy Inc; 2016.

Thio LC, Hawkins C. Hepatitis B Virus and Hepatitis Delta Virus. In: Bennett JE, Dolin R, Blaser MJ, eds. *Principles and Practice of Infectious Diseases*. 8th ed. Philadelphia: Elsevier Saunders; 2015:1815-1839.

HEPATITIS E

Gilbert DN, Chambers HF, Eliopoulos GM, et al., eds. *The Sanford Guide to Antimicrobial Therapy*. 46th ed. Sperryville, VA: Antimicrobial Therapy Inc; 2016.

Teshal EH. Hepatitis E. In: Brunette GW, ed. *CDC Yellow Book 2018 Health Information for International Travel*. Oxford, United Kingdom: Oxford University Press; 2017:198-199.

Walsh SR. Hepatitis E Virus. In: Bennett JE, Dolin R, Blaser MJ, eds. *Principles and Practice of Infectious Diseases*. 8th ed. Philadelphia: Elsevier Saunders; 2015:2131-2141.

INFECTIOUS DIARRHEA: BACTERIAL

SHIGELLOSIS

Acheson DWK. Shigella. In: Schlossberg D, ed. *Clinical Infectious Disease*. 2nd ed. Cambridge, United Kingdom: Cambridge University Press; 2015:1004-1006.

Bowen A. Shigellosis. In: Brunette GW, ed. *CDC Yellow Book 2018 Health Information for International Travel*. Oxford, United Kingdom: Oxford University Press; 2017: 319-321.

DuPomt HL. Bacillary Dysentery: Shigella and Enteroinvasive Escherichia coli. In: Bennett JE, Dolin R, Blaser MJ, eds. *Principles and Practice of Infectious Diseases*. 8th ed. Philadelphia: Elsevier Saunders; 2015:2569-2574.

Gilbert DN, Chambers HF, Eliopoulos GM, et al., eds. *The Sanford Guide to Antimicrobial Therapy*. 46th ed. Sperryville, VA: Antimicrobial Therapy Inc; 2016.

SALMONELLOSIS

Gilbert DN, Chambers HF, Eliopoulos GM, et al., eds. *The Sanford Guide to Antimicrobial Therapy*. 46th ed. Sperryville, VA: Antimicrobial Therapy Inc; 2016.

Hunter JC, Francois Watkins LK. Salmonellosis (Nontyphoidal). In: Brunette GW, ed. *CDC Yellow Book 2018 Health Information for International Travel*. Oxford, United Kingdom: Oxford University Press; 2017:304-306.

Lima AAM, Warren CA, Guerrant RL. Bacterial Inflammatory Enteritides. In: Bennett JE, Dolin R, Blaser MJ, eds. *Principles and Practice of Infectious Diseases*. 8th ed. Philadelphia: Elsevier Saunders; 2015:1263-1269.

Ribner BS. Salmonella. In: Schlossberg D, ed. *Clinical Infectious Disease*. 2nd ed. Cambridge, United Kingdom: Cambridge University Press; 2015:979-984.

CHOLERA

Gilbert DN, Chambers HF, Eliopoulos GM, et al., eds. *The Sanford Guide to Antimicrobial Therapy*. 46th ed. Sperryville, VA: Antimicrobial Therapy Inc; 2016.

Vugia DJ. Vibrios. In: Schlossberg D, eds. *Clinical Infectious Disease*. 2nd ed. Cambridge, United Kingdom: Cambridge University Press; 2015:1030-1033.

Waldor MK, Ryan ET. Vibrio Cholerae. In: Bennett JE, Dolin R, Blaser MJ, eds. *Principles and Practice of Infectious Diseases*. 8th ed. Philadelphia: Elsevier Saunders; 2015: 2471-2479.

Wong KK, Burdette E, Mintz ED. Cholera. In: Brunette GW, ed. *CDC Yellow Book 2018 Health Information for International Travel*. Oxford, United Kingdom: Oxford University Press; 2017:153-156.

CAMPYLOBACTERIOSIS

Acheson DWK. Campylobacter. In: Schlossberg D, ed. *Clinical Infectious Disease*. 2nd ed. Cambridge, United Kingdom: Cambridge University Press; 2015:870-872.

Allos BM, Iovine NM, Blaser MJ. Campylobacter jejuni and Related Species. In: Bennett JE, Dolin R, Blaser MJ, eds. *Principles and Practice of Infectious Diseases*. 8th ed. Philadelphia: Elsevier Saunders; 2015:2485-2493.

Geissler AL, Mahon BE, Fitzgerlad C. Campylobacteriosis. In: Brunette GW, ed. *CDC Yellow Book 2018 Health Information for International Travel*. Oxford, United Kingdom: Oxford University Press; 2017:14-150.

Gilbert DN, Chambers HF, Eliopoulos GM, et al., eds. *The Sanford Guide to Antimicrobial Therapy*. 46th ed. Sperryville, VA: Antimicrobial Therapy Inc; 2016.

ENTEROHEMORRHAGIC *ESCHERICHIA COLI*

Escherichia coli O26 Infections Linked to Chipotle Mexican Grill Restaurants (Final Update). November 2015. | E. coli | CDC. Available at: https://www.cdc.gov/ecoli/2015/o26-11-15/index.html. Accessed October 6, 2017.

Gilbert DN, Chambers HF, Eliopoulos GM, et al., eds. *The Sanford Guide to Antimicrobial Therapy*. 46th ed. Sperryville, VA: Antimicrobial Therapy Inc; 2016.

O'Reilly CE, Iwamoto M, Griffin PM. Escherichia coli, Diarrheagenic. In: Brunette GW, ed. *CDC Yellow Book 2018 Health Information for International Travel*. Oxford, United Kingdom: Oxford University Press; 2017: 147-177.

Update: Multistate Outbreak of Escherichia coli O157:H7 Infections from Hamburgers – Western United States, 1992-1993. Available at: https://www.cdc.gov/mmwr/preview/mmwrhtml/00020219.htm. Accessed October 6, 2017.

ENTEROTOXIGENIC *ESCHERICHIA COLI*

Gilbert DN, Chambers HF, Eliopoulos GM, et al., eds. *The Sanford Guide to Antimicrobial Therapy*. 46th ed. Sperryville, VA: Antimicrobial Therapy Inc; 2016.

O'Reilly CE, Iwamoto M, Griffin PM. Escherichia coli, Diarrheagenic. In: Brunette GW, ed. *CDC Yellow Book 2018 Health Information for International Travel*. Oxford, United Kingdom: Oxford University Press; 2017:147-177.

YERSINIOSIS

Gilbert DN, Chambers HF, Eliopoulos GM, et al., eds. *The Sanford Guide to Antimicrobial Therapy*. 46th ed. Sperryville, VA: Antimicrobial Therapy Inc; 2016.

Gould LH, Friedman CR. Yersiniosis. In: Brunette GW, ed. *CDC Yellow Book 2018 Health Information for International Travel*. Oxford, United Kingdom: Oxford University Press; 2017:368-369.

Johnson RH, Heidari A. Yersinia. In: Schlossberg D, ed. *Clinical Infectious Disease*. 2nd ed. Cambridge, United Kingdom: Cambridge University Press; 2015:1034-1036.

Lima AAM, Warren CA, Guerrant RL. Bacterial Inflammatory Enteritides. In: Bennett JE, Dolin R, Blaser MJ, eds. *Principles and Practice of Infectious Diseases*. 8th ed. Philadelphia: Elsevier Saunders; 2015:1263-1269.

CLOSTRIDIUM DIFFICILE INFECTION

Gerding DN, Young VB. Clostridium difficile Infection. In: Bennett JE, Dolin R, Blaser MJ, eds. *Principles and Practice of Infectious Diseases*. 8th ed. Philadelphia: Elsevier Saunders; 2015:2744-2756.

Gilbert DN, Chambers HF, Eliopoulos GM, et al., eds. *The Sanford Guide to Antimicrobial Therapy*. 46th ed. Sperryville, VA: Antimicrobial Therapy Inc; 2016.

VIBRIOSIS

Gilbert DN, Chambers HF, Eliopoulos GM, et al., eds. *The Sanford Guide to Antimicrobial Therapy*. 46th ed. Sperryville, VA: Antimicrobial Therapy Inc; 2016.

Lima AAM, Warren CA, Guerrant RL. Bacterial Inflammatory Enteritides. In: Bennett JE, Dolin R, Blaser MJ, eds. *Principles and Practice of Infectious Diseases*. 8th ed. Philadelphia: Elsevier Saunders; 2015:1263-1269.

Vugia DJ. Vibrios. In: Schlossberg D, ed. *Clinical Infectious Disease*. 2nd ed. Cambridge, United Kingdom: Cambridge University Press; 2015:1030-1033.

INFECTIOUS DIARRHEA: VIRAL

NOROVIRUS

CDC – Vessel Sanitation Program – Cruise Ship Outbreak Updates. Available at: https://www.cdc.gov/nceh/vsp/surv/gilist.htm. Published July 26, 2017. Accessed October 6, 2017.

Davis CR, Pavia AT. Food poisoning. In: Schlossberg D, ed. *Clinical Infectious Disease*. 2nd ed. Cambridge, United Kingdom: Cambridge University Press; 2015: 342-348.

Dolin R, Treanor JJ. Noroviruses and Sapoviruses (Caliciviruses). In: Bennett JE, Dolin R, Blaser MJ, eds. *Principles and Practice of Infectious Diseases*. 8th ed. Philadelphia: Elsevier Saunders; 2015:2122-2127.

Hall AJ, Lopman B. Norovirus. In: Brunette GW, ed. *CDC Yellow Book 2018 Health Information for International Travel*. Oxford, United Kingdom: Oxford University Press; 2017:269-271.

ROTAVIRUS

Dormitzer RR. Rotaviruses. In: Bennett JE, Dolin R, Blaser MJ, eds. *Principles and Practice of Infectious Diseases*. 8th ed. Philadelphia: Elsevier Saunders; 2015:1854-1864.

Kroger AT, Strikas RA. General Recommendations for Vaccination & Immunoprophylaxis. In: Brunette GW, ed. *CDC Yellow Book 2018 Health Information for International Travel*. Oxford, United Kingdom: Oxford University Press; 2017:32-43.

Morgan DR, Chidi V, Owen RL. Gastroenteritis. In: Schlossberg D, ed. *Clinical Infectious Disease*. 2nd ed. Cambridge, United Kingdom: Cambridge University Press; 2015:334-341.

INFECTIOUS DIARRHEA: PROTOZOAN

GIARDIASIS

Fullerton KE, Yoder JS. Giardiasis. In: Brunette GW, ed. *CDC Yellow Book 2018 Health Information for International Travel*. Oxford, United Kingdom: Oxford University Press; 2017:179-180.

Gilbert DN, Chambers HF, Eliopoulos GM, et al., eds. *The Sanford Guide to Antimicrobial Therapy*. 46th ed. Sperryville, VA: Antimicrobial Therapy Inc; 2016.

Hill DR, Nash TE. Giardia Iamblia. In: Bennett JE, Dolin R, Blaser MJ, eds. *Principles and Practice of Infectious Diseases*. 8th ed. Philadelphia: Elsevier Saunders; 2015:3154-3160.

Weber DJ, Huliano JJ, Rutala WA. Systemic infection from animals. In: Schlossberg D, ed. *Clinical Infectious Disease*. 2nd ed. Cambridge, United Kingdom: Cambridge University Press; 2015:790-796.

CRYPTOSPORIDIOSIS

Cryptosporidia Adult and Adolescent Opportunistic Infection. AIDSinfo. Available at: https://aidsinfo.nih.gov/guidelines/html/4/adult-and-adolescent-opportunistic-infection/323/cryptosporidia. Accessed October 10, 2017.

Gilbert DN, Chambers HF, Eliopoulos GM, et al., eds. *The Sanford Guide to Antimicrobial Therapy*. 46th ed. Sperryville, VA: Antimicrobial Therapy Inc; 2016.

Hlavsa MC, Xiao L. Cryptosporidiosis. In: Brunette GW, ed. *CDC Yellow Book 2018 Health Information for International Travel*. Oxford, United Kingdom: Oxford University Press; 2018:157-159.

Kelly P. Intestinal protozoa. In: Schlossberg D, ed. *Clinical Infectious Disease*. 2nd ed. Cambridge, United Kingdom: Cambridge University Press; 2015:1313-1317.

White Jr AC. Cryptosporidiosis (Cryptosporidium Species). In: Bennett JE, Dolin R, Blaser MJ, eds. *Principles and Practice of Infectious Diseases*. 8th ed. Philadelphia: Elsevier Saunders; 2015:3173-3183.

AMEBIASIS

Cope JR. Amebiasis. In: Brunette GW, ed. *CDC Yellow Book 2018 Health Information for International Travel*. Oxford, United Kingdom: Oxford University Press; 2017:139-140.

Gilbert DN, Chambers HF, Eliopoulos GM, et al., eds. *The Sanford Guide to Antimicrobial Therapy*. 46th ed. Sperryville, VA: Antimicrobial Therapy Inc; 2016.

Kelly P. Intestinal protozoa. In: Schlossberg D, ed. *Clinical Infectious Disease*. 2nd ed. Cambridge, United Kingdom: Cambridge University Press; 2015:1313-1317.

Petri Jr WA, Haque R. Entamoeba Species, Including Amebic Colitis and Liver Abscess. In: Bennett JE, Dolin R, Blaser MJ, eds. *Principles and Practice of Infectious Diseases*. 8th ed. Philadelphia: Elsevier Saunders; 2015:3047-3058.

CHILDHOOD ILLNESSES

MEASLES

Chirch LM, Dieckhaus KD, Grant-Kels JM. Classic viral exanthems. In: Schlossberg D, ed. *Clinical Infectious Disease*. 2nd ed. Cambridge, United Kingdom: Cambridge University Press; 2015:133-138.

Gastanaduy PA, Goodson JL. Measles (Rubeola). In: Brunette GW, ed. *CDC Yellow Book 2018 Health Information for International Travel*. Oxford, United Kingdom: Oxford University Press; 2017:256-259.

Gershon AA. Measles Virus (Rubeola). In: Bennett JE, Dolin R, Blaser MJ, eds. *Principles and Practice of Infectious Diseases*. 8th ed. Philadelphia: Elsevier Saunders; 2015:1967-1973.

Measles Outbreak — California, December 2014–February 2015. Available at: https://www.cdc.gov/mmwr/preview/mmwrhtml/mm6406a5.htm. Accessed October 6, 2017.

MUMPS

Alhamal Z, Jordan M, Raad I. *Infection of the salivary and lacrimal glands*. In: Schlossberg D, ed. *Clinical Infectious Disease*. 2nd ed. Cambridge, United Kingdom: Cambridge University Press; 2015:68-74.

Cardemil CV, Clemmons NS. Mumps. In: Brunette GW, ed. *CDC Yellow Book 2018 Health Information for International Travel*. Oxford, United Kingdom: Oxford University Press; 2017:268-269.

Jong EC. Immunizations. In: Schlossberg D, ed. *Clinical Infectious Disease*. 2nd ed. Cambridge, United Kingdom: Cambridge University Press; 2015:763-776.

Litman N, Baum SG. Mumps Virus. In: Bennett JE, Dolin R, Blaser MJ, eds. *Principles and Practice of Infectious Diseases*. 8th ed. Philadelphia: Elsevier Saunders; 2015: 1942-1947.

RUBELLA

Chirch LM, Dieckhaus KD, Grant-Kels JM. Classic viral exanthems. In: Schlossberg D, ed. *Clinical Infectious Disease*. 2nd ed. Cambridge, United Kingdom: Cambridge University Press; 2015:133-138.

Gershon AA. Rubella Virus (German Measles). In: Bennett JE, Dolin R, Blaser MJ, eds. *Principles and Practice of Infectious Diseases*. 8th ed. Philadelphia: Elsevier Saunders; 2015:1875-1879.

Lebo EJ, Cardemil CV, Reef SE. Rubella. In: Brunette GW, ed. *CDC Yellow Book 2018 Health Information for International Travel*. Oxford, United Kingdom: Oxford University Press; 2017:303-304.

ERYTHEMA INFECTIOSUM

Weber DJ, Cohen MS, Rutala WA. The Acutely Ill Patient with Fever and Rash. In: Bennett JE, Dolin R, Blaser MJ, eds.

Principles and Practice of Infectious Diseases. 8th ed. Philadelphia: Elsevier Saunders; 2015:732-747.

EXANTHEM SUBITUM

Chirch LM, Dieckhaus KD, Grant-Kels JM. Classic viral exanthems. In: Schlossberg D, ed. *Clinical Infectious Disease*. 2nd ed. Cambridge, United Kingdom: Cambridge University Press; 2015:133-138.

Cohen JI. Human Herpesvirus Types 6 and 7 (Exanthem Subitum). In: Bennett JE, Dolin R, Blaser MJ, eds. *Principles and Practice of Infectious Diseases*. 8th ed. Philadelphia: Elsevier Saunders; 2015:1172-1776.

CHICKENPOX

Marin M, Lopez AS. Varicella (Chickenpox). In: Brunette GW, ed. *CDC Yellow Book 2018 Health Information for International Travel*. Oxford, United Kingdom: Oxford University Press; 2017: 346-349.

Weinberg, JM. Varicella-zoster virus. In: Schlossberg D, ed. *Clinical Infectious Disease*. 2nd ed. Cambridge, United Kingdom: Cambridge University Press; 2015: 1226-1233.

Whitley RJ. Chickenpox and Herpes Zoster (Varicella-Zoster Virus). In: Bennett JE, Dolin R, Blaser MJ, eds. *Principles and Practice of Infectious Diseases*. 8th ed. Philadelphia: Elsevier Saunders; 2015:1731-1737.

CONGENITAL AND PERINATAL INFECTIONS

Batteiger BE, Tan M. Chlamydia trachomatis (Trachoma, Genital Infections, Perinatal Infections, and Lymphogranuloma Venereum). In: Bennett JE, Dolin R, Blaser MJ, eds. *Principles and Practice of Infectious Diseases*. 8th ed. Philadelphia: Elsevier Saunders; 2015:2154-2170.

CDC – Toxoplasmosis – General Information – Pregnant Women. Available at: https://www.cdc.gov/parasites/toxoplasmosis/gen_info/pregnant.html. Published August 25, 2017. Accessed October 11, 2017.

CDC. Prenatal Infections. Centers for Disease Control and Prevention. Available at: https://www.cdc.gov/features/prenatalinfections/. Published June 5, 2017. Accessed October 11, 2017.

CMV | Congenital CMV Infection | Cytomegalovirus | CDC. Available at: https://www.cdc.gov/cmv/congenital-infection.html. Accessed October 11, 2017.

Congenital Varicella Syndrome – NORD (National Organization for Rare Disorders). NORD (National Organization for Rare Disorders). Available at: https://rarediseases.org/rare-diseases/congenital-varicella-syndrome/. Accessed October 11, 2017.

Current Trends Update: Lyme Disease and Cases Occurring during Pregnancy – United States. Available at: https://www.cdc.gov/mmwr/preview/mmwrhtml/00000569.htm. Accessed October 11, 2017.

Ford-Jones EL, Kellner JD. "Cheap torches": an acronym for congenital and perinatal infections. *Pediatr Infect Dis J*. 1995;14(7):638-640.

Gershon AA. Rubella Virus (German Measles). In: Bennett JE, Dolin R, Blaser MJ, eds. *Principles and Practice of Infectious Diseases*. 8th ed. Philadelphia: Elsevier Saunders; 2015:1875-1879.

Marrazzo JM, Apicella MA. Neisseria gonorrhoeae (Gonorrhea). In: Bennett JE, Dolin R, Blaser MJ, eds. *Principles and Practice of Infectious Diseases*. 8th ed. Philadelphia: Elsevier Saunders; 2015:2446-2462.

Non-Polio Enterovirus | Pregnancy and Non-Polio Enterovirus | CDC. Available at: https://www.cdc.gov/non-polio-enterovirus/pregnancy.html. Accessed October 11, 2017.

Parvovirus B19 | Pregnancy and Fifth Disease | Human Parvovirus B19 | CDC. Available at: https://www.cdc.gov/parvovirusb19/pregnancy.html. Accessed October 11, 2017.

Pregnant Women, Infants, and Children | Gender | HIV by Group | HIV/AIDS | CDC. Available at: https://www.cdc.gov/hiv/group/gender/pregnantwomen/index.html. Published September 14, 2017. Accessed October 11, 2017.

Radolf JD, Tramont EC, Salazar JC. Syphilis (Treponema pallidum). In: Bennett JE, Dolin R, Blaser MJ, eds. *Principles and Practice of Infectious Diseases*. 8th ed. Philadelphia: Elsevier Saunders; 2015:2684-2709.

Ray SC, Thomas DL. Hepatitis C. In: Bennett JE, Dolin R, Blaser MJ, eds. *Principles and Practice of Infectious Diseases*. 8th ed. Philadelphia: Elsevier Saunders; 2015:1904-1927.

U.S. Preventive Service Task Force. Screening for Syphilis Infection in Pregnancy: Reaffirmation Recommendation Statement. *Am Fam Physician*. 2010;81(2):1-3. Available at: http://www.aafp.org/afp/2010/0115/od1.html. Accessed October 11, 2017.

STD Facts – Congenital Syphilis. Available at: https://www.cdc.gov/std/syphilis/stdfact-congenital-syphilis.htm. Published September 20, 2017. Accessed October 11, 2017.

STD Screening Recommendations – 2015 STD Treatment Guidelines. Available at: https://www.cdc.gov/std/tg2015/screening-recommendations.htm. Accessed October 11, 2017.

Syphilis in Pregnancy – 2015 STD Treatment Guidelines. Available at: https://www.cdc.gov/std/tg2015/syphilis-pregnancy.htm. Accessed October 11, 2017.

Thio LC, Hawkins C. Hepatitis B Virus and Hepatitis Delta Virus. In: Bennett JE, Dolin R, Blaser MJ, eds. *Principles and Practice of Infectious Diseases*. 8th ed. Philadelphia: Elsevier Saunders; 2015:1815-1839.

Whitley RJ. Chickenpox and Herpes Zoster (Varicella-Zoster Virus). In: Bennett JE, Dolin R, Blaser MJ, eds. *Principles and Practice of Infectious Diseases*. 8th ed. Philadelphia: Elsevier Saunders; 2015:1731-1737.

Zika Virus. CDC. Available at: https://www.cdc.gov/zika/healtheffects/birth_defects.html. Published November 5, 2014. Accessed October 11, 2017.

PERTUSSIS

Gilbert DN, Chambers HF, Eliopoulos GM, et al., eds. *The Sanford Guide to Antimicrobial Therapy*. 46th ed. Sperryville, VA: Antimicrobial Therapy Inc; 2016.

Long SS. Bordetella. In: Schlossberg D, ed. *Clinical Infectious Disease*. 2nd ed. Cambridge, United Kingdom: Cambridge University Press; 2015:859-862.

Skoff TH, Liang JL. Pertussis. In: Brunette GW, ed. *CDC Yellow Book 2018 Health Information for International Travel*. Oxford, United Kingdom: Oxford University Press; 2017:272-274.

Waters V, Halperin SA. Bordetella pertussis. In: Bennett JE, Dolin R, Blaser MJ, eds. *Principles and Practice of Infectious Diseases*. 8th ed. Philadelphia: Elsevier Saunders; 2015:2619-2628.

HAND, FOOT, AND MOUTH DISEASE

Oxman MN. Enteroviruses. In: Schlossberg D, ed. *Clinical Infectious Disease*. 2nd ed. Cambridge, United Kingdom: Cambridge University Press; 2015:1172-1182.

Romero JR, Modlin JF. Coxsackieviruses, Echoviruses, and Numbered Enteroviruses. In: Bennett JE, Dolin R, Blaser MJ, eds. *Principles and Practice of Infectious Diseases*. 8th ed. Philadelphia: Elsevier Saunders; 2015: 2080-2090.

Schneider E. Hand foot, & mouth disease. In: Brunette GW, ed. *CDC Yellow Book 2018 Health Information for International Travel*. Oxford, United Kingdom: Oxford University Press; 2017:180-181.

BRONCHIOLITIS

Bower J, McBride JT. Bronchiolitis. In: Bennett JE, Dolin R, Blaser MJ, eds. *Principles and Practice of Infectious Diseases*. 8th ed. Philadelphia: Elsevier Saunders; 2015:818-822.

Gilbert DN, Chambers HF, Eliopoulos GM, et al., eds. *The Sanford Guide to Antimicrobial Therapy*. 46th ed. Sperryville, VA: Antimicrobial Therapy Inc; 2016.

Poole P, Hobbs M. Acute bronchitis and acute exacerbations of chronic airways disease. In: Schlossberg D, ed. *Clinical Infectious Disease*. 2nd ed. Cambridge, United Kingdom: Cambridge University Press; 2015:193-198.

KAWASAKI DISEASE

Assimacopoulos AP, Salgado-Pabon W, Schlievert PM. Staphylococcal and streptococcal toxic shock and Kawasaki syndromes. In: Schlossberg D, ed. *Clinical Infectious Disease*. 2nd ed. Cambridge, United Kingdom: Cambridge University Press; 2015:127-132.

Burns JC. Kawasaki Disease. In: Bennett JE, Dolin R, Blaser MJ, eds. *Principles and Practice of Infectious Diseases*. 8th ed. Philadelphia: Elsevier Saunders; 2015: 3280-3285.

Gilbert DN, Chambers HF, Eliopoulos GM, et al., eds. *The Sanford Guide to Antimicrobial Therapy*. 46th ed. Sperryville, VA: Antimicrobial Therapy Inc; 2016.

CROUP

Behlau I. Croup, supraglottitis, and laryngitis. In: Schlossberg D, ed. *Clinical Infectious Disease*. 2nd ed. Cambridge, United Kingdom: Cambridge University Press; 2015: 199-204.

Bower J, McBride JT. Croup in Children (Acute Laryngotracheobronchitis). In: Bennett JE, Dolin R, Blaser MJ, eds. *Principles and Practice of Infectious Diseases*. 8th ed. Philadelphia: Elsevier Saunders; 2015:762-766.

TICK-BORNE ILLNESSES

TICK-BORNE ILLNESS AND TICKS AS VECTORS

Diaz JH. Ticks, Including Tick Paralysis. In: Bennett JE, Dolin R, Blaser MJ, eds. *Principles and Practice of Infectious Diseases*. 8th ed. Philadelphia: Elsevier Saunders; 2015:3266-3279.

ROCKY MOUNTAIN SPOTTED FEVER

Gilbert DN, Chambers HF, Eliopoulos GM, et al., eds. *The Sanford Guide to Antimicrobial Therapy*. 46th ed. Sperryville, VA: Antimicrobial Therapy Inc; 2016.

Holtom PD. Richettsial infections. In: Schlossberg D, ed. *Clinical Infectious Disease*. 2nd ed. Cambridge, United Kingdom: Cambridge University Press; 2015: 1093-1097.

Keystone JS. Skin & Soft Tissue Infections in Returned Travelers. In: Brunette GW, ed. *CDC Yellow Book 2018 Health Information for International Travel*. Oxford, United Kingdom: Oxford University Press; 2017:507-512.

Sensakovic JW, Smith LG. Fever and rash. In: Schlossberg D, ed. *Clinical Infectious Disease*. 2nd ed. Cambridge, United Kingdom: Cambridge University Press; 2015: 122-126.

Walker DH, Blanton LS. Rickettsia richettsii and Other Spotted Fever Group Rickettsiae (Rocky Mountain Spotted Fever and Other Spotter Fevers). In: Bennett JE, Dolin R, Blaser MJ, eds. *Principles and Practice of Infectious Diseases*. 8th ed. Philadelphia: Elsevier Saunders; 2015: 2198-2205.

LYME DISEASE

Evans J. Lyme disease. In: Schlossberg D, ed. *Clinical Infectious Disease*. 2nd ed. Cambridge, United Kingdom: Cambridge University Press; 2015:1060-1067.

Gilbert DN, Chambers HF, Eliopoulos GM, et al., eds. *The Sanford Guide to Antimicrobial Therapy*. 46th ed. Sperryville, VA: Antimicrobial Therapy Inc; 2016.

Mead PS. Lyme Disease. In: Brunette GW, ed. *CDC Yellow Book 2018 Health Information for International Travel*. Oxford, United Kingdom: Oxford University Press; 2017:232.

Steere AC. Lyme Disease (Lyme Borreliosis) Due to Borrelia burgdoferi. In: Bennett JE, Dolin R, Blaser MJ, eds. *Principles and Practice of Infectious Diseases*. 8th ed. Philadelphia: Elsevier Saunders; 2015:2725-2735.

Weber JW, Juliano JJ, Rutala WA. Systemic infection from animals. In: Schlossberg D, ed. *Clinical Infectious Disease*. 2nd ed. Cambridge, United Kingdom: Cambridge University Press; 2015:794-796.

EHRLICHIOSIS

Bakken JS, Dumler JS. Ehrlichiosis and anaplasmosis. In: Schlossberg D, ed. *Clinical Infectious Disease*. 2nd ed. Cambridge, United Kingdom: Cambridge University Press; 2015:1098-1099.

Gilbert DN, Chambers HF, Eliopoulos GM, et al., eds. *The Sanford Guide to Antimicrobial Therapy*. 46th ed. Sperryville, VA: Antimicrobial Therapy Inc; 2016.

Nicholson WL, Paddock CD. Rickettsial (Spotted & Typhus Fevers) & Related Infections, Including Anaplasmosis & Ehrlichiosis. In: Brunette GW, ed. *CDC Yellow Book 2018 Health Information for International Travel*. Oxford, United Kingdom: Oxford University Press; 2017:297-303.

Raoult D. Rickettsioses, Ehrlichioses, and Anaplasmosis. In: Bennett JE, Dolin R, Blaser MJ, eds. *Principles and Practice of Infectious Diseases*. 8th ed. Philadelphia: Elsevier Saunders; 2015:2194-2197.

ANAPLASMOSIS

Bakken JS, Dumler JS. Ehrlichiosis and anaplasmosis. In: Schlossberg D, ed. *Clinical Infectious Disease*. 2nd ed.

Cambridge, United Kingdom: Cambridge University Press; 2015:1098-1099.

Dumler JS, Walker DH. Ehrlichia chaffeensis (Human Monocyto-tropic Ehrlichiosis), Anaplasma phagocytophilum (Human Granulocytotropic Anaplasmosis), and Other Anaplasmataceae. In: Bennett JE, Dolin R, Blaser MJ, eds. *Principles and Practice of Infectious Diseases*. 8th ed. Philadelphia: Elsevier Saunders; 2015:2227-2233.

Gilbert DN, Chambers HF, Eliopoulos GM, et al., eds. *The Sanford Guide to Antimicrobial Therapy*. 46th ed. Sperryville, VA: Antimicrobial Therapy Inc; 2016.

Nicholson WL, Paddock CD. Rickettsial (Spotted & Typhus Fevers) & Related Infections, Including Anaplasmosis & Ehrlichiosis. In: Brunette GW, ed. *CDC Yellow Book 2018 Health Information for International Travel*. Oxford, United Kingdom: Oxford University Press; 2017:297-303.

BABESIOSIS

Chen TK, Mamoun CB, Krause PJ. Human babesiosis. In: Bakken JS, Dumler JS, Schlossberg D, eds. *Ehrlichiosis and anaplasmosis Clinical Infectious Disease*. 2nd ed. Cambridge, United Kingdom: Cambridge University Press; 2015:1295-1301.

Gilbert DN, Chambers HF, Eliopoulos GM, et al., eds. *The Sanford Guide to Antimicrobial Therapy*. 46th ed. Sperryville, VA: Antimicrobial Therapy Inc; 2016.

White Jr AC. Cryptosporidiosis (Cryptosporidium Species). In: Bennett JE, Dolin R, Blaser MJ, eds. *Principles and Practice of Infectious Diseases*. 8th ed. Philadelphia: Elsevier Saunders; 2015:3173-3183.

TULAREMIA

Gilbert DN, Chambers HF, Eliopoulos GM, et al., eds. *The Sanford Guide to Antimicrobial Therapy*. 46th ed. Sperryville, VA: Antimicrobial Therapy Inc; 2016.

Neemann KA, Snowden JN. Tularemia. In: Bakken JS, Dumler JS, Schlossberg D, eds. *Ehrlichiosis and anaplasmosis Clinical Infectious Disease*. 2nd ed. Cambridge, United Kingdom: Cambridge University Press; 2015:1007-1009.

Penn RL. Francisella tularensis (Tularemia). In: Bennett JE, Dolin R, Blaser MJ, eds. *Principles and Practice of Infectious*

Diseases. 8th ed. Philadelphia: Elsevier Saunders; 2015: 2590-2602.

CRIMEAN-CONGO HEMORRHAGIC FEVER

Bente DA. California Encephalitis, Hantavirus Pulmonary Syndrome, and Bunyavirus Hemorrhagic Fevers. In: Bennett JE, Dolin R, Blaser MJ, eds. *Principles and Practice of Infectious Diseases.* 8th ed. Philadelphia: Elsevier Saunders; 2015:2025-2030.

Crimean-Congo Hemorrhagic Fever (CCHF) | CDC. Available at: https://www.cdc.gov/vhf/crimean-congo/index. html. Accessed October 6, 2017.

COLORADO TICK FEVER

Colorado Tick Fever | Colorado Tick Fever | CDC. Available at: https://www.cdc.gov/coloradotickfever/. Accessed October 6, 2017.

Debiasi RL, Tyler KL. Coltiviruses and Seadornaviruses. In: Bennett JE, Dolin R, Blaser MJ, eds. *Principles and Practice of Infectious Diseases.* 8th ed. Philadelphia: Elsevier Saunders; 2015:1851-1853.

WORMS: ROUNDWORMS

ASCARIASIS

Gilbert DN, Chambers HF, Eliopoulos GM, et al., eds. *The Sanford Guide to Antimicrobial Therapy.* 46th ed. Sperryville, VA: Antimicrobial Therapy Inc; 2016.

Maguire JH. Intestinal Nematodes (Roundworms). In: Bennett JE, Dolin R, Blaser MJ, eds. *Principles and Practice of Infectious Diseases.* 8th ed. Philadelphia: Elsevier Saunders; 2015:3199-3207.

Suh KN, Keystone JS. Intestinal roundworms. In: Schlossberg D, ed. *Clinical Infectious Disease.* 2nd ed. Cambridge, United Kingdom: Cambridge University Press; 2015:1250-1257.

FILARIASIS

Fox LM. Filariasis, Lymphatic. In: Brunette GW, ed. *CDC Yellow Book 2018 Health Information for International Travel.* Oxford, United Kingdom: Oxford University Press; 2017:178-179.

Gilbert DN, Chambers HF, Eliopoulos GM, et al., eds. *The Sanford Guide to Antimicrobial Therapy.* 46th ed. Sperryville, VA: Antimicrobial Therapy Inc; 2016.

Kazura JW. Tissue Nematodes (Trichinellosis, Dracunculiasis, Filariasis, Loiasis, and Onchocerciasis). In: Bennett JE, Dolin R, Blaser MJ, eds. *Principles and Practice of Infectious Diseases.* 8th ed. Philadelphia: Elsevier Saunders; 2015:3208-3215.

Moore TA. Tissue nematodes. In: Schlossberg D, ed. *Clinical Infectious Disease.* 2nd ed. Cambridge, United Kingdom: Cambridge University Press; 2015:1258-1267.

ONCHOCERCIASIS

Cantey PT. Onchocerciasis (River Blindness). In: Brunette GW, ed. *CDC Yellow Book 2018 Health Information for International Travel.* Oxford, United Kingdom: Oxford University Press; 2017:271-272.

Gilbert DN, Chambers HF, Eliopoulos GM, et al., eds. *The Sanford Guide to Antimicrobial Therapy.* 46th ed. Sperryville, VA: Antimicrobial Therapy Inc; 2016.

Kazura JW. Tissue Nematodes (Trichinellosis, Dracunculiasis, Filariasis, Loiasis, and Onchocerciasis). In: Bennett JE, Dolin R, Blaser MJ, eds. *Principles and Practice of Infectious Diseases.* 8th ed. Philadelphia: Elsevier Saunders; 2015:3208-3215.

Vinelli GL, Koestenblatt KV, Weinberg JM. Superficial fungal diseases of the hair, skin, and nails. In: Schlossberg D, ed. *Clinical Infectious Disease.* 2nd ed. Cambridge, United Kingdom: Cambridge University Press; 2015:171-179.

PINWORM

Dubray C. Pinworm (Enterobiasis, Oxyuriasis, Threadworm). In: Brunette GW, ed. *CDC Yellow Book 2018 Health Information for International Travel.* Oxford, United Kingdom: Oxford University Press; 2017:275-276.

Gilbert DN, Chambers HF, Eliopoulos GM, et al., eds. *The Sanford Guide to Antimicrobial Therapy.* 46th ed. Sperryville, VA: Antimicrobial Therapy Inc; 2016.

Suh KN, Keystone JS. Intestinal roundworms. In: Schlossberg D, ed. *Clinical Infectious Disease.* 2nd ed. Cambridge, United Kingdom: Cambridge University Press; 2015: 1250-1257.

HOOKWORM

Dubray C. Helminths, Soil-Transmitted. In: Brunette GW, ed. *CDC Yellow Book 2018 Health Information for International Travel*. Oxford, United Kingdom: Oxford University Press; 2017:182-183.

Gilbert DN, Chambers HF, Eliopoulos GM, et al., eds. *The Sanford Guide to Antimicrobial Therapy*. 46th ed. Sperryville, VA: Antimicrobial Therapy Inc; 2016.

Maguire JH. Intestinal Nematodes (Roundworms). In: Bennett JE, Dolin R, Blaser MJ, eds. *Principles and Practice of Infectious Diseases*. 8th ed. Philadelphia: Elsevier Saunders; 2015:3199-3207.

Suh KN, Keystone JS. Intestinal roundworms. In: Schlossberg D, ed. *Clinical Infectious Disease*. 2nd ed. Cambridge, United Kingdom: Cambridge University Press; 2015: 1250-1257.

WHIPWORM

Dubray C. Helminths, Soil-Transmitted. In: Brunette GW, ed. *CDC Yellow Book 2018 Health Information for International Travel*. Oxford, United Kingdom: Oxford University Press; 2017:182-183.

Gilbert DN, Chambers HF, Eliopoulos GM, et al., eds. *The Sanford Guide to Antimicrobial Therapy*. 46th ed. Sperryville, VA: Antimicrobial Therapy Inc; 2016.

Moore TA. Tissue nematodes. In: Schlossberg D, ed. *Clinical Infectious Disease*. 2nd ed. Cambridge, United Kingdom: Cambridge University Press; 2015:1258-1267.

TRICHINOSIS

Gilbert DN, Chambers HF, Eliopoulos GM, et al., eds. *The Sanford Guide to Antimicrobial Therapy*. 46th ed. Sperryville, VA: Antimicrobial Therapy Inc; 2016.

Moore TA. Tissue nematodes. In: Schlossberg D, ed. *Clinical Infectious Disease*. 2nd ed. Cambridge, United Kingdom: Cambridge University Press; 2015:1258-1267.

Pasternack MS, Swartz MN. Myositis and Myonecrosis. In: Bennett JE, Dolin R, Blaser MJ, eds. *Principles and Practice of Infectious Diseases*. 8th ed. Philadelphia: Elsevier Saunders; 2015:1216-1225.

DRACUNCULIASIS

Gilbert DN, Chambers HF, Eliopoulos GM, et al., eds. *The Sanford Guide to Antimicrobial Therapy*. 46th ed. Sperryville, VA: Antimicrobial Therapy Inc; 2016.

Kazura JW. Tissue Nematodes (Trichinellosis, Dracunculiasis, Filariasis, Loiasis, and Onchocerciasis). In: Bennett JE, Dolin R, Blaser MJ, eds. *Principles and Practice of Infectious Diseases*. 8th ed. Philadelphia: Elsevier Saunders; 2015: 3208-3215.

Moore TA. Tissue nematodes. In: Schlossberg D, ed. *Clinical Infectious Disease*. 2nd ed. Cambridge, United Kingdom: Cambridge University Press; 2015:1258-1267.

CUTANEOUS LARVA MIGRANS

Gilbert DN, Chambers HF, Eliopoulos GM, et al., eds. *The Sanford Guide to Antimicrobial Therapy*. 46th ed. Sperryville, VA: Antimicrobial Therapy Inc; 2016.

Montgomery S. Cutaneous Larva Migrans. In: Brunette GW, ed. *CDC Yellow Book 2018 Health Information for International Travel*. Oxford, United Kingdom: Oxford University Press; 2017:159-160.

Moore TA. Tissue nematodes. In: Schlossberg D, ed. *Clinical Infectious Disease*. 2nd ed. Cambridge, United Kingdom: Cambridge University Press; 2015:1258-1267.

Nash TE. Visceral Larva Migrans and Other Uncommon Helminth Infections. In: Bennett JE, Dolin R, Blaser MJ, eds. *Principles and Practice of Infectious Diseases*. 8th ed. Philadelphia: Elsevier Saunders; 2015:3237-3242.

THREADWORM

Dubray C. Pinworm (Enterobiasis, Oxyuriasis, Threadworm). In: Brunette GW, ed. *CDC Yellow Book 2018 Health Information for International Travel*. Oxford, United Kingdom: Oxford University Press; 2017:275-276.

Gilbert DN, Chambers HF, Eliopoulos GM, et al., eds. *The Sanford Guide to Antimicrobial Therapy*. 46th ed. Sperryville, VA: Antimicrobial Therapy Inc; 2016.

Suh KN, Keystone JS. Intestinal roundworms. In: Schlossberg D, ed. *Clinical Infectious Disease*. 2nd ed. Cambridge, United Kingdom: Cambridge University Press; 2015:1250-1257.

WORMS: TAPEWORMS

PORK TAPEWORM AND CYSTICERCOSIS

CDC – Parasites – Taeniasis. Available at: https://www.cdc.gov/parasites/taeniasis/index.html. Published January 10, 2013. Accessed October 11, 2017.

Gilbert DN, Chambers HF, Eliopoulos GM, et al., eds. *The Sanford Guide to Antimicrobial Therapy.* 46th ed. Sperryville, VA: Antimicrobial Therapy Inc; 2016.

King CH, Fairley JK. Tapeworms (Cestodes). In: Bennett JE, Dolin R, Blaser MJ, eds. *Principles and Practice of Infectious Diseases.* 8th ed. Philadelphia: Elsevier Saunders; 2015:3227-3236.

Pawlowski ZS. Tapeworms (cestodes). In: Schlossberg D, ed. *Clinical Infectious Disease.* 2nd ed. Cambridge, United Kingdom: Cambridge University Press; 2015:1274-1278.

BROAD FISH TAPEWORM

CDC – Parasites – Diphyllobothrium Infection. Available at: https://www.cdc.gov/parasites/diphyllobothrium/. Published January 10, 2012. Accessed October 11, 2017.

Gilbert DN, Chambers HF, Eliopoulos GM, et al., eds. *The Sanford Guide to Antimicrobial Therapy.* 46th ed. Sperryville, VA: Antimicrobial Therapy Inc; 2016.

King CH, Fairley JK. Tapeworms (Cestodes). Bennett JE, Dolin R, Blaser MJ, eds. *Principles and Practice of Infectious Diseases.* 8th ed. Philadelphia: Elsevier Saunders; 2015:3227-3236.

BEEF TAPEWORM

Cantey PT, Jones JL. Taeniasis. In: Brunette GW, ed. *CDC Yellow Book 2018 Health Information for International Travel.* Oxford, United Kingdom: Oxford University Press; 2017:325.

CDC – Parasites – Taeniasis. Available at: https://www.cdc.gov/parasites/taeniasis/index.html. Published January 10, 2013. Accessed October 11, 2017.

Gilbert DN, Chambers HF, Eliopoulos GM, et al., eds. *The Sanford Guide to Antimicrobial Therapy.* 46th ed. Sperryville, VA: Antimicrobial Therapy Inc; 2016.

King CH, Fairley JK. Tapeworms (Cestodes). In: Bennett JE, Dolin R, Blaser MJ, eds. *Principles and Practice of Infectious Diseases.* 8th ed. Philadelphia: Elsevier Saunders; 2015:3227-3236.

ECHINOCOCCOSIS

CDC – Parasites – Echinococcosis. Available at: https://www.cdc.gov/parasites/echinococcosis/. Published December 12, 2012. Accessed October 11, 2017.

Gilbert DN, Chambers HF, Eliopoulos GM, et al., eds. *The Sanford Guide to Antimicrobial Therapy.* 46th ed. Sperryville, VA: Antimicrobial Therapy Inc; 2016.

King CH, Fairley JK. Tapeworms (Cestodes). In: Bennett JE, Dolin R, Blaser MJ, eds. *Principles and Practice of Infectious Diseases.* 8th ed. Philadelphia: Elsevier Saunders; 2015: 3227-3236.

DWARF TAPEWORM

CDC – Parasites – Hymenolepiasis (also known as Hymenolepis nana infection). Available at: https://www.cdc.gov/parasites/hymenolepis/. Published January 10, 2012. Accessed October 11, 2017.

Gilbert DN, Chambers HF, Eliopoulos GM, et al., eds. *The Sanford Guide to Antimicrobial Therapy.* 46th ed. Sperryville, VA: Antimicrobial Therapy Inc; 2016.

King CH, Fairley JK. Tapeworms (Cestodes). In: Bennett JE, Dolin R, Blaser MJ, eds. *Principles and Practice of Infectious Diseases.* 8th ed. Philadelphia: Elsevier Saunders; 2015:3227-3236.

WORMS: FLATWORMS

SCHISTOSOMIASIS

Gilbert DN, Chambers HF, Eliopoulos GM, et al., eds. *The Sanford Guide to Antimicrobial Therapy.* 46th ed. Sperryville, VA: Antimicrobial Therapy Inc; 2016.

Maguire JH. Schistosomes and other trematodes. In: Schlossberg D, ed. *Clinical Infectious Disease.* 2nd ed. Cambridge, United Kingdom: Cambridge University Press; 2015:1268-1273.

Maguire JH. Trematodes (Schistosomes and Liver Intestinal, and Lung Flukes). In: Bennett JE, Dolin R, Blaser MJ, eds. *Principles and Practice of Infectious Diseases.* 8th ed. Philadelphia: Elsevier Saunders; 2015:3216-3226.

Montgomery S. Schistosomiasis. In: Brunette GW, ed. *CDC Yellow Book 2018 Health Information for International Travel*. Oxford, United Kingdom: Oxford University Press; 2018:309-313.

LIVER FLUKE

Gilbert DN, Chambers HF, Eliopoulos GM, et al., eds. *The Sanford Guide to Antimicrobial Therapy*. 46th ed. Sperryville, VA: Antimicrobial Therapy Inc; 2016.

Maguire JH. Trematodes (Schistosomes and Liver Intestinal, and Lung Flukes). In: Bennett JE, Dolin R, Blaser MJ, eds. *Principles and Practice of Infectious Diseases*. 8th ed. Philadelphia: Elsevier Saunders; 2015:3216-3226.

LUNG FLUKE

Gilbert DN, Chambers HF, Eliopoulos GM, et al., eds. *The Sanford Guide to Antimicrobial Therapy*. 46th ed. Sperryville, VA: Antimicrobial Therapy Inc; 2016.

Maguire JH. Trematodes (Schistosomes and Liver Intestinal, and Lung Flukes). In: Bennett JE, Dolin R, Blaser MJ, eds. *Principles and Practice of Infectious Diseases*. 8th ed. Philadelphia: Elsevier Saunders; 2015:3216-3226.

FUNGAL

SPOROTRICHOSIS

Gilbert DN, Chambers HF, Eliopoulos GM, et al., eds. *The Sanford Guide to Antimicrobial Therapy*. 46th ed. Sperryville, VA: Antimicrobial Therapy Inc; 2016.

Greenfield RA. Sporotrichum. In: Schlossberg D, ed. *Clinical Infectious Disease*. 2nd ed. Cambridge, United Kingdom: Cambridge University Press; 2015:1124-1127.

Rex JH, Okhuysen PA. Sporothrix schenckii. In: Bennett JE, Dolin R, Blaser MJ, eds. *Principles and Practice of Infectious Diseases*. 8th ed. Philadelphia: Elsevier Saunders; 2015:2920-2924.

PARACOCCIDIOMYCOSIS

Gilbert DN, Chambers HF, Eliopoulos GM, et al., eds. *The Sanford Guide to Antimicrobial Therapy*. 46th ed. Sperryville, VA: Antimicrobial Therapy Inc; 2016.

Restrepo A, Tobon AM, Cano LE. Paracoccidioidomycosis. In: Bennett JE, Dolin R, Blaser MJ, eds. *Principles and Practice of Infectious Diseases*. 8th ed. Philadelphia: Elsevier Saunders; 2015:2995-3002.

COCCIDIOMYCOSIS

Chiller TM. Armstrong PA, McCotter OZ. Coccidioidomycosis. In: Brunette GW, ed. *CDC Yellow Book 2018 Health Information for International Travel*. Oxford, United Kingdom: Oxford University Press; 2017:156-157.

Galgiani JN. Coccidioidomycosis (Coccidioides Species). In: Bennett JE, Dolin R, Blaser MJ, eds. *Principles and Practice of Infectious Diseases*. 8th ed. Philadelphia: Elsevier Saunders; 2015:2974-2984.

Gilbert DN, Chambers HF, Eliopoulos GM, et al., eds. *The Sanford Guide to Antimicrobial Therapy*. 46th ed. Sperryville, VA: Antimicrobial Therapy Inc; 2016.

Mirels LF, Deresinski S. Coccidioidomycosis. In: Schlossberg D, ed. *Clinical Infectious Disease*. 2nd ed. Cambridge, United Kingdom: Cambridge University Press; 2015: 1141-1150.

BLASTOMYCOSIS

Bradsher Jr RW. Blastomucosis. In: Bennett JE, Dolin R, Blaser MJ, eds. *Principles and Practice of Infectious Diseases*. 8th ed. Philadelphia: Elsevier Saunders; 2015:2963-2973.

Gilbert DN, Chambers HF, Eliopoulos GM, et al., eds. *The Sanford Guide to Antimicrobial Therapy*. 46th ed. Sperryville, VA: Antimicrobial Therapy Inc; 2016.

Pappas PG. Blastomycosis. In: Schlossberg D, ed. *Clinical Infectious Disease*. 2nd ed. Cambridge, United Kingdom: Cambridge University Press; 2015:1138-1140.

HISTOPLASMOSIS

Deepe Jr GS. Histoplasma capsulatum (Histoplasmosis). In: Bennett JE, Dolin R, Blaser MJ, eds. *Principles and Practice of Infectious Diseases*. 8th ed. Philadelphia: Elsevier Saunders; 2015:2949-2962.

Gilbert DN, Chambers HF, Eliopoulos GM, et al., eds. *The Sanford Guide to Antimicrobial Therapy*. 46th ed. Sperryville, VA: Antimicrobial Therapy Inc; 2016.

Goldman M, Lapitz A. Histoplasmosis. In: Schlossberg D, ed. *Clinical Infectious Disease*. 2nd ed. Cambridge, United Kingdom: Cambridge University Press; 2015:1134-1137.

Jackson BR, Chiller TM. Histoplasmosis. In: Brunette GW, ed. *CDC Yellow Book 2018 Health Information for International Travel*. Oxford, United Kingdom: Oxford University Press; 2017:199-202.

TINEA INFECTIONS OF THE SKIN

Gilbert DN, Chambers HF, Eliopoulos GM, et al., eds. *The Sanford Guide to Antimicrobial Therapy*. 46th ed. Sperryville, VA: Antimicrobial Therapy Inc; 2016.

Hay RJ. Dermatophytosis (Ringworm) and Other Superficial Mycoses. In: Bennett JE, Dolin R, Blaser MJ, eds. *Principles and Practice of Infectious Diseases*. 8th ed. Philadelphia: Elsevier Saunders; 2015:2985-2994.

Keystone JS. Skin & Soft Tissue Infections in Returned Travelers. In: Brunette GW, ed. *CDC Yellow Book 2018 Health Information for International Travel*. Oxford, United Kingdom: Oxford University Press; 2017:507-512.

Vinelli GL, Koestenblatt KV, Weinberg JM. Superficial fungal diseases of the hair, skin, and nails. In: Schlossberg D, ed. *Clinical Infectious Disease*. 2nd ed. Cambridge, United Kingdom: Cambridge University Press; 2015:171-179.

TINEA VERSICOLOR

Gilbert DN, Chambers HF, Eliopoulos GM, et al., eds. *The Sanford Guide to Antimicrobial Therapy*. 46th ed. Sperryville, VA: Antimicrobial Therapy Inc; 2016.

Hay RJ. Dermatophytosis (Ringworm) and Other Superficial Mycoses. In: Bennett JE, Dolin R, Blaser MJ, eds. *Principles and Practice of Infectious Diseases*. 8th ed. Philadelphia: Elsevier Saunders; 2015:2985-2994.

Keystone JS. Skin & Soft Tissue Infections in Returned Travelers. In: Brunette GW, ed. *CDC Yellow Book 2018 Health Information for International Travel*. Oxford, United Kingdom: Oxford University Press; 2017:507-512.

Vinelli GL, Koestenblatt KV, Weinberg JM. Superficial fungal diseases of the hair, skin, and nails. In: Schlossberg D, ed. *Clinical Infectious Disease*. 2nd ed. Cambridge, United Kingdom: Cambridge University Press; 2015:171-179.

ASPERGILLOSIS

Gilbert DN, Chambers HF, Eliopoulos GM, et al., eds. *The Sanford Guide to Antimicrobial Therapy*. 46th ed. Sperryville, VA: Antimicrobial Therapy Inc; 2016.

Patterson TF. Aspergillus Species. In: Bennett JE, Dolin R, Blaser MJ. eds. *Principles and Practice of Infectious Diseases*. 8th ed. Philadelphia: Elsevier Saunders; 2015: 2895-2908.

Ram S, Levitz SM. Aspergillosis. In: Schlossberg D, ed. *Clinical Infectious Disease*. 2nd ed. Cambridge, United Kingdom: Cambridge University Press; 2015:1113-1118.

MUCORMYCOSIS

Durand ML. Periocular infections. In: Schlossberg D, ed. *Clinical Infectious Disease*. 2nd ed. Cambridge, United Kingdom: Cambridge University Press; 2015:116-120.

Gilbert DN, Chambers HF, Eliopoulos GM, et al., eds. *The Sanford Guide to Antimicrobial Therapy*. 46th ed. Sperryville, VA: Antimicrobial Therapy Inc; 2016.

Kontoyiannis DP, Lewis RE. Agents of Mucormycosis and Entomophthoramycosis. In: Bennett JE, Dolin R, Blaser MJ, eds. *Principles and Practice of Infectious Diseases*. 8th ed. Philadelphia: Elsevier Saunders; 2015:2909-2919.

SEXUALLY TRANSMITTED DISEASES

GONORRHEA

2015 STD Treatment Guidelines. Available at: https://www.cdc.gov/std/tg2015/default.htm. Accessed October 6, 2017.

Gilbert DN, Chambers HF, Eliopoulos GM, et al., eds. *The Sanford Guide to Antimicrobial Therapy*. 46th ed. Sperryville, VA: Antimicrobial Therapy Inc; 2016.

Marrazzo JM, Apicella MA. Neisseria gonorrhoeae (Gonorrhea). In: Bennett JE, Dolin R, Blaser MJ, eds. *Principles and Practice of Infectious Diseases*. 8th ed. Philadelphia: Elsevier Saunders; 2015:2446-2462.

Mathers AJ, Rein MF. Gonococcus: Neisseria gonorrhoeae. In: Schlossberg D, ed. *Clinical Infectious Disease*. 2nd ed. Cambridge, United Kingdom: Cambridge University Press; 2015:915-919.

CONDYLOMA ACUMINATA

2015 STD Treatment Guidelines. Available at: https://www.cdc.gov/std/tg2015/default.htm. Accessed October 6, 2017.

Bonnez W. Papillomaviruses. In: Bennett JE, Dolin R, Blaser MJ, eds. *Principles and Practice of Infectious Diseases*. 8th ed. Philadelphia: Elsevier Saunders; 2015:1794-1806.

Gilbert DN, Chambers HF, Eliopoulos GM, et al., eds. *The Sanford Guide to Antimicrobial Therapy*. 46th ed. Sperryville, VA: Antimicrobial Therapy Inc; 2016.

Kakuda TN, Tomaka FL. Antiviral therapy. In: Schlossberg D, ed. *Clinical Infectious Disease*. 2nd ed. Cambridge, United Kingdom: Cambridge University Press; 2015:1353-1365.

PUBIC LICE

2015 STD Treatment Guidelines. Available at: https://www.cdc.gov/std/tg2015/default.htm. Accessed October 6, 2017.

Diaz JH. Lice (Pediculosis). In: Bennett JE, Dolin R, Blaser MJ, eds. *Principles and Practice of Infectious Diseases*. 8th ed. Philadelphia: Elsevier Saunders; 2015:3246-3249.

Gilbert DN, Chambers HF, Eliopoulos GM, et al., eds. *The Sanford Guide to Antimicrobial Therapy*. 46th ed. Sperryville, VA: Antimicrobial Therapy Inc; 2016.

Monsel G, Chosidow O. Scabies, lice, and myiasis. In: Schlossberg D, ed. *Clinical Infectious Disease*. 2nd ed. Cambridge, United Kingdom: Cambridge University Press; 2015:162-166.

SYPHILIS

2015 STD Treatment Guidelines. Available at: https://www.cdc.gov/std/tg2015/default.htm. Accessed October 6, 2017.

Gilbert DN, Chambers HF, Eliopoulos GM, et al., eds. *The Sanford Guide to Antimicrobial Therapy*. 46th ed. Sperryville, VA: Antimicrobial Therapy Inc; 2016.

Radolf JD, Tramont EC, Salazar JC. Syphilis (Treponema pallidum). In: Bennett JE, Dolin R, Blaser MJ, eds. *Principles and Practice of Infectious Diseases*. 8th ed. Philadelphia: Elsevier Saunders; 2015:2684-2709.

Sena AC, Adimora AA. Syphilis and other treponematoses. In: Schlossberg D, ed. *Clinical Infectious Disease*. 2nd ed. Cambridge, United Kingdom: Cambridge University Press; 2015:1053-1059.

Staat MA, Burke H. International Adoption. In: Brunette GW, ed. *CDC Yellow Book 2018 Health Information for International Travel*. Oxford, United Kingdom: Oxford University Press; 2017:550-555.

CHLAMYDIA

2015 STD Treatment Guidelines. Available at: https://www.cdc.gov/std/tg2015/default.htm. Accessed October 6, 2017.

Bacon III AE. Chlamydia psittaci (psittacosis). In: Schlossberg D, ed. *Clinical Infectious Disease*. 2nd ed. Cambridge, United Kingdom: Cambridge University Press; 2015:1089-1091.

Batteiger BE, Tan M. Chlamydia trachomatis (Trachoma, Genital Infections, Perinatal Infections, and Lymphogranuloma Venereum). In: Bennett JE, Dolin R, Blaser MJ, eds. *Principles and Practice of Infectious Diseases*. 8th ed. Philadelphia: Elsevier Saunders; 2015:2154-2170.

Gilbert DN, Chambers HF, Eliopoulos GM, et al., eds. *The Sanford Guide to Antimicrobial Therapy*. 46th ed. Sperryville, VA: Antimicrobial Therapy Inc; 2016.

TRACHOMA

2015 STD Treatment Guidelines. Available at: https://www.cdc.gov/std/tg2015/default.htm. Accessed October 6, 2017.

Batteiger BE, Tan M. Chlamydia trachomatis (Trachoma, Genital Infections, Perinatal Infections, and Lymphogranuloma Venereum). In: Bennett JE, Dolin R, Blaser MJ, eds. *Principles and Practice of Infectious Diseases*. 8th ed. Philadelphia: Elsevier Saunders; 2015:2154-2170.

Gilbert DN, Chambers HF, Eliopoulos GM, et al., eds. *The Sanford Guide to Antimicrobial Therapy*. 46th ed. Sperryville, VA: Antimicrobial Therapy Inc; 2016.

Tu EY. Conjunctivitis. In: Schlossberg D, ed. *Clinical Infectious Disease*. 2nd ed. Cambridge, United Kingdom: Cambridge University Press; 2015:81-87.

WHO | Trachoma. WHO. Available at: http://www.who.int/trachoma/en/. Accessed October 6, 2017.

REACTIVE ARTHRITIS

Augenbraun MH, McCormack WM. Urethritis. In: Bennett JE, Dolin R, Blaser MJ, eds. *Principles and Practice of Infectious Diseases*. 8th ed. Philadelphia: Elsevier Saunders; 2015:1349-1357.

Dao KH, Cush JJ. Polyarthritis and fever. In: Schlossberg D, ed. *Clinical Infectious Disease*. 2nd ed. Cambridge, United Kingdom: Cambridge University Press; 2015:454-459.

HERPES SIMPLEX

2015 STD Treatment Guidelines. Available at: https://www.cdc.gov/std/tg2015/default.htm. Accessed October 6, 2017.

Gilbert DN, Chambers HF, Eliopoulos GM, et al., eds. *The Sanford Guide to Antimicrobial Therapy*. 46th ed. Sperryville, VA: Antimicrobial Therapy Inc; 2016.

Palmore TN, Henderson DK. Nosocomial Herpesvirus Infections. In: Bennett JE, Dolin R, Blaser MJ, eds. *Principles and Practice of Infectious Diseases*. 8th ed. Philadelphia: Elsevier Saunders; 2015:3376-3383.

Schmid DS. B Virus. In: Brunette GW, ed. *CDC Yellow Book 2018 Health Information for International Travel*. Oxford, United Kingdom: Oxford University Press; 2017:144-146.

Whitley RJ. Herpes simplex viruses 1 and 2. In: Schlossberg D, ed. *Clinical Infectious Disease*. 2nd ed. Cambridge, United Kingdom: Cambridge University Press; 2015:1193-1198.

TRICHOMONIASIS

2015 STD Treatment Guidelines. Available at: https://www.cdc.gov/std/tg2015/default.htm. Accessed October 6, 2017.

Gilbert DN, Chambers HF, Eliopoulos GM, et al., eds. *The Sanford Guide to Antimicrobial Therapy*. 46th ed. Sperryville, VA: Antimicrobial Therapy Inc; 2016.

Pappas G, Bliziotis IA, Falagas ME. Urethritis and dysuria. In: Schlossberg D, ed. *Clinical Infectious Disease*. 2nd ed. Cambridge, United Kingdom: Cambridge University Press; 2015:386-391.

Schwebke JR. Trichomonas vaginalis. In: Bennett JE, Dolin R, Blaser MJ, eds. *Principles and Practice of Infectious Diseases*. 8th ed. Philadelphia: Elsevier Saunders; 2015:3161-3164.

SCABIES

2015 STD Treatment Guidelines. Available at: https://www.cdc.gov/std/tg2015/default.htm. Accessed October 6, 2017.

Diaz JH. Scabies. In: Bennett JE, Dolin R, Blaser MJ, eds. *Principles and Practice of Infectious Diseases*. 8th ed. Philadelphia: Elsevier Saunders; 2015:3250-3254.

Gilbert DN, Chambers HF, Eliopoulos GM, et al., eds. *The Sanford Guide to Antimicrobial Therapy*. 46th ed. Sperryville, VA: Antimicrobial Therapy Inc; 2016.

Martin D. Scabies. In: Brunette GW, ed. *CDC Yellow Book 2018 Health Information for International Travel*. Oxford, United Kingdom: Oxford University Press; 2017:308-309.

Monsel G, Chosidow O. Scabies, lice and myiasis. In: Schlossberg D, ed. *Clinical Infectious Disease*. 2nd ed. Cambridge, United Kingdom: Cambridge University Press; 2015:162-166.

CHANCROID

2015 STD Treatment Guidelines. Available at: https://www.cdc.gov/std/tg2015/default.htm. Accessed October 6, 2017.

Gilbert DN, Chambers HF, Eliopoulos GM, et al., eds. *The Sanford Guide to Antimicrobial Therapy*. 46th ed. Sperryville, VA: Antimicrobial Therapy Inc; 2016.

Murphy TF. *Haemophilus Species, Including H. influenza and H. ducreyi (Chancroid)*. In: Bennett JE, Dolin R, Blaser MJ, eds. *Principles and Practice of Infectious Diseases*. 8th ed. Philadelphia: Elsevier Saunders; 2015:2575-2593.

Ronald A. Genital ulcer adenopathy syndrome. In: Schlossberg D, ed. *Clinical Infectious Disease*. 2nd ed. Cambridge, United Kingdom: Cambridge University Press; 2015:406-412.

DONOVANOSIS

2015 STD Treatment Guidelines. Available at: https://www.cdc.gov/std/tg2015/default.htm. Accessed October 6, 2017.

Ballard RC. Klebsiella granulomatis (Donovanosis, Granuloma Inguinale). In: Bennett JE, Dolin R, Blaser MJ, eds. *Principles and Practice of Infectious Diseases*. 8th ed. Philadelphia: Elsevier Saunders; 2015:2664-2666.

Gilbert DN, Chambers HF, Eliopoulos GM, et al., eds. *The Sanford Guide to Antimicrobial Therapy*. 46th ed. Sperryville, VA: Antimicrobial Therapy Inc; 2016.

Ronald A. Genital ulcer adenopathy syndrome. In: Schlossberg D, ed. *Clinical Infectious Disease*. 2nd ed. Cambridge, United Kingdom: Cambridge University Press; 2015: 406-412.

VAGINITIS

2015 STD Treatment Guidelines. Available at: https:// www.cdc.gov/std/tg2015/default.htm. Accessed October 6, 2017.

Edwards Jr JE. Candida Species. In: Bennett JE, Dolin R, Blaser MJ, eds. *Principles and Practice of Infectious Diseases*. 8th ed. Philadelphia: Elsevier Saunders; 2015: 2879-2894.

Faro S. Vaginitis and cervicitis. In: Schlossberg D, ed. *Clinical Infectious Disease*. 2nd ed. Cambridge, United Kingdom: Cambridge University Press; 2015:392-400.

Gilbert DN, Chambers HF, Eliopoulos GM, et al., eds. *The Sanford Guide to Antimicrobial Therapy*. 46th ed. Sperryville, VA: Antimicrobial Therapy Inc; 2016.

McCormack WM, Augenbraun MH. Vulvovaginitis and Cervicitis. In: Bennett JE, Dolin R, Blaser MJ, eds. *Principles and Practice of Infectious Diseases*. 8th ed. Philadelphia: Elsevier Saunders; 2015:1358-1371.

MOLLUSCUM CONTAGIOSUM

2015 STD Treatment Guidelines. Available at: https:// www.cdc.gov/std/tg2015/default.htm. Accessed October 6, 2017.

Gilbert DN, Chambers HF, Eliopoulos GM, et al., eds. *The Sanford Guide to Antimicrobial Therapy*. 46th ed. Sperryville, VA: Antimicrobial Therapy Inc; 2016.

Ogedegbe A, Glesby MJ. Differential diagnosis and management of HIV-associated opportunistic infections. In: Schlossberg D, ed. *Clinical Infectious Disease*. 2nd ed. Cambridge, United Kingdom: Cambridge University Press; 2015: 676-687.

Petersen BW, Damon IK. Other Poxviruses That Infect Humans: Parapoxviruses (Including Orf Virus), Molluscum Contagiosum, and Yatapoxviruses. In: Bennett JE, Dolin R, Blaser MJ, eds. *Principles and Practice of Infectious Diseases*. 8th ed. Philadelphia: Elsevier Saunders; 2015: 1703-1706.

LYMPHOGRANULOMA VENEREUM

2015 STD Treatment Guidelines. Available at: https://www. cdc.gov/std/tg2015/default.htm. Accessed October 6, 2017.

Batteiger BE, Tan M. Chlamydia trachomatis (Trachoma, Genital Infections, Perinatal Infections, and Lymphogranuloma Venereum). In: Bennett JE, Dolin R, Blaser MJ, eds. *Principles and Practice of Infectious Diseases*. 8th ed. Philadelphia: Elsevier Saunders; 2015:2154-2170.

Gilbert DN, Chambers HF, Eliopoulos GM, et al., eds. *The Sanford Guide to Antimicrobial Therapy*. 46th ed. Sperryville, VA: Antimicrobial Therapy Inc; 2016.

Ronald A. Genital ulcer adenopathy syndrome. In: Schlossberg D, ed. *Clinical Infectious Disease*. 2nd ed. Cambridge, United Kingdom: Cambridge University Press; 2015: 406-412.

PULMONARY

MIDDLE EASTERN RESPIRATORY SYNDROME

McIntosh K, Perlman S. Coronaviruses, Including Severe Acute Respiratory Syndrome (SARS) and Middle East Respiratory Syndrome (MERS). In: Bennett JE, Dolin R, Blaser MJ, eds. *Principles and Practice of Infectious Diseases*. 8th ed. Philadelphia: Elsevier Saunders; 2015: 1928-1936.

MERS-CoV | Home | Middle East Respiratory Syndrome | Coronavirus | CDC. Available at: https://www.cdc.gov/ coronavirus/mers/index.html. Published September 14, 2017. Accessed October 6, 2017.

Vyas KS. Community-acquired pneumonia. In: Schlossberg D, ed. *Clinical Infectious Disease*. 2nd ed. Cambridge, United Kingdom: Cambridge University Press; 2015: 214-220.

Watson JT, Gerber SI. Middle East Respiratory Syndrome (MERS). In: Brunette GW, ed. *CDC Yellow Book 2018 Health Information for International Travel*. Oxford, United Kingdom: Oxford University Press; 2017:267-268.

WHO | *Middle East respiratory syndrome coronavirus (MERS-CoV). WHO.* Available at: http://www.who.int/emergencies/mers-cov/en/. Accessed October 6, 2017.

TUBERCULOSIS

Fitzgerald DW, Sterling TR, Haas DW. Mycobacterium tuberculosis. In: Bennett JE, Dolin R, Blaser MJ, eds. *Principles and Practice of Infectious Diseases.* 8th ed. Philadelphia: Elsevier Saunders; 2015:2787-2818.

Gilbert DN, Chambers HF, Eliopoulos GM, et al., eds. *The Sanford Guide to Antimicrobial Therapy.* 46th ed. Sperryville, VA: Antimicrobial Therapy Inc; 2016.

LoBue P. Tuberculosis. In: Brunette GW, ed. *CDC Yellow Book 2018 Health Information for International Travel.* Oxford, United Kingdom: Oxford University Press; 2017: 334-341.

Mehta JB, Dutt AK. Tuberculosis. In: Schlossberg D, ed. *Clinical Infectious Disease.* 2nd ed. Cambridge, United Kingdom: Cambridge University Press; 2015:1010-1019.

LEGIONNAIRES' DISEASE

Edelstein PH, Roy CR. Legionnaires' Disease and Pontiac Fever. In: Bennett JE, Dolin R, Blaser MJ, eds. *Principles and Practice of Infectious Diseases.* 8th ed. Philadelphia: Elsevier Saunders; 2015:2633-2644.

Gilbert DN, Chambers HF, Eliopoulos GM, et al., eds. *The Sanford Guide to Antimicrobial Therapy.* 46th ed. Sperryville, VA: Antimicrobial Therapy Inc; 2016.

Kutty PK, Garrison LE. Legionellosis (Legionnaires' Disease & Pontiac Fever). In: Brunette GW, ed. *CDC Yellow Book 2018 Health Information for International Travel.* Oxford, United Kingdom: Oxford University Press; 2017: 224-225.

Marrie TJ. Legionellosis. In: Schlossberg D, ed. *Clinical Infectious Disease.* 2nd ed. Cambridge, United Kingdom: Cambridge University Press; 2015:924-930.

PSITTACOSIS

Gilbert DN, Chambers HF, Eliopoulos GM, et al., eds. *The Sanford Guide to Antimicrobial Therapy.* 46th ed. Sperryville, VA: Antimicrobial Therapy Inc; 2016.

Schlossberg D. Psittacosis (Due to Chlamydia psittaci). In: Bennett JE, Dolin R, Blaser MJ, eds. *Principles and Practice of Infectious Diseases.* 8th ed. Philadelphia: Elsevier Saunders; 2015:2171-2173.

Vyas KS. Community-acquired pneumonia. In: Schlossberg D, ed. *Clinical Infectious Disease.* 2nd ed. Cambridge, United Kingdom: Cambridge University Press; 2015:214-220.

AVIAN INFLUENZA

Appiah G, Bresee J. Influenza. In: Brunette GW, ed. *CDC Yellow Book 2018 Health Information for International Travel.* Oxford, United Kingdom: Oxford University Press; 2017:206-214.

CDC. *Information on Avian Influenza. Centers for Disease Control and Prevention.* Available at: https://www.cdc.gov/flu/avianflu/index.htm. Published April 13, 2017. Accessed October 6, 2017.

File TM. Atypical pneumonia. In: Schlossberg D, ed. *Clinical Infectious Disease.* 2nd ed. Cambridge, United Kingdom: Cambridge University Press; 2015:205-213.

Gilbert DN, Chambers HF, Eliopoulos GM, et al., eds. *The Sanford Guide to Antimicrobial Therapy.* 46th ed. Sperryville, VA: Antimicrobial Therapy Inc; 2016.

Treanor JJ. Influenza (Including Avian Influenza and Swine Influenza). In: Bennett JE, Dolin R, Blaser MJ, eds. *Principles and Practice of Infectious Diseases.* 8th ed. Philadelphia: Elsevier Saunders; 2015:2000-2024.

INFLUENZA

Appiah G, Bresee J. Influenza. In: Brunette GW, ed. *CDC Yellow Book 2018 Health Information for International Travel.* Oxford, United Kingdom: Oxford University Press; 2017:206-214.

Gilbert DN, Chambers HF, Eliopoulos GM, et al., eds. *The Sanford Guide to Antimicrobial Therapy.* 46th ed. Sperryville, VA: Antimicrobial Therapy Inc; 2016.

Herati RS, Friedman HM. Influenza. In: Schlossberg D, ed. *Clinical Infectious Disease.* 2nd ed. Cambridge, United Kingdom: Cambridge University Press; 2015:1205-1210.

Treanor JJ. Influenza (Including Avian Influenza and Swine Influenza). In: Bennett JE, Dolin R, Blaser MJ, eds. *Principles and Practice of Infectious Diseases.* 8th ed. Philadelphia: Elsevier Saunders; 2015:2000-2024.

SEVERE ACUTE RESPIRATORY SYNDROME

Gilbert DN, Chambers HF, Eliopoulos GM, et al., eds. *The Sanford Guide to Antimicrobial Therapy.* 46th ed. Sperryville, VA: Antimicrobial Therapy Inc; 2016.

LaRocque RC, Ryan ET. Respiratory Infections. In: Brunette GW, ed. *CDC Yellow Book 2018 Health Information for International Travel.* Oxford, United Kingdom: Oxford University Press; 2017:66-69.

McIntosh K, Perlman S. Coronaviruses, Including Severe Acute Respiratory Syndrome (SARS) and Middle East Respiratory Syndrome (MERS). In: Bennett JE, Dolin R, Blaser MJ, eds. *Principles and Practice of Infectious Diseases.* 8th ed. Philadelphia: Elsevier Saunders; 2015: 1928-1936.

SARS | Home | Severe Acute Respiratory Syndrome | SARS-CoV Disease | CDC. Available at: https://www.cdc.gov/sars/index.html. Accessed October 6, 2017.

Vyas KS. Community-acquired pneumonia. In: Schlossberg D, ed. *Clinical Infectious Disease.* 2nd ed. Cambridge, United Kingdom: Cambridge University Press; 2015: 214-220.

WHO | Severe acute respiratory syndrome. WHO. Available at: http://www.who.int/topics/sars/en/. Accessed October 6, 2017.

MOSQUITO-BORNE DISEASES

ZIKA FEVER

Chen TA, Staples JE, Fischer M. Zika. In: Brunette GW, ed. *CDC Yellow Book 2018 Health Information for International Travel.* Oxford, United Kingdom: Oxford University Press; 2017:369-371.

Gilbert DN, Chambers HF, Eliopoulos GM, et al., eds. *The Sanford Guide to Antimicrobial Therapy.* 46th ed. Sperryville, VA: Antimicrobial Therapy Inc; 2016.

Thomas SJ, Endy TP, Rothman AL, Barrett AD. Flaviviruses (Dengue, Yellow Fever, Japanese Encephalitis, West Nile Encephalitis, St. Louis Encephalitis, Tick-Borne Encephalitis, Kyasanur Forest Disease, Alkhurma Hemorrhagic Fever, Zika). In: Bennett JE, Dolin R, Blaser MJ, eds. *Principles and*

Practice of Infectious Diseases. 8th ed. Philadelphia: Elsevier Saunders; 2015:1881-1903.

Zika Virus. CDC. Available at: https://www.cdc.gov/zika/index.html. Published November 5, 2014. Accessed October 6, 2017.

DENGUE

Dengue | CDC. Available at: https://www.cdc.gov/dengue/index.html. Accessed October 6, 2017.

Gilbert DN, Chambers HF, Eliopoulos GM, et al., eds. *The Sanford Guide to Antimicrobial Therapy.* 46th ed. Sperryville, VA: Antimicrobial Therapy Inc; 2016.

Hung NT. Dengue. In: Schlossberg D, ed. *Clinical Infectious Disease.* 2nd ed. Cambridge, United Kingdom: Cambridge University Press; 2015:1168-1171.

Sharp TM, Perez-Padilla J, Waterman SH. Dengue. In: Brunette GW, ed. *CDC Yellow Book 2018 Health Information for International Travel.* Oxford, United Kingdom: Oxford University Press; 2017:162-169.

Thomas SJ, Endy TP, Rothman AL, Barrett AD. Flaviviruses (Dengue, Yellow Fever, Japanese Encephalitis, West Nile Encephalitis, St. Louis Encephalitis, Tick-Borne Encephalitis, Kyasanur Forest Disease, Alkhurma Hemorrhagic Fever, Zika). In: Bennett JE, Dolin R, Blaser MJ, eds. *Principles and Practice of Infectious Diseases.* 8th ed. Philadelphia: Elsevier Saunders; 2015:1881-1903.

YELLOW FEVER

Gershman MD, Staples JE. Yellow Fever. In: Brunette GW, ed. *CDC Yellow Book 2018 Health Information for International Travel.* Oxford, United Kingdom: Oxford University Press; 2017:352-368.

Gilbert DN, Chambers HF, Eliopoulos GM, et al., eds. *The Sanford Guide to Antimicrobial Therapy.* 46th ed. Sperryville, VA: Antimicrobial Therapy Inc; 2016.

Thomas SJ, Endy TP, Rothman AL, Barrett AD. Flaviviruses (Dengue, Yellow Fever, Japanese Encephalitis, West Nile Encephalitis, St. Louis Encephalitis, Tick-Borne Encephalitis, Kyasanur Forest Disease, Alkhurma Hemorrhagic Fever, Zika). In: Bennett JE, Dolin R, Blaser MJ, eds. *Principles and Practice of Infectious Diseases.* 8th ed. Philadelphia: Elsevier Saunders; 2015:1881-1903.

Wu HM, Fairley JK. Advice for travelers. In: Schlossberg D, ed. *Clinical Infectious Disease.* 2nd ed. Cambridge, United Kingdom: Cambridge University Press; 2015:778-784.

MALARIA

CDC – Malaria. Available at: https://www.cdc.gov/malaria/. Published September 29, 2017. Accessed October 6, 2017.

Fairhurst RM, Wellems TE. Malaria (Plasmodium Species). In: Bennett JE, Dolin R, Blaser MJ, eds. *Principles and Practice of Infectious Diseases.* 8th ed. Philadelphia: Elsevier Saunders; 2015:3070-3090.

Fairley JK, Wu HM. Malaria. In: Schlossberg D, ed. *Clinical Infectious Disease.* 2nd ed. Cambridge, United Kingdom: Cambridge University Press; 2015:1285-1294.

Gershman MD, Jentes ES, Stoney RJ, Tan KR, Arguin PM, Steele SF. In: Brunette GW, ed. *CDC Yellow Book 2018 Health Information for International Travel.* Oxford, United Kingdom: Oxford University Press; 2017:372-424.

Gilbert DN, Chambers HF, Eliopoulos GM, et al., eds. *The Sanford Guide to Antimicrobial Therapy.* 46th ed. Sperryville, VA: Antimicrobial Therapy Inc; 2016.

MOSQUITO-BORNE ENCEPHALITIS

Estrada-Franco JG, Navarro-Lopez R, Freier JE, et al. Venezuelan Equine Encephalitis Virus, Southern Mexico. *Emerg Infect Dis.* 2004;10:12.

Eastern Equine Encephalitis | CDC. Available at: https://www.cdc.gov/easternequineencephalitis/index.html. Accessed October 6, 2017.

Gilbert DN, Chambers HF, Eliopoulos GM, et al., eds. *The Sanford Guide to Antimicrobial Therapy.* 46th ed. Sperryville, VA: Antimicrobial Therapy Inc; 2016.

Irani DN. Acute viral encephalitis. In: Schlossberg D, ed. *Clinical Infectious Disease.* 2nd ed. Cambridge, United Kingdom: Cambridge University Press; 2015:487-494.

Japanese Encephalitis | CDC. Available at: https://www.cdc.gov/japaneseencephalitis/. Accessed October 6, 2017.

La Crosse Encephalitis | CDC. Available at: https://www.cdc.gov/lac/index.html. Accessed October 6, 2017.

Murray Valley Encephalitis virus | Disease Directory | Travelers' Health | CDC. Available at: https://wwwnc.cdc.gov/travel/diseases/murray-valley-encephalitis-virus. Accessed October 6, 2017.

Rift Valley Fever | CDC. Available at: https://www.cdc.gov/vhf/rvf/index.html. Accessed October 6, 2017.

St Louis Encephalitis | CDC. Available at: https://www.cdc.gov/sle/. Accessed October 6, 2017.

Tunkel AR. Approach to the Patient with Central Nervous System Infection. In: Bennett JE, Dolin R, Blaser MJ, eds. *Principles and Practice of Infectious Diseases.* 8th ed. Philadelphia: Elsevier Saunders; 2015:1091-1096.

West Nile virus | West Nile Virus | CDC. Available at: https://www.cdc.gov/westnile/index.html. Published October 3, 2017. Accessed October 6, 2017.

CHIKUNGUNYA

Chikungunya virus | CDC. Available at: https://www.cdc.gov/chikungunya/index.html. Published August 29, 2017. Accessed October 6, 2017.

Gilbert DN, Chambers HF, Eliopoulos GM, et al., eds. *The Sanford Guide to Antimicrobial Therapy.* 46th ed. Sperryville, VA: Antimicrobial Therapy Inc; 2016.

Markoff L. Alphaviruses. In: Bennett JE, Dolin R, Blaser MJ, eds. *Principles and Practice of Infectious Diseases.* 8th ed. Philadelphia: Elsevier Saunders; 2015:1865-1874.

Staples JE, Hills SK, Powers AM. Chikungunya. In: Brunette GW, ed. *CDC Yellow Book 2018 Health Information for International Travel.* Oxford, United Kingdom: Oxford University Press; 2017:151-153.

Wu HM, Fairley JK. Advice for travelers. In: Schlossberg D, ed. *Clinical Infectious Disease.* 2nd ed. Cambridge, United Kingdom: Cambridge University Press; 2015:778-784.

RAT-, FLEA-, LOUSE-, AND CHIGGER-BORNE ILLNESSES

HEMORRHAGIC FEVER WITH RENAL SYNDROME

Bente DA. *California Encephalitis, Hantavirus Pulmonary Syndrome, and Bunyavirus Hemorrhagic Fevers.* In: Bennett JE, Dolin R, Blaser MJ, eds. *Principles and*

Practice of Infectious Diseases. 8th ed. Philadelphia: Elsevier Saunders; 2015:2025-2030.

HANTAVIRUS PULMONARY SYNDROME

Bente DA. California Encephalitis, Hantavirus Pulmonary Syndrome, and Bunyavirus Hemorrhagic Fevers. In: Bennett JE, Dolin R, Blaser MJ, eds. *Principles and Practice of Infectious Diseases.* 8th ed. Philadelphia: Elsevier Saunders; 2015:2025-2030.

Mertz GJ, Iandiorio MJ. Hantavirus cardiopulmonary syndrome in the Americas. In: Schlossberg D, ed. *Clinical Infectious Disease.* 2nd ed. Cambridge, United Kingdom: Cambridge University Press; 2015:1190-1192.

PLAGUE

Gilbert DN, Chambers HF, Eliopoulos GM, et al., eds. *The Sanford Guide to Antimicrobial Therapy.* 46th ed. Sperryville, VA: Antimicrobial Therapy Inc; 2016.

Mead PS. Yersinia Species (Including Plague). In: Bennett JE, Dolin R, Blaser MJ. eds. *Principles and Practice of Infectious Diseases.* 8th ed. Philadelphia: Elsevier Saunders; 2015:2607-2618.

Mead PS. Plague (Bubonic, Pneumonic, Septicemic). In: Brunette GW, ed. *CDC Yellow Book 2018 Health Information for International Travel.* Oxford, United Kingdom: Oxford University Press; 2017:276-277.

Weber DJ, Juliano JJ, Rutala WA. Systemic infection from animals. In: Schlossberg D, ed. *Clinical Infectious Disease.* 2nd ed. Cambridge, United Kingdom: Cambridge University Press; 2015:790-796.

LEPTOSPIROSIS

Galloway RL, Stoffard RA, Schafer IJ. Leptospirosis. In: Brunette GW, ed. *CDC Yellow Book 2018 Health Information for International Travel.* Oxford, United Kingdom: Oxford University Press; 2017:230-231.

Gilbert DN, Chambers HF, Eliopoulos GM, et al., eds. *The Sanford Guide to Antimicrobial Therapy.* 46th ed. Sperryville, VA: Antimicrobial Therapy Inc; 2016.

Haake DA, Levett PN. Leptospira Species (Leptospirosis). In: Bennett JE, Dolin R, Blaser MJ, eds. *Principles and Practice of Infectious Diseases.* 8th ed. Philadelphia: Elsevier Saunders; 2015:2714-2720.

Huston CD. Leptospirosis. In: Schlossberg D, ed. *Clinical Infectious Disease.* 2nd ed. Cambridge, United Kingdom: Cambridge University Press; 2015:1072-1074.

RAT BITE FEVER

Gilbert DN, Chambers HF, Eliopoulos GM, et al., eds. *The Sanford Guide to Antimicrobial Therapy.* 46th ed. Sperryville, VA: Antimicrobial Therapy Inc; 2016.

Lipma NS. Rat-bite fevers. In: Schlossberg D, ed. *Clinical Infectious Disease.* 2nd ed. Cambridge, United Kingdom: Cambridge University Press; 2015:975-978.

Washburn RG. Rat-Bite Fever: Streptobacillus moniliformis and Spirillum minus. In: Bennett JE, Dolin R, Blaser MJ, eds. *Principles and Practice of Infectious Diseases.* 8th ed. Philadelphia: Elsevier Saunders; 2015:2629-2632.

TRENCH FEVER

Gilbert DN, Chambers HF, Eliopoulos GM, et al., eds. *The Sanford Guide to Antimicrobial Therapy.* 46th ed. Sperryville, VA: Antimicrobial Therapy Inc; 2016.

Schwartzman WA. Cat scratch disease and other Bartonella infections. In: Schlossberg D, ed. *Clinical Infectious Disease.* 2nd ed. Cambridge, United Kingdom: Cambridge University Press; 2015:853-858.

SCRUB TYPHUS

Gilbert DN, Chambers HF, Eliopoulos GM, et al., eds. *The Sanford Guide to Antimicrobial Therapy.* 46th ed. Sperryville, VA: Antimicrobial Therapy Inc; 2016.

Holtom PD. Rickettsial infections. In: Schlossberg D, ed. *Clinical Infectious Disease.* 2nd ed. Cambridge, United Kingdom: Cambridge University Press; 2015:1093-1097.

Nicholson WL, Paddock CD. Rickettsial (Spotted & Typhus Fevers) & Related Infections, Including Anaplasmosis & Ehrlichiosis. In: Brunette GW, ed. *CDC Yellow Book 2018 Health Information for International Travel.* Oxford, United Kingdom: Oxford University Press; 2017:297-303.

Raoult D. Orientia tsutsugamushi (Scrub Typhus). In: Bennett JE, Dolin R, Blaser MJ, eds. *Principles and Practice of Infectious Diseases*. 8th ed. Philadelphia: Elsevier Saunders; 2015:2225-2226.

EPIDEMIC TYPHUS

Blanton LS, Walker DH. Rickettsia prowazekii (Epidemic or Louse-Borne Typhus). In: Bennett JE, Dolin R, Blaser MJ, eds. *Principles and Practice of Infectious Diseases*. 8th ed. Philadelphia: Elsevier Saunders; 2015:2217-2220.

Gilbert DN, Chambers HF, Eliopoulos GM, et al., eds. *The Sanford Guide to Antimicrobial Therapy*. 46th ed. Sperryville, VA: Antimicrobial Therapy Inc; 2016.

Nicholson WL, Paddock CD. Rickettsial (Spotted & Typhus Fevers) & Related Infections, Including Anaplasmosis & Ehrlichiosis. In: Brunette GW, ed. *CDC Yellow Book 2018 Health Information for International Travel*. Oxford, United Kingdom: Oxford University Press; 2017:297-303.

ENDEMIC TYPHUS

Blanton LS, Dumler S, Walker DH. Rickettsia typhi (Murine Typhus). In: Bennett JE, Dolin R, Blaser MJ, eds. *Principles and Practice of Infectious Diseases*. 8th ed. Philadelphia: Elsevier Saunders; 2015:2221-2224.

Gilbert DN, Chambers HF, Eliopoulos GM, et al., eds. *The Sanford Guide to Antimicrobial Therapy*. 46th ed. Sperryville, VA: Antimicrobial Therapy Inc; 2016.

Holtom PD. Rickettsial infections. In: Schlossberg D, ed. *Clinical Infectious Disease*. 2nd ed. Cambridge, United Kingdom: Cambridge University Press; 2015:1093-1097.

Nicholson WL, Paddock CD. Rickettsial (Spotted & Typhus Fevers) & Related Infections, Including Anaplasmosis & Ehrlichiosis. In: Brunette GW, ed. *CDC Yellow Book 2018 Health Information for International Travel*. Oxford, United Kingdom: Oxford University Press; 2017: 297-303.

ARENAVIRIDAE

Arenaviridae | Viral Hemorrhagic Fevers (VHFs) | CDC. Available at: https://www.cdc.gov/vhf/virus-families/arenaviridae.html. Accessed October 6, 2017.

Knust B, Choi M. Viral Hemorrhagic Fevers. In: Brunette GW, ed. *CDC Yellow Book 2018 Health Information for International Travel*. Oxford, United Kingdom: Oxford University Press; 2017:349-352.

Seregin A, Yun N, Paessler S. Lymphocytic Choriomeningitis, Lassa Fever, and the South American Hemorrhagic Fevers (Arenaviruses). In: Bennett JE, Dolin R, Blaser MJ, eds. *Principles and Practice of Infectious Diseases*. 8th ed. Philadelphia: Elsevier Saunders; 2015:2031-2037.

OROPHARYNGEAL INFECTIONS

PERITONSILLAR ABSCESS

Bryant AE, Stevens DL. Streptococcus pyogenes. In: Bennett JE, Dolin R, Blaser MJ, eds. *Principles and Practice of Infectious Diseases*. 8th ed. Philadelphia: Elsevier Saunders; 2015:2285-2299.

Gilbert DN, Chambers HF, Eliopoulos GM, et al., eds. *The Sanford Guide to Antimicrobial Therapy*. 46th ed. Sperryville, VA: Antimicrobial Therapy Inc; 2016.

Slavoski LA, Levison ME. Peritonitis. In: Schlossberg D, ed. *Clinical Infectious Disease*. 2nd ed. Cambridge, United Kingdom: Cambridge University Press; 2015: 375-380.

DIPHTHERIA

Gilbert DN, Chambers HF, Eliopoulos GM, et al., eds. *The Sanford Guide to Antimicrobial Therapy*. 46th ed. Sperryville, VA: Antimicrobial Therapy Inc; 2016.

MacGregor RR. Corynebacterium diphtheriae (Diphtheria). In: Bennett JE, Dolin R, Blaser MJ, eds. *Principles and Practice of Infectious Diseases*. 8th ed. Philadelphia: Elsevier Saunders; 2015:2366-2372.

Ramirez-Ronda CH, Ramirez-Ramirez CR. Corynebacteria. In: Schlossberg D, ed. *Clinical Infectious Disease*. 2nd ed. Cambridge, United Kingdom: Cambridge University Press; 2015:881-887.

Tiwari TSP. Diphtheria. In: Brunette GW, ed. *CDC Yellow Book 2018 Health Information for International Travel*. Oxford, United Kingdom: Oxford University Press; 2017: 169-170.

HERPANGINA

Gilbert DN, Chambers HF, Eliopoulos GM, et al., eds. *The Sanford Guide to Antimicrobial Therapy*. 46th ed. Sperryville, VA: Antimicrobial Therapy Inc; 2016.

Oxman MN. Enteroviruses. In: Schlossberg D, ed. *Clinical Infectious Disease*. 2nd ed. Cambridge, United Kingdom: Cambridge University Press; 2015:1172-1182.

Romero JR, Modlin JF. Coxsackieviruses, Echoviruses, and Numbered Enteroviruses. In: Bennett JE, Dolin R, Blaser MJ, eds. *Principles and Practice of Infectious Diseases*. 8th ed. Philadelphia: Elsevier Saunders; 2015:2080-2090.

THRUSH

Edwards Jr JE. Candida Species. In: Bennett JE, Dolin R, Blaser MJ, eds. *Principles and Practice of Infectious Diseases*. 8th ed. Philadelphia: Elsevier Saunders; 2015: 2879-2894.

Gilbert DN, Chambers HF, Eliopoulos GM, et al., eds. *The Sanford Guide to Antimicrobial Therapy*. 46th ed. Sperryville, VA: Antimicrobial Therapy Inc; 2016.

Ogedegbe A, Glesby MJ. Differential diagnosis and management of HIV-associated opportunistic infections. In: Schlossberg D, ed. *Clinical Infectious Disease*. 2nd ed. Cambridge, United Kingdom: Cambridge University Press; 2015:676-687.

STREPTOCOCCAL PHARYNGITIS

Bradley SF. Staphylococcus. In: Schlossberg D, ed. *Clinical Infectious Disease*. 2nd ed. Cambridge, United Kingdom: Cambridge University Press; 2015:985-990.

Bryant AE, Stevens DL. Streptococcus pyogenes. In: Bennett JE, Dolin R, Blaser MJ, eds. *Principles and Practice of Infectious Diseases*. 8th ed. Philadelphia: Elsevier Saunders; 2015:2285-2299.

Centor RM, Witherspoon JM, Dalton HP, Brody CE, Link K. The diagnosis of strep throat in adults in the emergency room. *Med Decis Making*. 1981;1(3):239-246.

Gilbert DN, Chambers HF, Eliopoulos GM, et al., eds. *The Sanford Guide to Antimicrobial Therapy*. 46th ed. Sperryville, VA: Antimicrobial Therapy Inc; 2016.

McIsaac WJ, White D, Tannenbaum D, Low DE. A clinical score to reduce unnecessary antibiotic use in patients with sore throat. *CMAJ*. 1998;158(1):75-83.

VIRAL

EBOLA

Bausch DG. Viral hemorrhagic fevers. In: Schlossberg D, ed. *Clinical Infectious Disease*. 2nd ed. Cambridge, United Kingdom: Cambridge University Press; 2015:1234-1248.

Choi M, Knust B. Ebola Virus Disease & Marburg Virus Disease. In: Brunette GW, ed. *CDC Yellow Book 2018 Health Information for International Travel*. Oxford, United Kingdom: Oxford University Press; 2017:170-172.

Ebola Hemorrhagic Fever | CDC. Available at: https://www.cdc.gov/vhf/ebola/index.html. Accessed October 6, 2017.

Geisbert TW. Marburg and Ebola Hemorrhagic Fevers (Filoviruses). In: Bennett JE, Dolin R, Blaser MJ, eds. *Principles and Practice of Infectious Diseases*. 8th ed. Philadelphia: Elsevier Saunders; 2015:1995-1999.

RABIES

Geldern GV, Mahadevan A, Shankar SK, Nath A. Rabies. In: Schlossberg D, ed. *Clinical Infectious Disease*. 2nd ed. Cambridge, United Kingdom: Cambridge University Press; 2015:1220-1225.

Gilbert DN, Chambers HF, Eliopoulos GM, et al., eds. *The Sanford Guide to Antimicrobial Therapy*. 46th ed. Sperryville, VA: Antimicrobial Therapy Inc; 2016.

Petersen BW, Wallace RM, Shlim DR. Rabies. In: Brunette GW, ed. *CDC Yellow Book 2018 Health Information for International Travel*. Oxford, United Kingdom: Oxford University Press; 2017:287-293.

Research C for BE and. Approved Products – Imovax | FDA. Available at: https://www.fda.gov/biologicsbloodvaccines/vaccines/approvedproducts/ucm180097.htm. Accessed October 6, 2017.

Singh K, Rupprecht CE, Bleck TP. Rabies (Rhabdoviruses). In: Bennett JE, Dolin R, Blaser MJ, eds. *Principles and Practice of Infectious Diseases*. 8th ed. Philadelphia: Elsevier Saunders; 2015:1984-1994.

AIDS: OPPORTUNISTIC INFECTIONS

Bacterial Respiratory Adult and Adolescent Opportunistic Infection. AIDSinfo. Available at: https://aidsinfo.nih.gov/guidelines/html/4/adult-and-adolescent-opportunistic-infection/327/bacterial-respiratory. Accessed October 10, 2017.

Bartonella Adult and Adolescent Opportunistic Infection. AIDSinfo. Available at: https://aidsinfo.nih.gov/guidelines/html/4/adult-and-adolescent-opportunistic-infection/329/bartonella. Accessed October 10, 2017.

Cocci Adult and Adolescent Opportunistic Infection. AIDSinfo. Available at: https://aidsinfo.nih.gov/guidelines/html/4/adult-and-adolescent-opportunistic-infection/335/cocci. Accessed October 10, 2017.

Cryptococcosis Adult and Adolescent Opportunistic Infection. AIDSinfo. Available at: https://aidsinfo.nih.gov/guidelines/html/4/adult-and-adolescent-opportunistic-infection/333/cryptococcosis. Accessed October 10, 2017.

Cryptosporidia Adult and Adolescent Opportunistic Infection. AIDSinfo. Available at: https://aidsinfo.nih.gov/guidelines/html/4/adult-and-adolescent-opportunistic-infection/323/cryptosporidia. Accessed October 10, 2017.

Gilbert DN, Chambers HF, Eliopoulos GM, et al., eds. *The Sanford Guide to Antimicrobial Therapy.* 46th ed. Sperryville, VA: Antimicrobial Therapy Inc; 2016.

Histo Adult and Adolescent Opportunistic Infection. AIDSinfo. Available at: https://aidsinfo.nih.gov/guidelines/html/4/adult-and-adolescent-opportunistic-infection/334/histo. Accessed October 10, 2017.

Hlavsa MC, Xiao L. Cryptosporidiosis. In: Brunette GW, ed. *CDC Yellow Book 2018 Health Information for International Travel.* Oxford, United Kingdom: Oxford University Press; 2017:157-159.

MAC Adult and Adolescent Opportunistic Infection. AIDSinfo. Available at: https://aidsinfo.nih.gov/guidelines/html/4/adult-and-adolescent-opportunistic-infection/326/mac. Accessed October 10, 2017.

Microsporidia Adult and Adolescent Opportunistic Infection. AIDSinfo. Available at: https://aidsinfo.nih.gov/guidelines/html/4/adult-and-adolescent-opportunistic-infection/324/microsporidia. Accessed October 10, 2017.

Ogedegbe A, Glesby MJ. Differential diagnosis and management of HIV-associated opportunistic infections. In: Schlossberg D, ed. *Clinical Infectious Disease.* 2nd ed. Cambridge, United Kingdom: Cambridge University Press; 2015: 676-687.

PCP Adult and Adolescent Opportunistic Infection. AIDSinfo. Available at: https://aidsinfo.nih.gov/guidelines/html/4/adult-and-adolescent-opportunistic-infection/321/pcp. Accessed October 10, 2017.

Rio C, Curran JW. Epidemiology and Prevention of Acquired Immunodeficiency Syndrome and Human Immunodeficiency Virus Infection. In: Bennett JE, Dolin R, Blaser MJ, eds. *Principles and Practice of Infectious Diseases.* 8th ed. Philadelphia: Elsevier Saunders; 2015:1483-1502.

Suh KN, Kozarsky P, Keystone JS. Cyclospora cayetanensis, Cystoisospora (Isospora) belli, Sarcocystis Species, Balantidium coli, and Blastocystis Species. In: Bennett JE, Dolin R, Blaser MJ, eds. *Principles and Practice of Infectious Diseases.* 8th ed. Philadelphia: Elsevier Saunders; 2015:3184-3191.

TB Adult and Adolescent Opportunistic Infection. AIDSinfo. Available at: https://aidsinfo.nih.gov/guidelines/html/4/adult-and-adolescent-opportunistic-infection/325/tb. Accessed October 10, 2017.

Toxo Adult and Adolescent Opportunistic Infection. AIDSinfo. Available at: https://aidsinfo.nih.gov/guidelines/html/4/adult-and-adolescent-opportunistic-infection/322/toxo. Accessed October 10, 2017.

Weiss LM. Microsporidiosis. In: Bennett JE, Dolin R, Blaser MJ, eds. *Principles and Practice of Infectious Diseases.* 8th ed. Philadelphia: Elsevier Saunders; 2015:3031-3044.

What's New Adult and Adolescent Opportunistic Infection. AIDSinfo. Available at: https://aidsinfo.nih.gov/guidelines/html/4/adult-and-adolescent-opportunistic-infection/0. Accessed October 6, 2017.

SMALLPOX

Artenstein AW. Bioterrorism. In: Schlossberg D, ed. *Clinical Infectious Disease.* 2nd ed. Cambridge, United Kingdom: Cambridge University Press; 2015:815-826.

McCollum AM. Smallbox & Other Orthopoxvirus-Associated Infections. In: Brunette GW, ed. *CDC Yellow Book 2018 Health Information for International Travel.* Oxford, United Kingdom: Oxford University Press; 2017: 321-323.

Petersen BW, Damon IK. Orthopoxviruses: Vaccinia (Smallpox Vaccine), Variola (Smallpox), Monkeypox, and Cowpox. In: Bennett JE, Dolin R, Blaser MJ, eds. *Principles and Practice of Infectious Diseases*. 8th ed. Philadelphia: Elsevier Saunders; 2015:1694-1702.

Smallpox | CDC. Available at: https://www.cdc.gov/smallpox/index.html. Published July 13, 2017. Accessed October 6, 2017.

MONONUCLEOSIS

Crumpacker II CS. Cytomegalovirus (CMV). In: Bennett JE, Dolin R, Blaser MJ, eds. *Principles and Practice of Infectious Diseases*. 8th ed. Philadelphia: Elsevier Saunders; 2015:1738-1753.

Meier JL. Epstein-Barr virus and other causes of the mononucleosis syndrome. In: Schlossberg D, ed. *Clinical Infectious Disease*. 2nd ed. Cambridge, United Kingdom: Cambridge University Press; 2015:1183-1189.

POLIO

Alexander JP, Patel M, Wassilak SGF. Poliomyelitis. In: Brunette GW, ed. *CDC Yellow Book 2018 Health Information for International Travel*. Oxford, United Kingdom: Oxford University Press; 2017:278-282.

CDC Global Health – Polio. Available at: https://www.cdc.gov/polio/. Published March 27, 2017. Accessed October 6, 2017.

Jong EC. Immunizations. In: Schlossberg D, ed. *Clinical Infectious Disease*. 2nd ed. Cambridge, United Kingdom: Cambridge University Press; 2015:763-776.

Pinkbook | Polio | Epidemiology of Vaccine Preventable Diseases | CDC. Available at: https://www.cdc.gov/vaccines/pubs/pinkbook/polio.html. Accessed October 6, 2017.

Romero JR, Modlin JF. Poliovirus. In: Bennett JE, Dolin R, Blaser MJ, eds. *Principles and Practice of Infectious Diseases*. 8th ed. Philadelphia: Elsevier Saunders; 2015:2073-2079.

PARASITES AND PRIONS

CHAGAS DISEASE

Gilbert DN, Chambers HF, Eliopoulos GM, et al., eds. *The Sanford Guide to Antimicrobial Therapy*. 46th ed. Sperryville, VA: Antimicrobial Therapy Inc; 2016.

Kirchhoff LV. Trypanosoma Species (American Trypanosomiasis, Chagas' Disease): Biology of Trypanosomes. In: Bennett JE, Dolin R, Blaser MJ, eds. *Principles and Practice of Infectious Diseases*. 8th ed. Philadelphia: Elsevier Saunders; 2015:3108-3115.

Montgomery S. Trypanosomiasis, American (Chagas Disease). In: Brunette GW, ed. *CDC Yellow Book 2018 Health Information for International Travel*. Oxford, United Kingdom: Oxford University Press; 2017:332-333.

Sousa ADQ, Jeronimo SMB, Pearson RD. Trypanosomiases and leishmaniases. In: Schlossberg D, ed. *Clinical Infectious Disease*. 2nd ed. Cambridge, United Kingdom: Cambridge University Press; 2015:1302-1312.

AFRICAN SLEEPING SICKNESS

Gilbert DN, Chambers HF, Eliopoulos GM, et al., eds. *The Sanford Guide to Antimicrobial Therapy*. 46th ed. Sperryville, VA: Antimicrobial Therapy Inc; 2016.

Kirchhoff LV. Agents of African Trypanosomiasis (Sleeping Sickness). In: Bennett JE, Dolin R, Blaser MJ, eds. *Principles and Practice of Infectious Diseases*. 8th ed. *Philadelphia*: Elsevier Saunders; 2015:3116-3121.

PEDICULOSIS

2015 STD Treatment Guidelines. Available at: https://www.cdc.gov/std/tg2015/default.htm. Accessed October 6, 2017.

Diaz JH. Lice (Pediculosis). In: Bennett JE, Dolin R, Blaser MJ, eds. *Principles and Practice of Infectious Diseases*. 8th ed. Philadelphia: Elsevier Saunders; 2015:3246-3249.

Gilbert DN, Chambers HF, Eliopoulos GM, et al., eds. *The Sanford Guide to Antimicrobial Therapy*. 46th ed. Sperryville, VA: Antimicrobial Therapy Inc; 2016.

Monsel G, Chosidow O, Quinn TC. Scabies, lice, and myiasis., Sexually transmitted enteric infections. In: Schlossberg D, ed. *Clinical Infectious Disease*. 2nd ed. Cambridge, United Kingdom: Cambridge University Press; 2015:162-166.

NAEGLERIASIS

Boggild AK, Wilson ME. Recreational water exposure. In: Schlossberg D, ed. *Clinical Infectious Disease*. 2nd ed.

Cambridge, United Kingdom: Cambridge University Press; 2015:800-809.

Gilbert DN, Chambers HF, Eliopoulos GM, et al., eds. *The Sanford Guide to Antimicrobial Therapy*. 46th ed. Sperryville, VA: Antimicrobial Therapy Inc; 2016.

Koshy AA, Blackburn BG, Singh U. Free-Living Amebae. In: Bennett JE, Dolin R, Blaser MJ, eds. *Principles and Practice of Infectious Diseases*. 8th ed. Philadelphia: Elsevier Saunders; 2015:3059-3069.

Primary Amebic Meningoencephalitis (PAM) – Naegleria fowleri | Parasites | CDC. Available at: https://www.cdc.gov/parasites/naegleria/index.html. Accessed October 6, 2017.

PRION DISEASES

Bosque PJ, Tyler KL. Prions and Prion Diseases of the Central Nervous System (Transmissible Neurodegenerative Diseases). In: Bennett JE, Dolin R, Blaser MJ, eds. *Principles and Practice of Infectious Diseases*. 8th ed. Philadelphia: Elsevier Saunders; 2015:2142-2153.

Johnson RT. Prion diseases. In: Schlossberg D, ed. *Clinical Infectious Disease*. 2nd ed. Cambridge, United Kingdom: Cambridge University Press; 2015:541-543.

Prion Diseases | CDC. Available at: https://www.cdc.gov/prions/index.html. Published August 17, 2017. Accessed October 6, 2017.

BACTERIAL

ANTHRAX

Gilbert DN, Chambers HF, Eliopoulos GM, et al., eds. *The Sanford Guide to Antimicrobial Therapy*. 46th ed. Sperryville, VA: Antimicrobial Therapy Inc; 2016.

Walters KH, Traxler RM, Marston CK. Anthrax. In: Brunette GW, ed. *CDC Yellow Book 2018 Health Information for International Travel*. Oxford, United Kingdom: Oxford University Press; 2017:141-144.

Zangeneh TT, Traeger M, Klotz SA. Anthrax and other Bacillus species. In: Schlossberg D, ed. *Clinical Infectious Disease*. 2nd ed. Cambridge, United Kingdom: Cambridge University Press; 2015:843-849.

BOTULISM

Gilbert DN, Chambers HF, Eliopoulos GM, et al., eds. *The Sanford Guide to Antimicrobial Therapy*. 46th ed. Sperryville, VA: Antimicrobial Therapy Inc; 2016.

Hodowanec A, Bleck TP. Botulism (Clostridium botulinum). In: Bennett JE, Dolin R, Blaser MJ, eds. *Principles and Practice of Infectious Diseases*. 8th ed. Philadelphia: Elsevier Saunders; 2015:2763-2767.

Percak JM, Hasbun R. Myelitis and peripheral neuropathy. In: Schlossberg D, ed. *Clinical Infectious Disease*. 2nd ed. Cambridge, United Kingdom: Cambridge University Press; 2015:510-523.

BRUCELLOSIS

Carrillo C, Gotuzzo E. Brucellosis. In: Schlossberg D, ed. *Clinical Infectious Disease*. 2nd ed. Cambridge, United Kingdom: Cambridge University Press; 2015:866-869.

Gilbert DN, Chambers HF, Eliopoulos GM, et al., eds. *The Sanford Guide to Antimicrobial Therapy*. 46th ed. Sperryville, VA: Antimicrobial Therapy Inc; 2016.

Gul HC, Erdem H. Brucellosis (Brucella Species). In: Bennett JE, Dolin R, Blaser MJ, eds. *Principles and Practice of Infectious Diseases*. 8th ed. Philadelphia: Elsevier Saunders; 2015:2584-2589.

Negron ME, Tiller R, Kharod GA. Brucellosis. In: Brunette GW, ed. *CDC Yellow Book 2018 Health Information for International Travel*. Oxford, United Kingdom: Oxford University Press; 2017:148-149.

TYPHOID FEVER

Gilbert DN, Chambers HF, Eliopoulos GM, et al., eds. *The Sanford Guide to Antimicrobial Therapy*. 46th ed. Sperryville, VA: Antimicrobial Therapy Inc; 2016.

Judd MC, Mintz ED. Typhoid & Paratyphoid Fever. In: Brunette GW, ed. *CDC Yellow Book 2018 Health Information for International Travel*. Oxford, United Kingdom: Oxford University Press; 2017:342-345.

Lima AAM, Warren CA, Guerrant RL. Bacterial Inflammatory Enteritides. In: Bennett JE, Dolin R, Blaser MJ, eds. *Principles and Practice of Infectious Diseases*. 8th ed. Philadelphia: Elsevier Saunders; 2015:1263-1269.

CAT SCRATCH FEVER

Bartonella Adult and Adolescent Opportunistic Infection. AIDSinfo. Available at: https://aidsinfo.nih.gov/guidelines/html/4/adult-and-adolescent-opportunistic-infection/329/bartonella. Accessed October 10, 2017.

Gandhi TN, Slater LN, Welch DF, Koehler JE. Bartonella, Including Cat-Scratch Disease. In: Bennett JE, Dolin R, Blaser MJ, eds. *Principles and Practice of Infectious Diseases.* 8th ed. Philadelphia: Elsevier Saunders; 2015:2649-2663.

Gilbert DN, Chambers HF, Eliopoulos GM, et al., eds. *The Sanford Guide to Antimicrobial Therapy.* 46th ed. Sperryville, VA: Antimicrobial Therapy Inc; 2016.

Nelson CA. Bartonella Infections. In: Brunette GW, ed. *CDC Yellow Book 2018 Health Information for International Travel.* Oxford, United Kingdom: Oxford University Press; 2017:146-147.

Schwartzman WA. Cat scratch disease and other Bartonella infections. In: Schlossberg D, ed. *Clinical Infectious Disease.* 2nd ed. Cambridge, United Kingdom: Cambridge University Press; 2015:853-858.

LEPROSY

Castro-Echeverry E, Lee T, Vandergriff T, Cockerell CJ. Leprosy. In: Schlossberg D, ed. *Clinical Infectious Disease.* 2nd ed. Cambridge, United Kingdom: Cambridge University Press; 2015:931-934.

Gilbert DN, Chambers HF, Eliopoulos GM, et al., eds. *The Sanford Guide to Antimicrobial Therapy.* 46th ed. Sperryville, VA: Antimicrobial Therapy Inc; 2016.

National Hansen's Disease (Leprosy) Program Caring and Curing Since 1894 | Official web site of the U.S. Health Resources & Services Administration. Available at: https://www.hrsa.gov/hansens-disease/index.html. Accessed October 6, 2017.

Recommended Treatment Regimens | Official web site of the U.S. Health Resources & Services Administration. Available at: https://www.hrsa.gov/hansens-disease/diagnosis/recommended-treatment.html. Accessed October 6, 2017.

Renault CA, Ernst JD. Mycobacterium leprae (Leprosy). In: Bennett JE, Dolin R, Blaser MJ, eds. *Principles and Practice of Infectious Diseases.* 8th ed. Philadelphia: Elsevier Saunders; 2015:2819-2831.

WHO | Leprosy. WHO. Available at: http://www.who.int/mediacentre/factsheets/fs101/en/. Accessed October 6, 2017.

WHO Model Prescribing Information: Drugs Used in Leprosy: Treatment of leprosy. Available at: http://apps.who.int/medicinedocs/en/d/Jh2988e/5.html. Accessed October 6, 2017.

INFECTIVE ENDOCARDITIS

Chowdhury MA, Michael AM. Endocarditis of natural and prosthetic valves: treatment and prophylaxis. In: Schlossberg D, ed. *Clinical Infectious Disease.* 2nd ed. Cambridge, United Kingdom: Cambridge University Press; 2015: 243-253.

Gilbert DN, Chambers HF, Eliopoulos GM, et al., eds. *The Sanford Guide to Antimicrobial Therapy.* 46th ed. Sperryville, VA: Antimicrobial Therapy Inc; 2016.

Levine DP, Brown PD. Infections in Injection Drug Users. In: Bennett JE, Dolin R, Blaser MJ, eds. *Principles and Practice of Infectious Diseases.* 8th ed. Philadelphia: Elsevier Saunders; 2015:3475-3491.

TETANUS

Gilbert DN, Chambers HF, Eliopoulos GM, et al., eds. *The Sanford Guide to Antimicrobial Therapy.* 46th ed. Sperryville, VA: Antimicrobial Therapy Inc; 2016.

Hodowanec A, Bleck TP. Tetanus (Clostridium tetani). In: Bennett JE, Dolin R, Blaser MJ, eds. *Principles and Practice of Infectious Diseases.* 8th ed. Philadelphia: Elsevier Saunders; 2015:2757-2762.

Percak JM, Hasbun R. Myelitis and peripheral neuropathy. In: Schlossberg D, ed. *Clinical Infectious Disease.* 2nd ed. Cambridge, United Kingdom: Cambridge University Press; 2015:510-523.

Tiwari TSP. Tetanus. In: Brunette GW, ed. *CDC Yellow Book 2018 Health Information for International Travel.* Oxford, United Kingdom: Oxford University Press; 2017: 325-326.

LISTERIOSIS

Gilbert DN, Chambers HF, Eliopoulos GM, et al., eds. *The Sanford Guide to Antimicrobial Therapy.* 46th ed. Sperryville, VA: Antimicrobial Therapy Inc; 2016.

Lorber B. Listeria. In: Schlossberg D, ed. *Clinical Infectious Disease*. 2nd ed. Cambridge, United Kingdom: Cambridge University Press; 2015:942-949.

Lorber B. Listeria monocytogenes. In: Bennett JE, Dolin R, Blaser MJ, eds. *Principles and Practice of Infectious Diseases*. 8th ed. Philadelphia: Elsevier Saunders; 2015:2383-2390.

Q FEVER

Gilbert DN, Chambers HF, Eliopoulos GM, et al., eds. *The Sanford Guide to Antimicrobial Therapy*. 46th ed. Sperryville, VA: Antimicrobial Therapy Inc; 2016.

Holtom PD. Rickettsial infections. In: Schlossberg D, ed. *Clinical Infectious Disease*. 2nd ed. Cambridge, United Kingdom: Cambridge University Press; 2015:1093-1097.

Kersh GJ. Q Fever. In: Brunette GW, ed. *CDC Yellow Book 2018 Health Information for International Travel*. Oxford, United Kingdom: Oxford University Press; 2017:286-287.

Marrie TJ, Raoult D. Coxiella burnetii (Q Fever). In: Bennett JE, Dolin R, Blaser MJ, eds. *Principles and Practice of Infectious Diseases*. 8th ed. Philadelphia: Elsevier Saunders; 2015:2208-2216.

MELIOIDOSIS

Blaney DD, Gee JE. Melioidosis. In: Brunette GW, ed. *CDC Yellow Book 2018 Health Information for International Travel*. Oxford, United Kingdom: Oxford University Press; 2017:260-261.

Boggild AK, Wilson ME. Recreational water exposure. In: Schlossberg D, ed. *Clinical Infectious Disease*. 2nd ed. Cambridge, United Kingdom: Cambridge University Press; 2015:800-809.

Currie BJ. Burkholderia pseudomallei and Burkholderia mallei: Melioidosis and Glanders. In: Bennett JE, Dolin R, Blaser MJ, eds. *Principles and Practice of Infectious Diseases*. 8th ed. Philadelphia: Elsevier Saunders; 2015: 2541-2551.

Gilbert DN, Chambers HF, Eliopoulos GM, et al., eds. *The Sanford Guide to Antimicrobial Therapy*. 46th ed. Sperryville, VA: Antimicrobial Therapy Inc; 2016.

INDEX